Improving Palliative Care for Cancer

DATE DUE

Kathleen M. Foley and Hellen Gelband, *Editors*

National Cancer Policy Board

INSTITUTE OF MEDICINE

and

NATIONAL RESEARCH COUNCIL

NATIONAL ACADEMY PRESS
Washington, D.C.

AUG 0 1 2002

NATIONAL ACADEMY PRESS • 2101 Constitution Avenue, N.W. • Washington, DC 20418

NOTICE: The project that is the subject of this report was approved by the Governing Board of the National Research Council, whose members are drawn from the councils of the National Academy of Sciences, the National Academy of Engineering, and the Institute of Medicine. The members of the Board responsible for the report were chosen for their special competences and with regard for appropriate balance.

Support for the National Cancer Policy Board is provided by the National Cancer Institute; the Centers for Disease Control and Prevention; Abbott Laboratories; the American Cancer Society; American Society of Clinical Oncology; Amgen, Inc.; Aventis; and United Health Care Foundation. The views presented in this report are those of the Institute of Medicine and the Division of Earth and Life Studies National Cancer Policy Board and are not necessarily those of the funding agencies.

International Standard Book Number 0-309-07402-9

Library of Congress Control Number: 2001094187

Additional copies of this report are available for sale from the National Academy Press, 2101 Constitution Avenue, N.W., Box 285, Washington, D.C. 20055. Call (800) 624-6242 or (202) 334-3313 (in the Washington metropolitan area), or visit the NAP home page at **www.nap.edu**. The full text of this report is available at **www.nap.edu**.

For more information about the Institute of Medicine, visit the IOM home page at: **www.iom.edu**.

Printed in the United States of America.

THE NATIONAL ACADEMIES

National Academy of Sciences
National Academy of Engineering
Institute of Medicine
National Research Council

The **National Academy of Sciences** is a private, nonprofit, self-perpetuating society of distinguished scholars engaged in scientific and engineering research, dedicated to the furtherance of science and technology and to their use for the general welfare. Upon the authority of the charter granted to it by the Congress in 1863, the Academy has a mandate that requires it to advise the federal government on scientific and technical matters. Dr. Bruce M. Alberts is president of the National Academy of Sciences.

The **National Academy of Engineering** was established in 1964, under the charter of the National Academy of Sciences, as a parallel organization of outstanding engineers. It is autonomous in its administration and in the selection of its members, sharing with the National Academy of Sciences the responsibility for advising the federal government. The National Academy of Engineering also sponsors engineering programs aimed at meeting national needs, encourages education and research, and recognizes the superior achievements of engineers. Dr. Wm. A. Wulf is president of the National Academy of Engineering.

The **Institute of Medicine** was established in 1970 by the National Academy of Sciences to secure the services of eminent members of appropriate professions in the examination of policy matters pertaining to the health of the public. The Institute acts under the responsibility given to the National Academy of Sciences by its congressional charter to be an adviser to the federal government and, upon its own initiative, to identify issues of medical care, research, and education. Dr. Kenneth I. Shine is president of the Institute of Medicine.

The **National Research Council** was organized by the National Academy of Sciences in 1916 to associate the broad community of science and technology with the Academy's purposes of furthering knowledge and advising the federal government. Functioning in accordance with general policies determined by the Academy, the Council has become the principal operating agency of both the National Academy of Sciences and the National Academy of Engineering in providing services to the government, the public, and the scientific and engineering communities. The Council is administered jointly by both Academies and the Institute of Medicine. Dr. Bruce M. Alberts and Dr. Wm. A. Wulf are chairman and vice chairman, respectively, of the National Research Council.

NATIONAL CANCER POLICY BOARD

Sandra Millon Underwood, ACS Oncology Nursing Professor, University of Wisconsin School of Nursing, Milwaukee

Frances Visco, President, National Breast Cancer Coalition, Washington, DC *(member through April 2001)*

Susan Weiner, President, The Children's Cause, Silver Spring, MD

Study Staff

Hellen Gelband, Study Director
Florence Poillon, Editor

NCPB Staff

Robert Cook-Deegan, Director, National Cancer Policy Board
  (through August 2000)
Roger Herdman, Director, National Cancer Policy Board
  (from September 2000)
Ellen Johnson, Administrator *(through July 2000)*
Nicci T. Dowd, Administrator *(from August 2000)*
Jennifer Cangco, Financial Associate

Reviewers

This report has been reviewed in draft form by individuals chosen for their diverse perspectives and technical expertise, in accordance with procedures approved by the NRC's Report Review Committee. The purpose of this independent review is to provide candid and critical comments that will assist the institution in making its published report as sound as possible and to ensure that the report meets institutional standards for objectivity, evidence, and responsiveness to the study charge. The review comments and draft manuscript remain confidential to protect the integrity of the deliberative process. We wish to thank the following individuals for their review of this report:

Susan Dale Block, Dana Farber Cancer Institute
Eduardo Bruera, MD Anderson Cancer Center
LaVera M. Crawley, Stanford University Center for Biomedical Ethics
Betty R. Ferrell, City of Hope National Medical Center
Priscilla Kissick, Philadelphia, Pennsylvania
Joseph S. Pagano, University of North Carolina at Chapel Hill
Thomas Smith, Medical College of Virginia
T. Declan Walsh, The Cleveland Clinic Foundation
George Wetherill, Carnegie Institution of Washington

Although the reviewers listed above have provided many constructive comments and suggestions, they were not asked to endorse the conclusions or recommendations nor did they see the final draft of the report before its release. The review of this report was overseen by Harold Sox of the Dartmouth-Hitchcock Medical Center, appointed by the NRC's Report Review Committee, who was responsible for making certain that an independent examination of this report was carried out in accordance with institutional procedures and that all review comments were carefully considered. Responsibility for the final content of this report rests entirely with the National Cancer Policy Board, the Institute of Medicine, and the National Research Council.

Preface

It is innately human to comfort and provide care to those suffering from cancer, particularly those close to death. Yet what seems self-evident at an individual, personal level has, by and large, not guided policy at the level of institutions in this country. There is no argument that palliative care should be integrated into cancer care from diagnosis to death. But significant barriers—attitudinal, behavioral, economic, educational, and legal—still limit access to care for a large proportion of those dying from cancer, and in spite of tremendous scientific opportunities for medical progress against all the major symptoms associated with cancer and cancer death, public research institutions have not responded. In accepting a single-minded focus on research toward cure, we have inadvertently devalued the critical need to care for and support patients with advanced disease, and their families.

This report builds on and takes forward an agenda set out by the 1997 IOM report *Approaching Death: Improving Care at the End of Life*, which came at a time when leaders in palliative care and related fields had already begun to air issues surrounding care of the dying. That report identified significant gaps in knowledge about care at the end of life and the need for serious attention from biomedical, social science, and health services researchers. Most importantly, it recognized that the impediments to good care could be identified and potentially remedied. The report itself catalyzed further public involvement in specific initiatives—mostly pilot and demonstration projects and programs funded by the nonprofit foundation community, which are now coming to fruition.

There are no villains in this piece but ourselves and our culture. Public institutions and policymakers reflect dominant societal values that still deny dying and death. Although it does occur, change to improve care of the suffering and dying is slow and conflicted with the tension between cure and care. This report encourages continued innovation and collaboration of foundations and others, but focuses on ways in which the government can embrace opportunities to improve existing palliative care, make access to it equitable for all, and help realize better palliative interventions by making research funds more available.

It is a truism that death—not just our own—affects all of us, even if it is a topic most people do not want to contemplate for long. Death is inevitable, but severe suffering is not. Willpower and determination will be required, but it is time to move our public institutions toward policies that emphasize the importance of improving palliative care for those who want and need it. This report identifies the special needs of cancer patients and the importance of the clinical and research establishment involved in cancer care to take a leadership role in modeling the best quality care from diagnosis to death for all Americans.

Kathleen M. Foley, M.D.
Director, Project on Death in America, The Open Society

Acronyms and Abbreviations

AAMC	American Association of Medical Colleges
ACoS	American College of Surgeons
ACS	American Cancer Society
ADL	activities of daily living
AHRQ	Agency for Healthcare Research and Quality
AMA	American Medical Association
APA	American Psychiatric Association
APS	American Pain Society
ASCO	American Society of Clinical Oncology
ASPHO	American Society of Pediatric Hematology/Oncology
BFI	Brief Fatigue Inventory
CAHPS	Consumer Assessment of Health Plans Survey
CIS	Cancer Information Service
CME	continuing medical education
CNS	central nervous system
COPD	Chronic Obstructive Pulmonary Disease
CPR	Cardiopulmonary resuscitation
CPT	Current Procedural Terminology
DCTD	Division of Cancer Treatment and Diagnosis
DNR	do not resuscitate

DSM-IV	*Diagnostic and Statistical Manual of Mental Disorders,* Fourth Edition
ECOG	Eastern Cooperative Oncology Group
HCFA	Health Care Financing Administration
HPCN	Harlem Palliative Care Network
HELP	Hospitalized Elderly Longitudinal Project
HRSA	Health Resources and Services Administration
ICD-9	International Classification of Diseases, 9th revision
ICU	intensive care unit
IL-6	interleukin-6
INF-α	alpha-interferon
IOM	Institute of Medicine
IV	intravenous
JCAHO	Joint Commission on Accreditation of Healthcare Organizations
LCME	Liaison Committee on Medical Education
MDS	Minimum Data Set
MedPAC	Medicare Payment Advisory Commission
MRI	magnetic resonance imaging
MSKCC	Memorial Sloan-Ketterin Cancer Center
NCCN	National Comprehensive Cancer Network
NCHS	National Center for Health Statistics
NCI	National Cancer Institute
NCPB	National Cancer Policy Board
NGH	North General Hospital
NHO	National Hospice Organization
NHPCO	National Hospice and Palliative Care Organization
NIA	National Institute on Aging
NIAID	National Institute of Allergy and Infectious Diseases
NIH	National Institutes of Health
NINR	National Institute of Nursing Research
NMFBS	National Mortality Followback Survey
OCD	obsessive-compulsive disorder
PCP	President's Cancer Panel

PDIA   Project on Death in America
PDQ   Physician Data Query
PSDA   Patient Self-Determination Act
PTSD   post-traumatic stress disorder
PVS   persistent vegetative state

QI   quality indicator

RFP   request for proposals
RWJF   Robert Wood Johnson Foundation

SEER   Surveillance, Epidemiology, and End Results Program
SIOP   International Society of Paediatric Oncology
SSRI   selective serotonin reuptake inhibitor
SUPPORT   Study to Understand Prognoses and Preferences for
            Outcomes and Risks of Treatment

THC   tetrahydrocannabinol

VA   Department of Veterans Affairs
VNSNY   Visiting Nurse Service of New York

WHO   World Health Organization

Contents

PART 2

Part 1

Executive Summary

Until the early part of the twentieth century, most Americans died of infectious diseases, many in childhood and middle age. Then, virtually every serious illness, including cancer, spelled a fairly rapid course to death. Those who survived to old age and developed the chronic diseases that the majority of people now die from had shorter trajectories until death, with few experiencing prolonged periods of illness. Malignancies were identified only when large or in a critical location, and most often, no treatments were available that substantially altered the course. Now, many patients with cancer live much longer, with periods of adaptation to cancer as a chronic debilitating disease. However, most still eventually die from the cancer.

Improvements in the development and delivery of symptom control and other aspects of palliative care needed in the late stages of cancer (and other chronic diseases) have not kept pace with the medical advances that have allowed people to live longer. For at least half of those dying from cancer, death entails a spectrum of symptoms, including pain, labored breathing, distress, nausea, confusion, and other physical and psychological conditions that go untreated or undertreated and vastly diminish the quality of their remaining days. Patients, their families, and caregivers all suffer from the inadequate care available to patients in pain and distress, although the magnitude of these burdens is only now being described.

This report defines the major barriers that keep people from receiving excellent palliative care, as needed, throughout the course of their illness with cancer and recommends a series of steps forward. It builds on the

1999 National Cancer Policy Board report *Ensuring Quality Cancer Care,* which included a recommendation to

> Ensure quality of care at the end of life, in particular, the management of cancer-related pain and timely referral to palliative and hospice care.

This report also takes forward the agenda outlined in a 1997 Institute of Medicine (IOM) report, *Approaching Death: Improving Care at the End of Life,* the first comprehensive, evidence-based, national report on these issues, which stimulated widespread interest and progress in some aspects of care for the dying. With the 1997 and 1999 reports as backdrop, the current effort focuses on specific areas in which the National Cancer Policy Board believes action still has to be catalyzed.

Barriers to Excellent Palliative and End-of-Life Care

Barriers throughout the health care and medical research systems stand in the way of many people receiving effective palliative care where and when they need it. These barriers include the following:

• the separation of palliative and hospice care from potentially life-prolonging treatment within the health care system, which is both influenced by and affects reimbursement policy;
• inadequate training of health care personnel in symptom management and other end-of-life care skills;
• inadequate standards of care and lack of accountability in caring for dying patients;
• disparities in care, even when available, for African Americans and other ethnic and socioeconomic segments of the population;
• lack of information resources for the public dealing with palliative and end-of-life care;
• lack of reliable data on the quality of life, and the quality of care of patients dying from cancer (as well as other chronic diseases); and
• low level of public sector investment in palliative and end-of-life care research and training.

Background papers (Part 2 of this report) were commissioned to explore the reasons for inadequacies in palliative and end-of-life care, and these (as well as consultation with additional experts and literature review) form the evidence base for the recommendations in this report. The background papers cover the following topics:

• Economic Issues and Barriers to Reliable, High-Quality, Efficient End of Life Care for Cancer Patients
• Quality Indicators for End-of-Life Cancer Care

- The Current State of Patient and Family Information About End-of-Life Care Issues
- Improving Access to and Quality of Palliative and End-of-Life Care: Issues in the African-American Community and Other Vulnerable Populations
- Special Issues in Pediatiric Oncology: End-of-Life Care
- Clinical Practice Guidelines for the Management of Psychosocial and Physical Symptoms of Cancer
- Cross-Cutting Research Issues: A Research Agenda for Reducing Distress of Patients with Cancer
- Professional Education in Palliative and End-of-Life Care for Physicians, Nurses, and Social Workers

CONCLUSIONS AND RECOMMENDATIONS

People with cancer suffer from an array of symptoms at all stages of the disease (and its treatment), though these are most frequent and severe in advanced stages. Much of the suffering could be alleviated if currently available symptom control measures were used more widely. For symptoms not amenable to relief by current measures, new approaches could be developed and tested, if even modest research resources were made available. Both the use of current interventions and the development of new ones are hindered by the barriers discussed earlier (and in the chapters that follow). The National Cancer Policy Board's recommendations are intended to break down or lower the barriers to excellent palliative care for people with cancer today, and those who will develop cancer in years to come. The recommendations describe a series of initiatives directed largely—though not exclusively—at the federal government, which should be playing a more powerful role than it does currently.

The conclusions and recommendations are not laid out in parallel to the barriers. They have been consolidated as "packages" for particular organizations and entities, and some address more than one barrier. Recommendation 1, in particular, which focuses on the role of National Cancer Institute (NCI)-designated cancer centers, contains elements that address all the barriers.

NCI-designated cancer centers should play a central role as agents of national policy in advancing palliative care research and clinical practice, with initiatives that address many of the barriers identified in this report.

Recommendation 1: NCI should designate certain cancer centers, as well as some community cancer centers, as centers of excellence in symptom control and palliative care for both adults and children. The centers will deliver the best available care, as well as carrying out research, training, and treatment aimed at developing portable model programs that can be adopted by other cancer centers and hospitals. Activities should include, but not be limited to the following:

- *formal testing and evaluation of new and existing practice guidelines for palliative and end-of-life care;*
- *pilot testing "quality indicators" for assessing end-of-life care at the level of the patient and the institution;*
- *incorporating the best palliative care into NCI-sponsored clinical trials;*
- *innovating in the delivery of palliative and end-of-life care, including collaboration with local hospice organizations;*
- *disseminating information about how to improve end-of-life care to other cancer centers and hospitals through a variety of media;*
- *uncovering the determinants of disparities in access to care by minority populations that should be served by the center, and developing specific programs and initiatives to increase access; these might include educational activities for health care providers and the community, setting up outreach programs, etc.;*
- *providing clinical and research training fellowships in medical and surgical oncology in end-of-life care for adult and pediatric patients;*
- *creating faculty development programs in oncology, nursing, and social work; and*
- *Providing in-service training for local hospice staff in new palliative care techniques.*

Recommendation 2: NCI should add the requirement of research in palliative care and symptom control for recognition as a "Comprehensive Cancer Center."

Practices and policies that govern payment for palliative care (in both public and private sectors) hinder delivery of the most appropriate mix of services for patients who could benefit from palliative care during the course of their illness and treatments.

Recommendation 3: The Health Care Financing Administration (HCFA) should fund demonstration projects for service delivery and reimbursement that integrate palliative care and potentially life-prolonging treatments throughout the course of disease.

Recommendation 4: Private insurers should provide adequate compensation for end-of-life care. The special circumstances of dying children— particularly the need for extended communication with children and par-

ents, *as well as health care team conferences—should be taken into account in setting reimbursement levels and in actually paying claims for these services when providers bill for them.*

Information on palliative and end-of-life care is largely absent from materials developed for the public about cancer treatment. In addition, reliable information about survival from different types and stages of cancer is not routinely included with treatment information.

Recommendation 5: Organizations that provide information about cancer treatment (NCI, the American Cancer Society, and other patient-oriented organizations [e.g., disease-specific groups], health insurers and pharmaceutical companies) should revise their inventories of patient-oriented material, as appropriate, to provide comprehensive, accurate information about palliative care throughout the course of disease. Patients would also be helped by having reliable information on survival by type and stage of cancer easily accessible. Attention should be paid to cultural relevance and special populations (e.g., children).

Practice guidelines for palliative care and for other end-of-life issues are in comparatively early stages of development, and quality indicators are even more embryonic. Progress toward their further development and implementation requires continued encouragement by professional societies, funding bodies, and payers of care.

Recommendation 6: Best available practice guidelines should dictate the standard of care for both physical and psychosocial symptoms. Care systems, payers, and standard-setting and accreditation bodies should strongly encourage their expedited development, validation, and use. Professional societies, particularly the American Society of Clinical Oncology, the Oncology Nursing Society, and the Society for Social Work Oncology, should encourage their members to facilitate the development and testing of guidelines and their eventual implementation, and should provide leadership and training for nonspecialists, who provide most of the care for cancer patients.

Recommendation 7: The recommendations in the NCPB report, Enhancing Data Systems to Improve the Quality of Cancer Care *(see Appendix B) should be applied equally to palliative and end-of-life care as to other aspects of cancer treatment. These recommendations include*

- *developing a core set of cancer care quality measures;*
- *increasing public and private support for cancer registries;*
- *supporting research and demonstration projects to identify new mechanisms to organize and finance the collection of data for cancer care quality studies;*

- *supporting the development of technologies, including computer-based patient record systems and intranet-based communication systems, to improve the availability, quality, and timeliness of clinical data relevant to assessing quality of cancer care;*
- *expanding support for training in health services research and other disciplines needed to measure quality of care;*
- *increasing support for health services research aimed toward improved quality of cancer care measures;*
- *developing models for linkage studies and the release of confidential data for research purposes that protect the confidentiality and privacy of health care information; and*
- *funding demonstration projects to assess the impact of quality monitoring programs within health care systems.*

Research on palliative care for cancer patients has had a low priority at NCI and as a result, few researchers have been attracted to the field and very few relevant studies have been funded over the past decades. NCI should continue to collaborate with the National Institute of Nursing Research on end-of-life research (the lead NIH institute for this topic), but cannot discharge its major responsibilities in cancer research through that mechanism.

Recommendation 8: NCI should convene a State of the Science Meeting[1] on palliative care and symptom control. It should invite other National Institutes of Health and other government research agencies with shared interests should be invited to collaborate. The meeting should result in a high-profile strategic research agenda that can be pursued by NCI and its research partners over the short and long terms.

Recommendation 9: NCI should establish the most appropriate institutional locus (or more than one) for palliative care, symptom control, and end-of-life research, possibly within the Division of Cancer Treatment and Diagnosis.

Recommendation 10: NCI should review the membership of its advisory bodies to ensure representation of experts in cancer pain, symptom management, and palliative care.

---

[1]In 1999, NCI initiated State of the Science Meetings focused on specific types of cancer "to bring together the Nation's leading multidisciplinary experts, to identify the important research questions for a given disease and help define the scientific research agenda that will assist us in addressing those questions."

1

Background and Recommendations

INTRODUCTION

The last half-century produced amazing advances in the treatment and early detection of a few types of cancer and at least modest gains in many others. Yet the reality is that at the beginning of the twenty-first century, half of all patients diagnosed with cancer will die of their disease within a few years. This translates into more than half a million people each year in the United States, and the annual toll will grow as the population ages and more people survive to get cancer over the coming decades.

The imperative in cancer research and treatment has been, understandably, an almost single-minded focus on attempts to cure every patient at every stage of disease. Recognition of the importance of symptom control and other aspects of palliative care from diagnosis through the dying process has been growing, however, and has reached the national health care agenda through the efforts of prominent bodies such as the President's Cancer Panel, the Medicare Payment Advisory Commission, the Institute of Medicine (IOM), and major health care foundations. All conclude that patients should not have to choose between treatment with curative intent *or* comfort care. There is a need for both, in varying degrees, throughout the course of cancer, whether the eventual outcome is long-term survival or death.

The goal is to maintain the best possible quality of life, allowing cancer patients the freedom to choose whatever treatments they so wish throughout the course of the disease, while also meeting the needs of patients with advanced disease through adequate symptom control. This goal is not met for most cancer patients in the United States today. We have words for "survivors" and those in active treatment, but even today, those with advanced disease who are not in active treatment and who are dying are nameless and faceless without a priority.

For at least half of those dying from cancer—most of them elderly and many vulnerable—death entails a spectrum of symptoms, including pain, labored breathing, distress, nausea, confusion and other physical and psychological conditions that go untreated or undertreated and vastly diminish the quality of their remaining days (Donnelly and Walsh, 1995; Phillips et al., 2000). The patient is not the only one who suffers during the dying process. The impact on families and caregivers is still poorly documented, but evidence has begun to be collected demonstrating a heavy and mostly unrelieved emotional and financial burden (Emanuel et al., 2000b). This cannot be ignored within the context of caring for people who are terminally ill.

A major problem in palliative care is the underrecognition, underdiagnosis, and thus undertreatment of patients with significant distress, ranging from existential anguish to anxiety and depression. This situation continues to exist despite the fact that when dying patients themselves have been asked their primary concerns about their care, three of their five concerns were psychosocial: (1) no prolongation of dying; (2) maintaining a sense of control; and (3) relieving burdens (conflicts) and strengthening ties (Singer et al., 1999).

All this is true at the same time that one-quarter of Medicare dollars are spent in the last year of life, and half of that is spent in the last month of life. Living with, and eventually dying from, a chronic illness runs up substantial costs for patient, family, and society, and costs for those dying from cancer are about 20 percent higher than average costs (Hogan et al., 2000). Dying patients are sick, dependent, changing, and needy. Most likely, high costs would be acceptable if patients and families were satisfied with the care provided for those with advanced disease, but few can count on being satisfied. In short, our society is spending a great deal and not getting what dying cancer patients need.

The current inadequacy of palliative and end-of-life care springs not from a single cause or sector of society, but from institutional and economic barriers, lack of information about what can be achieved, lack of training and education of health care professionals, and minuscule public sector investments in research to improve the situation. This is not to suggest that there is no ongoing research on relevant questions or training programs— there are—but the efforts are not coordinated, and there is no locus for these activities in any federal agency. What has resulted is underfunding, a lack of appropriate training, and a lack of research leadership, with no sustained programs for developing and disseminating palliative treatments. Despite the enormous health care expenditures for the dying, less than 1 percent of the National Cancer Institute (NCI) budget is spent on any aspect of symptom control, palliative care, or end-of-life research or training.

WHAT IS PALLIATIVE CARE?

The World Health Organization (WHO) defines palliative care in cancer as the "active total care of patients whose disease is not responsive to curative treatment." The definition is extended in an important way with the statement, "Many aspects of palliative care are also applicable earlier in the course of the illness, in conjunction with anticancer treatment" (WHO, 1990). Palliative care focuses on addressing the control of pain and other symptoms, as well as psychological, social, and spiritual distress. In its recommendation to member governments, WHO states that any national cancer control program should address the needs of its citizens for palliative care. This National Cancer Policy Board report adopts the WHO definition and position, focusing on the importance of palliative care beginning at the time of a cancer diagnosis and increasing in amount and intensity throughout the course of a patient's illness, until death.

In a practical sense, 6 major skill sets comprise complete palliative care:

1. communication,
2. decisionmaking,
3. management of complications of treatment and the disease,
4. symptom control,
5. psychosocial care of patient and family, and
6. care of the dying.

Some of these skills—communication, decisionmaking, psychosocial care of patient and family—are important throughout the trajectory of illness. Others emerge and recede in importance at different times. Treatment and prevention of complications caused by primary cancer treatments are generally episodic, though some require long-term management. Disease complications may require a variety of interventions (including surgery and radiation) that, for many, do not fit neatly into a palliative care definition. The need for symptom control unrelated to treatment generally increases as a person approaches death, but at least for some patients, it begins much earlier. Symptom control is never, however, a substitute for primary cancer care that is desired by a patient.

INTENT OF THIS REPORT

The National Cancer Policy Board (NCPB) recognized that excellent palliative care is possible but is not being delivered to a large number of those living with and dying from cancer. In its 1999 report *Ensuring Quality Cancer Care*, one of the Board's recommendations was:

> Ensure quality of care at the end of life, in particular, the management of cancer-related pain and timely referral to palliative and hospice care.

The current report delves into and expands on that mandate, addressing not only what can be done for people now nearing the end of life, but also setting a course for the development of better treatments and better ways of delivering and paying for them. This report also takes forward the agenda outlined in an influential 1997 IOM report *Approaching Death: Improving Care at the End of Life*, the first comprehensive, evidence-based, national report on these issues, which stimulated widespread interest and progress in some aspects of care for the dying. With the 1997 and 1999 reports as backdrop, the current effort focuses on specific areas in which the Board believes action still has to be catalyzed.

To accomplish this, eight papers were commissioned, which comprise Part II of this report. This chapter summarizes the current state of affairs, drawing on those papers and other sources, and ends with a set of broad-based recommendations supported by the evidence supplied in the commissioned papers. The papers themselves should be consulted for many more suggestions of specific activities and actions to be considered. The titles and authors are as follows:

- *Chapter 2: Reliable, High-Quality, Efficient End-of-Life Care for Cancer Patients: Economic Issues and Barriers*, Joanne Lynn and Ann O'Mara
- *Chapter 3: Quality of Life and Quality Indicators for End-of-Life Cancer Care: Hope for the Best, Yet Prepare for the Worst*, Joan M. Teno
- *Chapter 4: The Current State of Patient and Family Information About End-of-Life Care*, Aaron S. Kesselheim
- *Chapter 5: Palliative Care for African Americans and Other Vulnerable Populations: Access and Quality Issues*, Richard Payne
- *Chapter 6: End-of-Life Care: Special Issues in Pediatric Oncology*, Joanne M. Hilden, Bruce P. Himelstein, David R. Freyer, Sarah Friebert, and Javier R. Kane
- *Chapter 7: Clinical Practice Guidelines for the Management of Psychosocial and Physical Symptoms of Cancer*, Jimmie C. Holland and Lisa Chertkov
- *Chapter 8: Cross-Cutting Research Issues: A Research Agenda for Reducing Distress of Patients with Cancer*, Charles S. Cleeland

• *Chapter 9: Professional Education in Palliative and End-of-Life Care for Physicians, Nurses, and Social Workers, Hellen Gelband*

This report focuses exclusively on deaths from cancer, despite the fact that the number of people in the United States dying from other chronic diseases exceeds the number dying from cancer. Many of the issues raised and recommendations made in the report should benefit people dying from all these conditions, and it is not the NCPB's intent to divert attention from the many people dying from congestive heart failure, kidney disease, or other diseases. There is a logic, however, to looking at cancer deaths alone, aside from the obvious point that this report is a product of the National Cancer Policy Board.

Cancer has been the "prototype" disease for organizing end-of-life care for several reasons: it has a more predictable trajectory from the point at which cure becomes unlikely until death than other chronic diseases; the most frequent and distressing symptoms are similar for many forms of cancer; there is a nationwide infrastructure of cancer centers carrying on cancer research, treating a significant minority of patients, and influencing the practice of oncology across the country; and the most generously funded of the National Institutes of Health (NIH)—NCI, approaching $4 billion in 2001—is focused on cancer.

This report points out deficiencies in the way patients with advanced cancer are treated, but this does not signify that oncology is behind other medical disciplines in palliative care in general or in care for dying patients. In fact, the cancer establishment has played a leading role in the area of pain management, using the cancer patient with pain as a model for other conditions and developing national guidelines and educational initiatives. Hospice care also developed around the needs of advanced cancer patients in close association with the cancer establishment. With that head start, cancer professionals are poised to take the lead in other areas of symptom control and the organization and delivery of excellent palliative care.

BARRIERS TO EXCELLENT PALLIATIVE AND END-OF-LIFE CARE

Barriers throughout the health care and medical research systems stand in the way of many people receiving effective palliative care where and when they need it. These barriers include

• the separation of palliative and hospice care from potentially life-prolonging treatment within the health care system, which is both influenced by and affects reimbursement policy;
• inadequate training of health care personnel in symptom management and other palliative care skills;

  • inadequate standards of care and lack of accountability in caring for dying patients;
  • disparities in care, even when available, for African Americans and other ethnic and socioeconomic segments of the population;
  • lack of information resources for the public dealing with palliative and end-of-life care;
  • lack of reliable data on the quality of life and the quality of care of patients dying from cancer (as well as other chronic diseases); and
  • low level of public sector investment in palliative and end-of-life care research and training.

Separation of Palliative and Hospice Care Within the Health Care System

A major barrier to adequate palliative care has been the institutionalization of a system that focuses on *either* active therapy *or* palliative or hospice care and does not allow the appropriate interface between these two approaches. Lynn and O'Mara (Chapter 2) describe the ways in which this split is reinforced by the rules governing hospice care under the Medicare program, the largest payer of care for dying Americans. In addition, Holland and Chertkov (Chapter 7) describe the lack of attention to psychosocial, existential, and spiritual needs even when palliative care is available, and Payne (Chapter 5) describes the unequal access and even poorer treatment often afforded African Americans and other special population groups.

Hospice is the most substantial innovation to serve dying Americans, and for most, it is paid for by the Medicare hospice benefit (using a per diem rate), which was created in 1982. Hospice services—which are predominantly home based—include many elements that are not typically part of Medicare coverage (e.g., an interdisciplinary team, care planning, personal care nursing, family and patient teaching and support, chaplaincy, medication [with a small copayment], medical equipment and supplies, counseling, symptomatic treatment, bereavement support). However, Medicare allows hospice enrollment only for patients with a "prognosis of less than six months" and it is only with difficulty that hospices deal with documentation requirements for longer stays. These requirements ensure that hospice enrollment is seen as a decision to pursue a death-accepting course, which is an obvious deterrent for many patients. Furthermore, hospices are prohibited from offering any of their services to patients who are not formally enrolled, but who might benefit from some aspects of hospice care.

In recent years, more than 60 percent of patients who have enrolled in the Medicare hospice benefit have had cancer, and more than half of all dying cancer patients have used some hospice services (Hogan et al., 2000). The creation of the Medicare benefit was a major step forward, but its strict and limiting rules have led to inappropriately short stays of patients in hospice care, depriving them of the full application of palliative care in the final days of their lives.

The interface of hospice services and nursing home care is also unsettled. Nursing home stays are reimbursed by Medicare for only a minority of patients, but for these patients, Medicare reimbursement is high enough that they are unlikely to be offered the opportunity to enroll in hospice (only either skilled nursing home care or hospice can be in effect at one time). Since most nursing home stays do not qualify for Medicare payment, patients in nursing homes are often eligible for hospice services, but administrative complications deter enrollment for a large proportion of them.

The hospice requirement of a "six-month" prognosis has never been defined and is the source of trouble. Is the "just barely qualified" patient simply "more likely than not" to die within six months, or should that patient be "virtually certain to die"? This may seem like an arcane issue, but the population of everyone who is more likely than not to die within six months is *two to three orders of magnitude* (100 to 1,000 times) larger than the population that is virtually certain to die. The uncertainty of definition affects the willingness of hospices to accept patients who might stabilize and live a long time. Well-publicized fraud investigations for long-stay hospice patients (e.g., Lagnado, 2000, in the *Wall Street Journal*) have increased the chances that these patients, who are chronically ill and have benefited from hospice care, are likely to be discharged.

A number of other issues that affect access to and use of hospice services cause concern for patients and hospice providers. Hospices have significant latitude in deciding what services to offer, and they can vary tremendously, so patients are faced with selecting among them to find the best fit. Hospices are bedeviled with short stays, which have gotten shorter in recent years (from an average of 90 days in 1990 [Christakis and Escarce, 1996] to 48 days in 1999 [National Hospice and Palliative Care Organization, 2000]). No reliable research has yet sorted out the sources of increasingly short stays, but the financial impact on hospices has been substantial. The first day or two and the last few days in hospice are always costly. When these days come close together, there can be too few "stable" days with lower costs to offset losses on the "expensive days."

Hospices struggle with a plethora of developments in palliative care. Twenty years ago, it was not much of an exaggeration to claim that the hospice physician could do most everything with little more than cheap opioid medications, steroids, diuretics, and antibiotics. Now, there are more technologically advanced interventions, more expensive medications, more use of radiation or surgery, and so on—and additional costs of keeping hospice staff trained in their use—yet the Medicare hospice payment is a fixed amount per day. Some hospice programs rely on philanthropic donations to cover expensive interventions that they would not otherwise be able to offer.

Not everyone dying of cancer is covered by Medicare. The special case of children, analyzed by Hilden and colleagues (Chapter 6), demonstrates severe problems in securing and being paid for adequate palliative care through private insurers. Holland and Chertkov (Chapter 7) add that reimbursement for professional psychosocial care is poor to absent even in major cancer centers and is often excluded from medical and behavioral health contracts.

Some small-scale innovative demonstration projects are under way to test new ways of providing and paying for good palliative care throughout the course of fatal illness (e.g., see Box 1-1), but it is too soon to recommend a comprehensive set of changes (particularly for Medicare) without further experience, experimentation, and evaluation. A period of innovation, with thoughtful evaluation and learning, is needed in order to shape the care system and payment arrangements that would better serve cancer patients coming to the end of life.

Inadequate Training of Health Care Personnel

Most U.S. physicians—oncologists, other specialists, and generalists alike—are not prepared by education or experience to satisfy the palliative care needs of dying cancer patients or even to help them get needed services from other providers (Emanuel, personal communication). The same holds for the other mainstays of end-of-life care: nurses and social workers. In a review of the education and training of professionals, Gelband (Chapter 9) reports that this finding is consistent with the lack of funding for end-of-life or palliative care educational initiatives, which has begun to change only recently. Needs in training and education were covered in depth in the IOM (1997) report *Approaching Death*, and some of the new programs have taken root from that report. Even in 2000, however, the programs are small and funded largely by private grant-making organizations, with little contribution by the federal government. Holland and Chertkov (Chapter 7) attribute much of the difficulty that patients find in getting adequate treatment to the fact that there are no training standards to prepare physicians to identify patients with distress, nor are there standards of competence for those who provide psychosocial and spiritual services at the end of life.

Most new physicians leave medical school and residency programs with little training or experience in caring for dying patients. In most cases, a few lectures are folded into other courses (in many cases in psychiatry and behavioral sciences, ethics, or the humanities). A few schools offer full-length courses on palliative care, but they are nearly all electives. Contact

BOX 1-1
Promoting Excellence in End-of-Life Care—
The Robert Wood Johnson Foundation

Typically, patients with incurable cancers do not receive palliative care in the form of hospice until all life-prolonging options have been exhausted, often within just two weeks of death. As part of its "Promoting Excellence in End-of-Life Care" program, the Robert Wood Johnson Foundation began, in 1999, funding three-year demonstration projects at four cancer centers around the country to test innovative, integrated models of palliative and cancer care. The projects, located in Michigan, New Hampshire, Ohio, and California, are independent and are organized differently, but with common themes. Using approaches designed to fit within their particular health systems, each project is striving to incorporate palliative care within the continuum of cancer treatment from diagnosis through the trajectory of illness, extending to bereavement support for patients' families. Interdisciplinary teams, which may include physicians, nurses, social workers, and pastoral care providers, respond to the needs of patients and families. Emphasis is accorded communication, advance care planning, symptom management, and coordination of medical and support services.

Disease-modifying therapy is provided, including available NCI clinical trials. Patients with advanced cancer, or those whose cancers are deemed incurable at onset, are eligible for enrollment in these demonstrations. Project evaluation focuses on the feasibility and acceptability of these new models to patients, their families, and the collaborating local health systems. Outcome measures include clinical parameters of longevity, symptom frequency and severity, patient-family satisfaction, and quality of life. Utilization of resources, including hospitalizations, intensive care unit admissions, use of hospice services, and hospice lengths of stay, are also being studied.

A key to all of the programs is laying out options for care at an earlier stage of illness than usually occurs. Particularly important is avoiding the "terrible choice" that the health care system now imposes between potentially life-prolonging treatment and pure palliative care ("active" treatment versus "hospice") and to smooth the transition from one to the other when necessary. Brief descriptions of the programs and some early results are presented here.

1. The Palliative Care Program—University of Michigan Comprehensive Cancer Center

Researchers at the University of Michigan's Comprehensive Cancer Center, in conjunction with Hospice of Michigan, are integrating hospice services into the care of patients with advanced breast, prostate, or lung cancer or advanced congestive heart failure, while potentially life-prolonging treatment continues. They are conducting a randomized trial that follows on a pilot study involving patients with advanced prostate cancer, which found improvements in patient comfort and satisfaction when palliative care was provided concomitant with disease-modifying treatments.

According to Dr. Kenneth J. Pienta, a principal investigator for the project, "Within this new system, the patient and family can appropriately begin the process of transition and we can provide an opportunity for patients and families to grow through the end of life."

box continued on next page

BOX 1-1 Continued

In the first year, 84 patients enrolled in the trial. In this early group, no overall difference is seen in standard quality-of-life measures two months after enrollment, but for those who functional status was poorer to begin with (Karnofsky score d70), the program appears to have improved quality of life in the intervention group compared with the usual care group, with the suggestion of a greater effect over time.

2. Project ENABLE: Educate, Nurture, Advise, Before Life Ends—
Dartmouth-Hitchcock Medical Center

The Dartmouth-Hitchcock Medical Center's ENABLE Project team has moved high-quality end-of-life care into New Hampshire's regional cancer center and beyond, into three rural communities. The ENABLE team assesses patients' needs and provides continuous palliative care throughout the course of cancer care. Patient education is a priority. The team travels to each town with a unique educational seminar, "Charting Your Course: A Whole Person's Approach to Living with Cancer," empowering cancer patients and their families to better navigate the health care system, engage in advanced care planning, and extending support to those confronting issues of life completion and closure. The goal is to help people retain control of their lives and key decisions.

Following diagnosis, a palliative care coordinator works with patients and families to develop a care plan, stressing continuity of care during the course of the illness. Each of the three communities has a palliative care team, consisting of a pain management specialist, a psychiatrist or psychologist, a hospice or home health liaison, a social worker or case manager, and a pastoral caregiver. Each team tailors its work to the specific health care system in the community.

"Project ENABLE will allow us to demonstrate that, regardless of geographic location, cultural identification, or clinical sophistication, patients need not be abandoned when a cure for their disease seems no longer possible," said E. Robert Greenberg, M.D., principal investigator for the project.

One early indication of the program's success at merging the cultures of hospice and oncology treatment is the commitment shown by six staff oncologists in sitting for—and passing—the certification exam in palliative medicine.

3. Project Safe Conduct—Ireland Cancer Center, Case Western Reserve University

Case Western Reserve University Hospitals of Cleveland has literally invited the palliative team into the Ireland Cancer Center. The Project Safe Conduct team's office is in the same building, and each member of the team wears an Ireland Cancer Center nametag. The team attends staff orientations and meets regularly with the therapeutic staff. Physician acceptance of the program is high, and patients have been recruited to the program faster than anticipated. This collaboration between the cancer center, Hospice of the Western Reserve, and Case Western Reserve University creates a system that allows patients to receive life-prolonging care—including experimental therapy protocols—integrated with palliative care. In Project Safe Conduct, patients and families are guided through the labyrinth of available treatments and services, emphasizing state-of-the-art symptom management as well as psychosocial and spiritual support.

Early results are encouraging. In the first year, 133 patients were enrolled, of whom 40 percent were members of ethnic or racial minorities. Pain assessment has been documented in 100 percent of Safe Conduct patients, compared to a historical control of just 3 percent. Quality-of-life scores remained steady or improved in Safe Conduct patients, despite concomitant decline in functional status. At baseline, only 13 percent of the center's patients were served by hospice and for an average of just 3 days before death. Now, only 18 months into the Safe Conduct Project, more than 80 percent of Ireland's patients have the benefits of hospice care, achieving an average length of stay of 18 days.

As part of the effort, Project Safe Conduct is also developing innovative palliative care curricula for the Case Western Reserve Schools of Medicine and Nursing, as well as postgraduate training for specialists in oncology.

4. Improvements in End-of-Life Care for Selected Populations—University of California-Davis Cancer Center

Researchers at the University of California-Davis (UC Davis) Medical Center and the West Coast Center for Palliative Education, Sacramento, California, have developed the Simultaneous Care project to extend palliative care to patients undergoing active, anticancer treatments (who would otherwise be ineligible for hospice care). In Simultaneous Care, palliative care staff work together with clinical oncologists to serve patients with advanced cancer, including those participating in experimental treatment protocols. In early results, quality of life as measured by the FACT (Functional Assessment of Cancer Therapy) shows a clear trend toward improvement for Simultaneous Care patients compared to patients receiving best customary care. There has also been a greater adherence to chemotherapy protocols for Simultaneous Care patients, a higher percentage of referrals to hospice, and improved length of stays in hospice. Finally, preliminary data suggest that the distress experienced by primary caregivers may be reduced, both during the illness and after the patient's death.

In another aspect of this project, some of California's hardest-to-serve populations are also being reached. The program expands and improves the level of palliative care available to people in three isolated, rural areas—Colusa, Tuolumne, and Plumas Counties—as well as the state women's prison population. According to the project's principal investigator, Dr. Frederick J. Meyers, although they are dissimilar in many ways, each of the targeted populations lacks access to palliative or hospice care.

In this project, palliative care experts have trained teams of health providers to work in the rural counties and to use teleconferencing links to UC Davis physicians for immediate assistance in the care of dying patients. Using remote television, UC Davis physicians consult with patients and offer suggestions for care. In a third component of the project, staff are working with California Department of Corrections and health care teams in the women's prison to offer palliative care training and begin development of a prison hospice program to serve inmates who are dying.

with dying patients, particularly for undergraduate medical students, if any, is limited.

Nurses are expected to provide physical, emotional, spiritual, and practical care for patients in every phase of life. They spend more time with patients near the end of life than do any other health professionals. Yet like physicians, most nurses in the United States do not receive the training and practical experience they need to carry out these duties in the best fashion. The nursing curriculum has been less studied than the medical curriculum, but this has been changing, particularly in response to debates about assisted suicide and euthanasia (Ferrell et al., 2000).

Social workers are central to counseling, case management, and advocacy services for the dying and for bereaved families. With their focus on the psychosocial aspects of the dying process, they work not only with patients but with those around them in making decisions about treatment options, marshaling resources, helping families cope with terminal illness and death of a relative, and generally encouraging the best quality of life for all concerned. Just as nursing and medicine have begun to do, the social work profession has been examining its education process for preparing practitioners to care for dying patients and their families. Efforts to improve undergraduate- and master's-level social work training in this area are just getting under way in the United States, in comparison to the more mature field in Canada and England and in comparison to medical and nursing education (Christ and Sormanti, 1999).

In medicine, nursing, and social work, the following are needed:

- faculty development,
- educational materials and curriculum development,
- coordination among training programs for the variety of professionals involved in the care of dying patients,
- guidelines for residency programs and increased palliative and end-of-life content in licensing and certifying examinations, and
- improving the research base for palliative care education.

Inadequate Standards of Care and Lack of Accountability in Caring for Dying Patients

Practice Guidelines

The process of developing standards of care for patients at the end of life is under way, but still at an early stage. Holland and Chertkov (Chapter 7) review the status of practice guidelines for care at the end of life, including both physical and psychosocial components (Table 1-1). The one aspect for which evidence-based guidelines for end-of-life care do exist is pain

TABLE 1-1 Clinical Practice Guidelines for End-of-Life Care: Status, Source, and Further Development Needed

Symptom	Status	Source	Further Development
Overall end-of-life care	NCCN Practice Guidelines (pending) (NCCN, 2001)	Evidence, consensus, or combination	Pilot testing; modify for end-of-life care
Doctor-patient communication	NCCN Practice Guidelines: breaking bad news (pending) (NCCN, 2001)	Evidence, consensus, or combination	Pilot testing; modify for end-of-life care
Distress	NCCN Practice Guidelines: ambulatory care		Algorithm for recognition and referral; modify for end-of-life care
	Definition— Psychosocial, existential or spiritual (NCCN, 1999)		
Delirium	APA Practice Guidelines: physically healthy (APA, 2000)	Evidence, consensus, or combination	Modify for medically ill and end-of-life care
	NCCN Practice Guidelines: ambulatory care (NCCN, 1999)	Evidence, consensus, or combination	Modify for end-of-life care; pilot test
Depressive disorders	APA Practice Guidelines: physically healthy (APA, 2000)	Evidence, consensus, or combination	Modify for end-of-life care
	NCCN Practice Guidelines: ambulatory care (NCCN, 1999)	Evidence, consensus, or combination	Modify for end-of-life care; pilot test

continued on next page

TABLE 1-1 Continued

Symptom	Status	Source	Further Development
Anxiety disorders	APA Practice Guidelines: panic disorder in healthy patients (APA, 2000)	Evidence, consensus, or combination	Modify for medically ill/ end-of-life care
	NCCN Practice Guidelines: ambulatory care (NCCN, 1999)	Evidence, consensus, or combination	Modify for end-of-life care; pilot test
Personality disorders	APA Practice Guidelines (APA, 2000)	Evidence, consensus, or combination	Modify for medically ill and end-of-life care
	NCCN Practice Guidelines: ambulatory care (NCCN, 1999)	Evidence, consensus, or combination	Modify for end-of-life care; pilot test
Social problems: practical or psychosocial	NCCN Guidelines for Social Work Services: Ambulatory (NCCN, 1999)	Evidence, consensus, or combination	Modify for end-of-life care; pilot test
Spiritual or religious problems	NCCN Guidelines for Clergy/ Pastoral Counselors: ambulatory (NCCN, 1999)	Evidence, consensus, or combination	Modify for end-of-life care; pilot test
Pain	AHCPR Guidelines (AHCPR, 1994)	Evidence, consensus, or combination	Modify for end-of-life care
	APS Guidelines (APS, 1995)	Evidence, consensus, or combination	Dissemination and implementation
	WHO Pain Management (WHO, 1996)	Evidence, consensus, or combination	Compliance and implementation

TABLE 1-1 Continued

Symptom	Status	Source	Further Development
	NCCN Guidelines (NCCN, 1999)	Evidence, consensus, or combination	Modify for end-of-life care; pilot test; dissemination and compliance
Fatigue	NCCN Practice Guidelines: guidelines for anemia-related fatigue management (NCCN, 1999)	Evidence, consensus, or combination	Modify for end-of-life care; pilot test
Nausea and vomiting	NCCN anti-emesis (for treatment-related nausea and vomiting) (NCCN, 1997)	Evidence, consensus, or combination	Modify for end-of-life care; pilot test
Dyspnea	Descriptive guides to care (Ahmedzai, 1998)	Literature	Develop guidelines; pilot test

NOTE: APA = American Psychiatric Association; APS = American Pain Society; AHCPR = Agency for Health Care Policy and Research; NCCN = National Comprehensive Cancer Network

management. In addition to general pain management guidelines (the Agency for Healthcare Research and Quality [AHRQ] and the National Comprehensive CancerNetwork [NCCN]), guidelines specifically for pain control at the end of life have been developed. Work is progressing on guidelines for some other common symptoms. NCCN guidelines exist for a variety of psychosocial conditions—distress, delirium, depression, anxiety, personality disorders, social problems, and spiritual and religious issues—but they are general and have to be modified for dying patients (a process that is under way through NCCN). A guideline for fatigue is in the same state, and one for nausea and vomiting has been developed for treatment-related symptoms, but not for end-of-life symptoms. No guidelines exist for managing dyspnea, a frequent and distressing symptom.

Various groups are working toward guidelines in these areas (despite, in many cases, a lack of evidence forcing reliance on consensus), but plans for validation and field testing are probably years off for most of them.

Accountability: Quality Indicators

It is not enough to define the best treatments and develop models of excellent palliative and end-of-life care, or even to educate health care providers about what works and what doesn't, although these are all necessary steps. What is important is that dying patients, in the variety of health care settings in which they receive care, actually get the best treatments. The NCPB report *Ensuring Quality Cancer Care* (IOM, 1999) outlined a vision for the development of "indicators" to cover the spectrum of cancer care—including the dying process—that could be used to hold health care providers, institutions, and health plans accountable for the quality of care given.

As Teno demonstrates in Chapter 3 of this report, we are not close to meeting this mandate for care at the end of life, either for cancer or for other conditions (Table 1-2). Research and demonstration programs will be needed before even a preliminary set of satisfactory indicators can be developed. The focus of early work will be on the development and validation of measurement tools based on administrative data, medical records, and interviews with patients, family members, and health care providers. These instruments must be developed and adapted for different cultures and ethnicities.

Quality indicators are needed for two main purposes: accountability (external use by regulators, health care purchasers, or consumers) and quality improvement (internal use for the purpose of monitoring or continuous quality improvement). The same types of indicators may serve both purposes, but for some aspects, they may have to be different.

At this early stage in development, there is a strong evidence base to support the use of quality indicators for pain management for the purpose of accountability, and in fact, a standard (not specific to end-of-life care or cancer) has just taken effect through the Joint Commission on Accreditation of Healthcare Organizations (JCAHO), requiring all participating hospitals to demonstrate that they adequately monitor and manage the pain of patients (JCAHO, 2000). However, more basic research and demonstration projects are needed to develop indicators for managing other common symptoms (e.g., emotional distress and depression, fatigue, gastrointestinal symptoms). An important aspect of demonstration and validation is monitoring for potential unintended consequences (e.g., patients are sedated contrary to their preferences to improve accountability statistics).

Besides the domain of symptom management, four other domains should be considered for early development and implementation of accountability measures: (1) patient satisfaction, (2) shared decisionmaking, (3) coordination, and (4) continuity of care. In each of these domains, indicators must validly represent the perceptions of the dying person and family members. This means investing in new survey methods that are patient centered and include questions that get at unmet needs.

TABLE 1-2 Status of Quality Indicator Development for End-of-Life Care

Domain	Proposed Indicators	Readiness
Pain	Frequency and severity of pain from Minimum Data Set	Proposed indicators require validation, but can be measured for all hospitalized cancer patients Major limitation: captures only health care provider perspective
	Patient and family perspective on pain management	Instruments available (e.g., from American Pain Society or Toolkit of Instruments to Measure End-of-Life Care)
Satisfaction	Measures of patient satisfaction, based on patient or surrogate responses New instruments include some questions relevant to people dying from cancer	New instruments have undergone reliability and validity testing. Additional questions are specific for cancer (e.g., whether patients are informed of recommended treatments, access to high-quality clinical trials) and incorporation into ongoing data collection efforts
Shared Decisionmaking	Questions from Toolkit of Instruments to Measure End-of-Life Care	Reliability and validity testing completed Examination of responsiveness not complete
Coordination and Continuity of Care	No indicators yet available	

Shared decisionmaking has been increasingly recognized as a key aspect throughout the continuum of care. Although the focus of research has been on resuscitation decisions, the most important decision for the majority of cancer patients is the one to stop active treatment, but there is little research that examines this decision.

Beyond those mentioned, there is debate over which other domains are important in the care of the dying. Various conceptual models have been proposed to examine the quality of end-of-life care, with different emphases. Research is now needed to examine the correlations among structures of the health care system, processes of care, and important outcomes to identify the most fruitful areas for developing new quality measures.

Ongoing national data collection efforts include little information to describe the quality of care of dying persons and their families. An occasional survey, the National Mortality Followback Survey (NMFBS), has collected information on access to care and functional status, but not on important domains that are central to the quality of care of the dying. A redesigned NMFBS could collect information on key domains to describe the quality of care for patients who died based on the perspective of the bereaved family member. There are no current plans for further iterations of the NMFBS, however.

Two national data collection systems warrant consideration for development of quality indicators: Medicare claims files and the Nursing Home Minimum Data Set (MDS). The NCPB has recommended previously that hospice enrollment and length of stay be examined as quality indicators (IOM, 1999). From a national perspective, the only source of that information is Medicare claims data. Other indicators based on administrative data have also been proposed. Work to develop and validate these indicators using claims data is still to be done.

The second national data collection effort is the MDS, which routinely collects extensive information on every nursing home resident in the United States. Nursing homes increasingly are providing end-of-life care for frail and older Americans. In 1998, an estimated 10 percent of cancer patients died in a nursing home. The Health Care Financing Administration (HCFA) is now embarking on a national program of examining nursing home quality performance. There are important lessons to be learned from the MDS, including concerns about the institutional response burden in implementing data collection and the potential for unintended consequences. In the nursing home setting, a concern is that quality indicators have been developed for the majority of nursing home residents (who are not dying imminently) where the main goals of care are to restore function, yet the same indicators will be applied to those who are dying. For example, the rates of dehydration and weight loss are now among the core quality indicators for nursing homes. With increased scrutiny of these indicators, there is concern that unintended consequences for the dying might include increased use of feeding tubes, which could be contrary to patient preferences.

Disparities in End-of-Life Care for Minority Groups

Cancer statistics for certain minority groups in the United States reveal substantial inequalities in health outcomes. African Americans represent the largest minority population, and the one for which there is the best documentation of unequal access to, and quality of, care. Cancer incidence and mortality rates are significantly higher, and survival rates significantly lower, for African Americans than for whites in the United States. African

Americans are also underrepresented in the use of hospice care. In recent years, only 5-7 percent of hospice patients have been African Americans, even though they make up about 14 percent of the total population. Payne (Chapter 5) describes the historical, cultural, and economic determinants of this pattern of underutilization of palliative and end-of-life care in the African-American population, which can be taken as a model for other medically underserved and vulnerable populations that are less well studied. Bias (conscious and unconscious) of health care providers, lack of economic access for many African-American and other minority group members, and a wide range of cultural factors place minority groups at a disadvantage in getting adequate palliative care.

Unequal treatment in the U.S. health care system has deep roots in the African-American community. The health care system, along with many other societal institutions, lacks credibility with many African Americans because of past abuses, which are commonly known: slavery, medical experimentation, Jim Crow laws, and so forth. Denial of death (even in the face of terminal illness) is seen—if unconsciously—as fighting back against past injustice; whereas accepting palliative care is viewed as giving up on care that the majority might receive.

Even when palliative care is wanted and needed, however, it may not be available. Hospice care may not be available in poor, inner-city areas, which are generally underserved for health care. A stark example comes from a recent study demonstrating that pharmacies in predominantly non-white communities do not stock opioids at all or have inadequate stocks (Morrison et al., 2000). In an accompanying editorial, the story is recounted of an elderly woman with unrelieved bone pain from metastatic cancer, whose daughter was unable to buy a prescribed morphine-based drug in any local pharmacy (Freeman and Payne, 2000). This is just an example of inequities that pervade the provision of palliative care for minority populations.

There is an urgent need for palliative care units in inner-city hospitals, which involves not only providing facilities, but training teams of providers to staff these units. Even more fundamental, research is required to understand the needs and preferences of African Americans and other minorities for end-of-life care and to elucidate the health policy and financial barriers that leave these groups with inadequate care during the dying process.

Lack of Information Resources for the Public on Palliative and End-of-Life Care

Faced with a diagnosis of cancer, people often respond by gathering information about the cause of their ailment, treatment options, and advances in medical research. Patients find information from any number of sources—health professionals, family, friends, religious leaders, printed materials, telephone hotlines, mail order, and increasingly, the World Wide Web. The materials available, however, emphasize curative treatment and living as a cancer survivor to the relative exclusion of information on palliative care and end-of-life issues. Kesselheim, in Chapter 4, analyzes the state of information available for those with advanced cancer who are likely to die from their disease.

Physicians are often the first, and remain the most important, source of information for a large proportion of patients about all aspects of a cancer diagnosis and treatment.

Information Producers: National Cancer Institute, American Cancer Society, and Others

NCI and the American Cancer Society (ACS) write the majority of educational materials for cancer patients, in the form of booklets, pamphlets, and fact sheets, and make them freely available in a variety of ways. Most of the materials deal with cancer prevention, descriptions of various cancers and their treatments, clinical trials, and survivorship concerns. Only recently have NCI and ACS begun publishing materials related to end-of-life issues.

NCI produces one publication, *Advanced Cancer: Living Each Day* (1998), aimed at dying patients and booklets for some specific end-of-life concerns: *Eating Hints for Cancer Patients* (1998), *Get Relief from Cancer Pain* (1994), and *Pain Control* (2000, published in conjunction with ACS). NCI's Physician Data Query (PDQ) has a section dealing with "Supportive Care Topics," covering the major symptoms at the end of life. There are also "Cancer Facts," information sheets about hospice care and national and local cancer support organizations.

Finally, NCI's Cancer Information Service (CIS) comprises 19 resource centers across the country that answer calls to "1-800-4-CANCER." CIS representatives mail patients NCI-produced and other approved materials, according to the type and stage of cancer and the caller's requests.

In addition to distributing NCI material, ACS offers its own booklets, including one directed at end-of-life care, called *Caring for the Patient with Cancer at Home* (1998).

Overall, the easily available information about palliative and end-of-life care is inadequate. The few publications mentioned are among hundreds of cancer-related publications that ignore the dimension of advanced disease and death from cancer. For instance, the NCI booklet *What You Need to Know About Ovarian Cancer* (1993) mentions nothing about the possibility that a patient might die of an ovarian tumor, despite the fact that this cancer often is diagnosed in late stages, with little hope for long-term survival. While the ACS document on lung cancer relays the generally low overall survival rates and suggests "supportive care" as a viable choice for patients diagnosed as Stage IV non-small cell lung cancer, these paragraphs are given less space than highly investigational treatments such as immunotherapy and gene therapy. The materials that NCI and ACS offer to deal with other end-of-life symptoms (e.g., pain, loss of appetite) also mention little about death and dying. A factor limiting the effective reach of even the few relevant NCI and ACS materials that exist is that most are currently available only in English.

Many other organizations issue educational materials and distribute NCI and ACS booklets, and a few organizations dedicate themselves specifically to end-of-life concerns in cancer care. In general, these organizations have low visibility, and even if they have good information, most patients will never hear about them. In addition, the organizations themselves have limited abilities to adapt information to the individual needs of patients. Most patients who call, no matter how advanced their condition is, receive the same introductory packet and pamphlets, which are likely to have little relevance for patients with advanced, recurrent, or terminal cancer.

Pharmaceutical companies have begun producing information about symptom control that, not surprisingly, concentrates on their own products. A pharmaceutical firm that produces an antiemetic has little reason to alert people to competing products or approaches, much less treatments for other symptoms.

End-of-Life Information from Health Care Providers

Physicians remain the primary source of information for patients about end-of-life care, but patients are often reluctant to bring up the topics of death and dying, so physicians themselves must initiate discussions if they are to take place (Pfeifer et al., 1994). Many physicians are not well prepared for this task, however, either by training or by experience. They may avoid it altogether, or if they attempt to inform and counsel patients, they may be unaware that the patient (and family members) may not fully understand the information or may be overwhelmed by too much information. Physicians and other health care providers, even at major cancer centers, may not have access to information resources that would facilitate informing their patients.

Another illustration relates to advance directives, mandated by law in some states and by hospital policy in some institutions. Many physicians and nurses will admit that these forms are often handed to newly admitted patients, among a large stack of paperwork, with little explanation.

Finally, even though many NCI-designated cancer centers might advertise themselves as extremely effective sources of patient education and information, the number of people who have access to these institutions is limited, both geographically and because most patients simply are not treated in cancer centers. Most of the centers are currently reluctant (or unable) to provide information to outsiders who are not patients at their institution.

Current deficiencies in communication between patients and their physicians about end-of-life issues have many other origins. Poor provider communication skills and knowledge of end-of-life issues, and a health care market that discourages referrals to hospice and rewards medical procedures and treatments over cognitive therapy, also can contribute to poor communication by health care providers.

End-of-Life Information from the World Wide Web

The Internet has emerged as a powerful influence in all information-gathering activities, and cancer and end-of-life information is no exception. The interactive nature of the World Wide Web allows people not only to access static sites, but also to communicate with counselors or support groups and watch or listen to audiovisual clips.

Nearly all of the cancer organizations that patients and their family members have traditionally contacted by phone or letter have now constructed Web pages to disseminate their resources. Exclusively Web-based sources of patient education and information have also emerged. A search for "end-of-life issues" leads to reviews of palliative care handbooks, hospice information sites, video downloads, and numerous articles and hyperlinks. NCI lists a number of links on its Web site, including major organizations and Web sites devoted to hospice.

The biggest hurdle to effective use of the Web is access. Surfing the Internet requires a computer, a modem, and a Web browser, as well as facility in navigating. A larger problem, in the long run, is the variable quality of information on the Internet, the accuracy of which is unregulated.

Lack of Reliable Data on Quality of Life and
Quality of Care at the End of Life

There is sufficient information from recent studies to demonstrate that cancer patients are consistently undertreated for pain, are underdiagnosed for their psychological distress, and have significant economic barriers to getting palliative care and that health care professionals identify their lack of both knowledge and training, as well as ability to obtain effective services for their patients, as major barriers to providing adequate care. At the same time, we have little understanding of the particular dying experiences of most patients with cancer—where they die, who cares for them as they are dying, what the quality of such care is, whether guidelines are in fact being followed, and whether these things are changing over time. This lack of information hampers our ability to develop a clear policy agenda and will, in the future, impede monitoring trends to determine whether interventions are having their intended effects.

Knowing how well we're doing or whether things are getting better in end-of-life care requires some routinely collected information, as well as specific studies. New data collection efforts might be necessary, but it may be possible to make better use of data already being collected, including those collected for other purposes. HCFA's claims for Medicare reimbursement constitute a major resource on their own, and because it is becoming increasingly feasible to link these "claims data" to those from other systems and surveys, they may prove an even more powerful data source.

The needs for an in-depth assessment of the information potential of current data sources and for an assessment of future needs are identified in this report but are not within the scope of work. The NCPB plans a comprehensive follow-on report to delve into this topic and will defer recommendations related to data collection until that report is complete.

Low Level of Public Investment in Palliative and End-of-Life Care Research

Despite billions of dollars spent on research in cancer biology and cancer therapeutics, there has been little investment in research that might significantly alleviate the physical and psychological distress of patients at the end of life. Cleeland (Chapter 8) reports that compared to the rest of the cancer research establishment, research directed at cancer-related symptom management is poorly organized, poorly conceptualized, underfunded, and dependent on an insufficient number of well-trained researchers.

The feasibility of symptom control research has been demonstrated. Studies of the epidemiology of symptoms, behavioral research, health services research, and basic research, as well as clinical trials, have already produced benefits that have been translated into better care. Although the amount of improvement has not been well studied, it is very possible that patients now experience less distress related to medical procedures, that pain is somewhat better managed, and that there is wider recognition of and attention to end-of-life issues such as patient preference for end-of-life decisionmaking. Research has also documented the gaps between current care and optimal care and has identified very specific obstacles that could be addressed to improve care.

Perhaps less obvious has been a maturation of research methods that should facilitate rapid progress of research in this area. Subjective reports of patients about quality of life and symptoms are increasingly accepted as reasonable measures for clinical and laboratory research. Quality-of-life outcomes—including aspects of symptom control—have become more accepted as clinical trial end points. New technologies offer unique opportunities to understand the nature, mechanisms, and expression of symptoms that were not possible a few years ago (e.g., new brain imaging techniques to study pain and depression) and, further, to see how treatment affects them. Developments in neurobiology have opened windows to a better understanding of end-of-life symptoms. Exciting new agents that could provide better control of most of the symptoms of the dying process have been and are being developed. There is a real possibility that individual variation in symptom expression may be better understood through progress in genetic science. It can no longer be said that tools to advance the area are lacking, and there is also no lack of research targets.

The understanding of pain, although more advanced than that of other symptoms, still has enormous gaps to be filled. This finding is confirmed and detailed in a January 2001 AHRQ Evidence Report/Technology Assessment, *Management of Cancer Pain* (AHRQ, 2001), which concludes:

> Randomized controlled trials establish that many current treatment modalities can individually reduce cancer pain. These trials constitute 1 percent of the published literature on cancer pain, enroll one in 10,000 patients at risk for cancer pain in industrialized countries, are often heterogeneous, and use poor methodology. Leading investigators in the area of cancer pain relief have repeatedly called for improving the quality of trials in this area. The quantity and quality of scientific evidence on cancer pain relief still, however, compare unfavorably with the great deal that is known about other high-impact conditions, including cancer itself. In the current era of patient-centered care, closing this gap should be a high research priority.

Our understanding of symptoms other than pain is much more limited. Research examining ways of improving the care given to patients with advanced cancer is just beginning. Methods for studying and providing for the more complex subjective needs of patients (spiritual, existential) have to be developed. Few of the common practices of caring for patients with advanced cancer have been subjected to careful randomized clinical trials, impeding the provision of evidence-based practice recommendations.

Cleeland has laid out a research agenda for the most important symptoms in the disciplines of basic science, epidemiology, social-behavioral research, health services research, and clinical trials. Specific opportunities and currently unmet research needs in symptom control are outlined in Table 1-3.

END-OF-LIFE AND PALLIATIVE CARE:
EVOLUTION OF THE ISSUE

Until the early part of the twentieth century, most Americans died of infectious diseases, many in childhood and middle age. Then, virtually every serious illness, including cancer, spelled a fairly rapid course to death. Those who survived to old age and developed the chronic diseases that the majority of people now die from had shorter trajectories until death, with few experiencing prolonged periods of critical illness leading up to death. Malignancies were identified only when large or in a critical location, and most often, no treatments were available that substantially altered the course. The fact that cancer patients often lingered a few months, often with disturbing appearance, odors, and suffering, undoubtedly contributed to cancer's special position of abhorrence in the popular mythology. Now, patients with cancer often live much longer because of better prevention, earlier diagnosis, and treatments that prolong survival, resulting in longer periods of adaptation to cancer as a chronic debilitating disease. However, most still eventually die from the cancer.

After World War II, the health care system grew rapidly, with hospitals assuming a place of prominence. The emphasis was on acute care, which led to what has been referred to as the "medicalization" of death, confining it largely to hospitals. By the late 1960s and early 1970s, a grassroots movement had taken hold in the United States that began focusing on the development of volunteer hospice programs, in an attempt to "demedicalize" death. This reached its peak in 1982, when the Medicare hospice benefit was developed. From 1982 to the present, hospice has become more and more available under Medicare (although with the problems alluded to earlier). Over the period 1994 through 1998, 45 percent of all beneficiaries who died from cancer used some hospice services, and for 1998 alone, more than half of all cancer patients who died used hospice services. Although use by people dying from other conditions has grown considerably, far fewer use hospice (e.g., 10 percent of beneficiaries dying of congestive heart failure from 1994 through 1998 used hospice, as did 20 percent of those dying of Alzheimer's and other dementias) (Hogan et al., 2000).

Even thoroughly tested, effective measures to improve the quality of life of dying patients through symptom control have not been widely adopted; in contrast, the most marginal improvements in chemotherapy to extend life—often at reduced quality—diffuse remarkably quickly. Our desire to evade and avoid the events associated with death pervades society. It could be argued that no institution mirrors society as well as the U.S. Congress. In their recommendations for funding the National Cancer Institute—approaching $4 billion for fiscal year 2001—the House of Representatives

TABLE 1-3 Symptom Control Research Opportunities and Unmet Needs

Symptom	Basic	Clinical or Health Services
Pain	• Elucidate basic mechanisms of visceral and neuropathic pain; identify new treatments • Identify modifications of nervous system involved in chronic pain perception • Find new compounds with more precise analgesic action and fewer side effects • Find molecular basis of pain signaling, receptor modification due to pain, and ways to modify • Identify forebrain structures that modulate responses to "painful" signals • Determine receptor affinities of different opioids	• Determine why so many patients have poorly controlled pain • Study ways to improve cancer pain management • Determine effectiveness of treatments for neuropathic pain • Determine effects of cancer on tolerance to opioid analgesics and how pain can be managed in already tolerant patients • Determine side-effect profiles of different opioids • Conduct trials of intrathecal delivery of novel analgesics
Anorexia or Cachexia	• Elucidate roles for various cytokines in cachexia • Elucidate roles of food regulatory peptides in cachexia	Conduct clinical trials of • Proinflammatory mediators • Appetite stimulants • Anticatabolic agents (e.g., neuropeptide agonists or antagonists, beta$_2$-adrenoceptor agonists) • Polyunsaturated fatty acids, n-3 fatty acids, fish oil • Anabolic agents (especially hormonal) • Anticytokines (e.g., megestrol acetate, medroxyprogesterone acetate, thalidomide, melatonin)

Cognitive failure: delirium, temporary and permanent cognitive impairment	• Elucidate underlying mechanisms of delirium and cognitive impairment
	• Identify role of cancer disease process in cognitive impairment
	• Determine how biological therapies (e.g., interferon alpha, interleukin-2) produce cognitive impairment
	• Find biological markers for patients most at risk of
		• Develop standardized assessment for delirium
		• Determine prevalence, nature, and current treatments for delirium and cognitive impairment
		• Conduct clinical trials of
		  – Drugs used empirically for delirium (haloperidol) and cognitive impairment (methylphenidate)
		  – stimulants for cognitive

TABLE 1-3 Continued

Symptom	Basic	Clinical or Health Services
	delirium or cognitive impairment	impairment • Require neuropsychological assessments in cancer treatment trials to determine whether drugs are causing cognitive impairment
Dyspnea	• Standardize measurement and assessment • Develop animal model • Determine relationship of dyspnea to anemia in chronic illness • Determine role of respiratory muscle metabolism and function • Elucidate link between cachexia, tumor necrosis factor, muscle fatigue or weakness, and dyspnea	• Study prevalence, severity, and current treatment • Conduct clinical trials of opioids by different routes of administration • Conduct clinical trials of other agents (e.g., corticosteroids)
Fatigue	• Explore new agents (e.g., anticytokines) • Develop animal models • Explore common pathways for fatigue and other symptoms	Conduct clinical trials of • Stimulant therapies • Current anticytokines • Selective serotonin receptor uptake inhibitors (SSRIs) • Exercise • Behavioral interventions
Gastrointestinal symptoms	• Study relationship of terminal nausea to other symptoms of advanced disease • Determine mechanisms of terminal and treatment-induced nausea	• Study prevalence, severity and current treatment of terminal nausea • Conduct clinical trials of agents for nausea of advanced disease and for bowel obstruction
Psychiatric or affective symptoms	• Develop animal model for cancer-related affective disturbances • Study mechanisms of depression unique to cancer and its treatment	• Describe current management in advanced disease • Conduct clinical trials of standard antidepressants, especially SSRIs; stimulant therapies (e.g., methyl-phenidate); and agents for terminal agitation or restlessness • Consider trials of novel agents: "empathogens"

and the Senate Appropriations Committees both detail a rich research agenda that covers many specific types of cancer, screening and early detection, and finding cures, but not a word about research to help alleviate the symptoms of cancer, either for those who survive or for those who die.

Societal attitudes have evolved, to some extent, as a result of public airing of the issues. Discussions about dying have become more acceptable, and patients and families have increasingly played greater roles in deciding on the goals and details of treatment. Yet the task of ensuring that the best care is available when people are dying and that avoidable distress is minimized to provide the best "quality of death" has to be accomplished even in the face of reluctance of the dying and those around them to grapple with key issues and necessary decisions. Fortunately, there is progress to report.

A constellation of factors has put palliative care on the agenda as a medical issue: the development of technology-intensive approaches for patients with advanced disease, advances in treatment for cancer patients and patients with AIDS, a large and aging elderly population, a growing population of patients with significant neurological and neurodegenerative diseases requiring continuous care, and limitations in health care resources. All of these issues have come together at a time when the country is trying to address how it cares for patients with serious life-threatening illness and the controversies of withholding and withdrawing care, physician-assisted suicide, euthanasia, and a U.S. Supreme Court decision on physician-assisted suicide that asserts a right to palliative care. It is also a time of medical advance and the potential for much greater advances.

The lead in tackling palliative care and improved end-of-life care has been taken largely by private foundations, in particular, the Robert Wood Johnson Foundation, the Nathan Cummings Foundation, the Fetzer Institute, the Commonwealth Fund, and the Project on Death in America, which together have underwritten a wide range of innovative research, training, and public awareness programs. They have laid the groundwork for moving forward, but the foundation focus does not represent a permanent presence in the field and is likely to be scaled back in the future.

Federal government efforts took shape in hospitals run by the Department of Veterans Affairs (VA), in their role as caregivers for elderly and dying veterans. VA developed a faculty scholars program in palliative care, the requirement that pain be recorded as a "fifth vital sign" for all patients, and hospice programs at all its major hospitals. Other early government steps include the Medicare hospice benefit and the efforts of the Health Resources and Services Administration (HRSA) in care provided within the prison system, as well as for patients with AIDS.

THE 1990S: SIGNAL EFFORTS AND EVENTS AROUND PALLIATIVE AND END-OF-LIFE CARE

Central among the early prime movers in palliative care has been the Robert Wood Johnson Foundation (RWJF), which funded the groundbreaking Study to Understand Prognoses and Preferences for Outcomes and Risks of Treatment. RWJF has continued to shine the spotlight on end-of-life needs through its "Last Acts" program, which encourages activities at local levels and other activities; its "Promoting Excellence in End-of-Life Care" program (see Box 1-2); and others, including sponsorship of a recent six-hour public television special on palliative and end-of-life care ("On Our Own Terms: Moyers on Dying," September 2000).

Some of the touchstone events in end-of-life and palliative care are described in the sections that follow.

The Study to Understand Prognoses and Preferences for Outcomes and Risks of Treatment

Asked to name the most influential phenomenon in moving end-of-life care in the 1990s, most who know the field would probably name SUPPORT—the Study to Understand Prognoses and Preferences for Outcomes and Risks of Treatment. SUPPORT was a two-stage research project, beginning with an observational study of aspects of end-of-life care, followed by a randomized intervention trial to try to improve the quality of care found in the first stage, with the emphasis on communication between caregivers and patients. A companion study, HELP—the Hospitalized Elderly Longitudinal Project—was similar to the first stage of SUPPORT, but included only the very old, people 80 years and over (see Box 1-2 for a description of the studies). SUPPORT and HELP were funded solely by the Robert Wood Johnson Foundation at more than $29 million, the largest project ever funded by RWJF (Phillips et al., 2000).

The SUPPORT randomized trial is "negative," in that the interventions did not improve quality of care in the hoped-for ways. The irony is that SUPPORT and HELP focused the attention of professionals and the public on care of the dying—stories about the project made front-page news in the national press—in a way that nothing else had. SUPPORT also catalyzed new thinking about the nature of the problems underlying care at the end of life and about what changes would be needed to fix them. Simplistically, we moved from hoping that doing A, B, and C to improve communication would result in better care (widely believed by experts to be the answer before SUPPORT), to an understanding that much broader system-wide and society-wide changes would have to take place. The depth and richness

BOX 1-2
SUPPORT

Although the Study to Understand Prognoses and Preferences for Outcomes and Risks of Treatment—SUPPORT—came to public attention in the 1990s, it was conceived in the early 1980s, at a time when costs for high-technology medical interventions were increasing rapidly and people had begun to question the appropriateness of using all available measures to extend briefly the lives of people with untreatable, soon fatal, conditions. The Robert Wood Johnson Foundation, sponsor of SUPPORT and HELP, held a meeting in 1985 to discuss this. Subsequently, it asked Drs. William Knaus and Joanne Lynn to propose a study to improve the care of critically ill, hospitalized adults, specifically through improving the match between what patients wanted and the care they actually received.

A two-stage process was planned: Phase I was observational, and Phase II was a randomized trial testing an intervention tailored to address problems identified in Phase I. Planning, pilot testing, and recruitment took several years. Defining which patients would be eligible for the study was pivotal. The investigators chose conditions that were common and often fatal; that required important decisions during hospitalization; and that had stable treatment possibilities, to ensure that prognostic estimates would be similar throughout the study (this is one reason HIV/AIDS was not selected). Patients' conditions had to be severe enough that about half would die within six months. The conditions selected were

- acute respiratory failure,
- chronic obstructive pulmonary disease,
- congestive heart failure,
- coma,
- cirrhosis,
- advanced colon or non-small cell lung cancer, and
- multiorgan system failure with sepsis or malignancy.

Between 1989 and 1991, a full complement of 4,301 patients had been recruited to Phase I at the five large hospitals around the country that had been selected (out of 55 applications) as study sites. The following are key Phase I findings:

- Patients with advanced life-threatening illnesses could be interviewed successfully about their treatment preferences.
- Physicians often misunderstood patient preferences, especially when patients did not want high-technology, life-extending care.
- Do-not-resuscitate (DNR) orders were often written very late—just before

of the studies, beyond this single finding, are hinted at by the 100 or so journal articles that have probed SUPPORT data (Phillips et al., 2000).

The failure of the planned interventions spurred the interested community to try to understand what went wrong and what could be done differ-

death—and many patients died after long stays in intensive care units (ICUs) either comatose or with mechanical ventilation.

• Survival time could be better predicted by a computerized model with appropriate data inputs than by an individual physician.

• An unexpectedly large percentage of patients experienced substantial pain across all diagnoses.

• The study participants were younger than anticipated (median age less than 65), which led to HELP, a companion study of patients more than 80 years of age.

The Phase II intervention employed a skilled nurse specialist to interact with patients and their families, staff, and the intervention physicians. Specifically,

• physicians were given detailed prognostic information for each patient on survival, outcome if cardiopulmonary resuscitation was used, and prospect of severe disability;

• nurse specialists talked to patients and families about their specific wishes regarding treatment and communicated that information to the physicians and nurses treating the patient; and

• physicians were given written information regarding each patient's wishes about treatment, including pain control and the use of technology-intensive measures (e.g., CPR).

All participating physicians also were given feedback on the overall results of the observational phase of the study, characterizing the shortcomings of physician-patient communication, pain, and the timing of DNR orders.

A form of "cluster randomization" (by physician specialty and study site) was used to assign patients to either the intervention or the usual-care groups (see SUPPORT Principal Investigators, 1995, for details). The evidence after enrollment of 4,804 patients in two years was examined for five outcomes:

1. median time until the DNR order was written,
2. agreement between patient and physician regarding the DNR order,
3. number of days spent in an "undesirable state" (e.g., comatose, on mechanical ventilation, in ICUs),
4. percentage of patients in substantial pain, and
5. median resource use (in 1993 dollars).

None of the outcomes was better for patients in the intervention group than for those in the control group.

ently. This led RWJF to begin its Last Acts campaign, an effort to improve end-of-life care at the grassroots level that now has more than 400 members (Schroeder, 1999), and funding of demonstration programs to reduce the identified barriers to high-quality care for those who are dying.

Other Key Foundation Commitments

The Project on Death in America (PDIA) (www.soros.org/death) has committed $30 million to improving end-of-life care through its Faculty Scholars Program, grant programs, and special initiatives. The 70 or so faculty scholars that have been funded by PDIA serve as role models and clinical researchers in academic medical centers around the United States (and a few in Canada). About one-third of them are oncologists involved in direct patient care and directing palliative care programs.

The Nathan Cummings Foundation, together with the Commonwealth Fund, supported a major study of nearly 1,000 dying patients (most with cancer, heart disease, or chronic lung disease) and their caregivers. This is one of eight major research projects designed to expand the nation's understanding of the dying experience and find ways to improve it.

The Milbank Foundation (www.milbank.org) sponsored the development and publication of *Principles for Care of Patients at the End of Life: An Emerging Consensus Among the Specialties of Medicine* (Cassel and Foley, 1999), a document now signed onto by at least 17 health professional societies that have agreed to incorporate its principles into their professional education activities and residency training programs.

The Institute of Medicine

Another milestone was the 1997 report *Approaching Death: Improving Care at the End of Life* from the Institute of Medicine (IOM, 1997). This was the first major national report covering the range of end-of-life issues, with evidence-based recommendations (see Box 1-3). It received widespread national attention and continues to be cited as a reference and source of guidance for improving end-of-life care. This report builds on the earlier report and its recommendations. (The reader is referred to the 1997 report for a thorough review of issues up to that time.) The 1999 National Cancer Policy Board report *Ensuring Quality Cancer Care* (IOM, 1999) has already been mentioned.

The President's Cancer Panel

The 1997-1998 report of the President's Cancer Panel[1] (PCP) was entitled *Cancer Care Issues in the United States: Quality of Care, Quality of Life*, with a major focus on the need for NCI to fund research and training

---

[1]The President's Cancer Panel, consisting of three individuals, was created by congressional charter in 1971 to "monitor the development and execution of the activities of the National Cancer Program, and ... report directly to the President."

BOX 1-3

RECOMMENDATIONS AND FUTURE DIRECTIONS—
From *Approaching Death: Improving Care at the End of Life*
(IOM, 1997)

Seven recommendations address different decisionmakers and different deficiencies in care at the end of life. Each applies generally to people approaching death including those for whom death is imminent and those with serious, eventually fatal illnesses who may live for some time. Each is intended to contribute to the achievement of a compassionate care system that dying people and those close to them can rely on for respectful and effective care.

Recommendation 1: People with advanced, potentially fatal illnesses and those close to them should be able to expect and receive reliable, skillful, and supportive care.

Recommendation 2: Physicians, nurses, social workers, and other health professionals must commit themselves to improving care for dying patients and to using existing knowledge effectively to prevent and relieve pain and other symptoms.

Recommendation 3: Because many problems in care stem from system problems, policymakers, consumer groups, and purchasers of health care should work with health care practitioners, organizations, and researchers to:

a) strengthen methods for measuring the quality of life and other outcomes of care for dying patients and those close to them;
b) develop better tools and strategies for improving the quality of care and holding health care organizations accountable for care at the end of life;
c) revise mechanisms for financing care so that they encourage rather than impede good end-of-life care and sustain rather than frustrate coordinated systems of excellent care; and
d) reform drug prescription laws, burdensome regulations, and state medical board policies and practices that impede effective use of opioids to relieve pain and suffering.

Recommendation 4: Educators and other health professionals should initiate changes in undergraduate, graduate, and continuing education to ensure that practitioners have relevant attitudes, knowledge, and skills to care well for dying patients.

Recommendation 5: Palliative care should become, if not a medical specialty, at least a defined area of expertise, education, and research.

Recommendation 6: The nation's research establishment should define and implement priorities for strengthening the knowledge base for end-of-life care.

Recommendation 7: A continuing public discussion is essential to develop a better understanding of the modern experience of dying, the options available to patients and families, and the obligations of communities to those approaching death.

across the spectrum of care, including cancer prevention, cancer control, rehabilitation, palliation, and end-of-life care (President's Cancer Panel, 1998). The report states:

> The quality of care provided to dying patients remains woefully inadequate and is a major failure of our health care system. Dying patients frequently face abandonment by their physicians and inadequate pain and other symptom control when treatment with curative intent is no longer tenable.

The PCP developed its report after a series of meetings around the country, at which a wide range of individuals—from the medical treatment and research communities, industry, the advocacy community, and the public at large—presented testimony about the quality of cancer care in the United States. Those who spoke about palliative and end-of-life care reinforced earlier findings (PCP, 1998):

> Speakers emphasized the need for a compassionate and humane system of care for cancer patients at the end of life, including improved financing of hospice care, expanding the availability of palliative care approaches from hospice programs to cancer centers (including offering palliative care as an option in all clinical trials), establishing a focal point for palliative care research at the NCI, improving health care professional education about palliative care, and fostering more honest health professional and public dialogue about dying. A number of respected organizations, including the American Society of Clinical Oncology, the Institute of Medicine, and the World Health Organization, have developed reports and accompanying recommendations to address the deeply ingrained obstacles to compassionate end of life care for people with cancer. However, implementation of these recommendations and their integration into the standard of care is slow.

Among the panel's recommendations, the following relate to training and research in end-of-life and palliative care:

> Training is needed to improve the ability of physicians and other health professionals to...:

> Acknowledge that death and end of life issues are a part of the cancer experience for some patients, and provide more comprehensive and compassionate care to dying patients and their families.

The panel also stated:

> Continued funding across the research spectrum is needed to continue the flow of discovery that leads to improvements in care across the cancer continuum. Research efforts should focus particularly on improving interventions in the areas of cancer prevention, cancer control, rehabilitation, palliation, and end of life care, and on outcomes research. In addition,

targeted funding may be needed for behavioral and other research to improve quality of care in vulnerable populations, including those with low income and/or educational levels, differing cultures, the elderly, and rural populations.

Medicare Payment Advisory Commission (MedPAC)

MedPAC is an independent federal organization that was established by Congress for advice on issues affecting the Medicare program. Chapters devoted to end-of-life care appeared in recent major reports (MedPAC, 1998, 1999) including, in 1999, recommendations for the Medicare program and the Department of Health and Human Services, more broadly. They directed the Secretary of Health and Human Services to

- make end-of-life care a national quality improvement priority for Medicare+Choice and traditional Medicare;
- support research on care at the end of life and work with nongovernmental organizations as they (1) educate the health care profession and the public about care at the end of life and (2) develop measures to accredit health care organizations and provide public accountability for the quality of end-of-life care;
- sponsor projects to develop and test measures of the quality of end-of-life care for Medicare beneficiaries, and enlist quality improvement organizations and Medicare+Choice plans to implement quality improvement programs for care at the end of life; and
- promote advance care planning by practitioners and patients well before terminal health crises occur.

As yet, neither the Congress nor the Secretary has responded to these MedPAC recommendations.

Other Organizations and Efforts

A variety of professional and trade organizations, consumer groups, pharmaceutical companies, and others have taken positive steps related to palliative and end-of-life care, only the most prominent of which are touched on here. The American Society of Clinical Oncology (ASCO) is the main professional organization for practicing oncologists. In 1998, it took two important steps. First, ASCO published a position statement on cancer care during the last phase of life (ASCO, 1998), outlining the role of the oncologist, identifying impediments to achieving the best care, and recommending solutions. The details of the position statement flow from the belief that "it is the oncologists' responsibility to care for their patients in a continuum that extends from the moment of diagnosis throughout the course of the illness." The statement goes on, "In addition to appropriate anticancer treatment, this includes symptom control and psychosocial support during all phases of care, including those during the last phase of life."

Also in 1998, ASCO surveyed its membership in the first nationwide inquiry into end-of-life practices. The survey asked about education and training, current practice, perceived barriers to the delivery of care, decisionmaking vignettes about the management of patients, and individual experiences with terminal patients. The results, which have been presented at meetings and have begun to appear in print, confirm many of the deficiencies that have been recognized in caring for dying patients, but coming from the oncology community, they have hit with added force (see Box 1-4 for key survey findings).

For the long term, ASCO has placed high priority on developing its program called "Optimizing Cancer Care: The Importance of Symptom Management." The curriculum consists of 32 modules covering specific symptoms and symptom control issues (e.g., ascites, breaking bad news, depression, lymphedema). Modules are designed to get information into manageable pieces for practicing oncologists in a way that is concise and information-dense. The program has been featured at national ASCO meetings and will be featured at all yearly state ASCO meetings. ASCO plans to make it available on CD-ROM, on-line, and in print.

The Joint Commission on the Accreditation of Healthcare Organizations is the first national accrediting body to develop mandatory standards for pain assessment and management. JCAHO, which accredits the majority of hospitals and other health care organizations (including hospices), will begin evaluating the hospitals, home care agencies, nursing homes, behavioral health facilities, outpatient clinics, and health plans it inspects for compliance with the new standards in 2001. The organizations will be required to

- recognize the right of patients to appropriate assessment and management of pain;
- assess the existence and, if so, the nature and intensity of pain in all patients;
- record the results of the assessment in a way that facilitates regular reassessment and follow-up;
- determine and ensure staff competency in pain assessment and management, and address pain assessment and management in the orientation of all new staff;
- establish policies and procedures that support the appropriate prescription or ordering of effective pain medications;
- educate patients and their families about effective pain management; and

- address patient needs for symptom management in the discharge planning process.

The standards were developed collaboratively with the University of Wisconsin-Madison Medical School, as part of a project funded by RWJF to make pain assessment and management a priority in the nation's health care system (JCAHO Web site, http://www.jcaho.org/news/nb207.html).

CURRENT NIH INVOLVEMENT IN PALLIATIVE AND END-OF-LIFE CARE

The National Institutes of Health responded to recommendations in the IOM (1997) report and to the widely publicized SUPPORT findings with an initiative in symptom control and palliative care at a meeting in November 1997. This was by no means NIH's first recognition of research needs in palliative care. A prominent earlier effort was a 1979 interdisciplinary meeting on pain, which provided some of the stimulus for advances in pain control in the 1980s and 1990s, and a follow-up meeting in the early 1990s. Despite these activities, no standing program was ever developed.

The main event of the 1997 effort was a workshop that was cosponsored by the National Institute of Nursing Research (NINR), the Division of AIDS Research of the National Institute of Allergy and Infectious Diseases (NIAID), NCI, and the Office of Alternative Medicine to target research needs in palliative care. The research workshop "Symptoms in Terminal Illness" had three principal goals:

1. to summarize the current state of knowledge concerning the most common symptoms associated with terminal illness;
2. to identify important needs and opportunities for research that would be appropriate for NIH funding; and
3. to initiate a process for enhancing interdisciplinary collaboration and interagency collaboration in research in palliative care.

The workshop was organized into four topic sessions that focused on specific symptom areas: pain, dyspnea, cognitive disturbances, and cachexia and wasting. A research agenda was developed from the workshop report (http://www.nih.gov/ninr/end-of-life.htm), and in 1998, the collaborating institutes issued a program announcement "Management of Symptoms at the End of Life," with a call for proposals addressing the following objectives:

- managing the transition to palliative care;
- understanding and managing pain and other symptoms, such as nausea and depression in the context of end-stage illness;

BOX 1-4
THE ASCO SURVEY

In 1998, American Society of Clinical Oncology conducted the first and only large-scale survey of U.S. oncologists about their experiences in providing care to dying patients. The questionnaire consisted of 118 questions about end-of-life care under eight headings (Hilden et al., 2001):

1. education and training,
2. current practice,
3. perceived barriers to the delivery of care,
4. decisionmaking,
5. vignettes about the management of patients,
6. individual experiences with terminal patients,
7. the role of ASCO in improving care, and
8. demographics and practice characteristics of the respondents.

All U.S. oncologists who reported that they managed patients at the end of life, and were ASCO members, were eligible for the survey, a total of 6,645 (the small number of ASCO members from England and Canada was also included). About 40 percent (2,645) responded (see table below) (Emanuel, 2000). No information is available to compare the characteristics of those who responded with those who did not.

This survey documented serious shortcomings in the training and current practices of a large proportion of oncologists. Among the key findings are the following:

• Most oncologists have not had adequate formal training in the key skills needed for them to provide excellent palliative and end-of-life care. Less than one-third reported their formal training "very helpful" in communicating with dying patients, coordinating their care, shifting to palliative care, or beginning hospice care. About 40 percent found their training very helpful in managing dying patients' symptoms.

• Slightly more than half (56 percent) reported "trial and error in clinical practice" as one important source of learning about end-of-life care. About 45 percent also ranked role models during fellowships and in practice as important. Traumatic patient experiences ranked higher as a source of learning than did lectures during fellowship, medical school role models, and clinical clerkships.

• Only 25 percent reported end-of-life care as highly satisfying; about 40 percent thought it intellectually satisfying; and 63 percent, emotionally satisfying. Substantial numbers reported a sense of failure when a patient becomes terminally ill (10 percent), and a similar proportion reported anxiety and strong emotions when faced with follow-up meetings with dying patients and managing difficult symptoms. About twice as many reported anxiety and strong emotions when they had to tell a patient that his or her condition would lead to death.

• The large majority of oncologists report that they are highly competent in managing patients' cancer-related end-of-life symptoms, including pain (95 percent report high competency), constipation (91 percent), nausea and vomiting (93 percent), fever, and neutropenia (89 percent); somewhat fewer report high competency in managing shortness of breath (79 percent), anorexia (63 percent), and depression (57 percent).

• Very few oncologists (6 percent) feel they can arrange for their patients to get all the services they need. About half report getting their patients "almost all" of what they need, but the rest report that their patients get less. More than half (56 percent) report that a palliative care team is either not available or not easy to access. Smaller but still substantial proportions report lack of availability or difficult access to hospital-based hospice (28 percent), a pain service (18 percent), outpatient case management (17 percent), and psychosocial support services (15 percent).

• The barriers to providing adequate end-of-life care most often cited are patient and family denial that death is approaching and unrealistic expectations for curative treatment. Other factors (e.g., laws restricting opioid usage) are reported as frequent problems by only 6 percent.

• Reimbursement practices are reported as frequent barriers to providing good care. Slightly more than one-quarter report insufficient reimbursement for time spent in discussion with patients and families as the "most troublesome" among reimbursement barriers. A much larger group (41 percent) reports lack of coverage for unskilled home health services as the most troublesome aspect. Also troublesome are restrictive referral networks and lack of appropriate coding categories (diagnosis-related groups) for end-of-life and palliative care.

• In answer to questions about a series of patient vignettes, respondents indicated what course of treatment they favored. As an example, for a patient with locally advanced lung cancer who "failed first line chemotherapy," 3 percent would recommend hospice and the rest would recommend additional chemotherapy (paclitaxel or a phase I trial); after failing paclitaxel, 19 percent would refer to hospice and the rest to additional chemotherapy; failing the third-line treatment, 80 percent would refer the patient to hospice care, but the remaining 20 percent would consider additional chemotherapy.

Attitudes and practices relating to euthanasia and "physician-assisted suicide" were elicited in various questions, with the following points emerging (Emanuel et al., 2000a):

• About one-third of the respondents had been asked to perform either euthanasia or "physician-assisted suicide" within the previous year, and nearly two-thirds had had such requests at some time during their career; 4 percent had performed one or both within the previous year, and 13 percent, at some time in their career. Most instances were physician-assisted suicide (11 percent of respondents) rather than euthanasia (4 percent).

• Concern among oncologists about performing euthanasia and physician-assisted suicide limits their willingness to prescribe adequate doses of opioids to control pain. Oncologists who do not support euthanasia or physician-assisted suicide are less willing than others to increase opioid dosages for severe pain.

• Better training in end-of-life care and the ability to obtain good palliative care for patients are associated with a lower likelihood of oncologists' performing euthanasia or physician-assisted suicide.

Response Rate Among Specialties

	Medical Oncologists	Surgical Oncologists	Radiation Oncologists	Pediatric Oncologists
Eligible	5010	499	703	371
Responders	2129	128	203	172
Response Rate, %	42.5	25.7	28.9	46.4

- measuring outcomes (e.g., relief of symptoms);
- measuring of quality of life in end-stage illness;
- investigating changes in patient status that influence nutrition and hydration choices in terminal illness; and
- documenting costs incurred by patients and family caregivers during end-stage illness.

About two dozen small grants were issued as a result of this program, most funded by NINR, and three by NCI. NINR, which is designated the lead institute for end-of-life care, maintains it as an area of special research interest and has issued "program announcements" calling for proposals in end-of-life care every year since 1998 (NCI is a cosponsor of these announcements but has no up-front financial commitment to funding projects). In 1999, NINR-awarded grants related to end-of-life care totaled $2.3 million, and an addition $1.7 million went to cancer-related research projects with some end-of-life component (Hudgings, 2000). While nursing-related research is needed, the bulk of research needs extend far beyond nursing and are closely allied with cancer treatment, the bailiwick of NCI.

Within NCI, control of pain and other symptoms, psychosocial distress, and end-of-life issues has been associated administratively with cancer control or cancer prevention, which may be limiting the opportunities for broader research. The portfolio of palliative and end-of-life projects is currently within the Division of Cancer Prevention, where it has a very low profile among the many other issues more clearly related to cancer prevention. In fact, no direct mention of palliative or end-of-life care appears on the NCI Web site in association with any unit within the institute (although pain and other symptoms are mentioned in various places). Although a more natural fit, palliative care research has never been included as a specific topic in the Division of Cancer Treatment and Diagnosis (DCTD), which takes in preclinical and clinical drug development and testing. While not specifically excluding drugs for symptom control, the language describing the Cancer Therapy Evaluation Program within DCTD refers to developing and evaluating "anticancer agents" (NCI Web site, October 2000), which would generally be understood as treatments aimed directly at the cancers themselves, not agents for palliative care.

NCI currently designates 37 centers as Comprehensive Cancer Centers (as of December 2000). The designation of "comprehensive" is awarded based on a strong and diverse research program, but current requirements do not include a program in palliative care research.

Researchers are not prohibited from applying to divisions other than the Division of Cancer Prevention for symptom control or end-of-life research (e.g., DCTD), but it appears that appropriate review mechanisms may be lacking, placing such researchers at a competitive disadvantage. For example, none of the established cooperative clinical trial groups have a specific mandate to conduct trials in symptom control, and there is no "coordinating center" for such trials, such as those that exist for other areas of treatment research.

NCI Funding for Palliative Care Research and Training

In this report, the Board recommends strongly that NCI step up its commitment to research toward improving end-of-life and palliative care—including symptom control, psychosocial issues, shared decisionmaking, and related topics. NCI has provided an accounting of its fiscal year 1999 extramural funding for all research with components related to palliative care or hospice, totaling $24.5 million (Colbert, 2000). (Most grants supported activities that were not focused exclusively on palliative care, so NCI has apportioned the dollar amounts attributed to this category as some percentage of the total grant.) Of that total, $18.3 million went to specific projects or programs (Appendix 1A, Table 1A-1), and $6.1 million represents fractions of institutional grants (Appendix 1A, Table 1A-2). Grants included in the list are those dealing with

• any and all aspects of cancer pain research, including mechanism, prevention, therapy, measurement tools, and so forth;
• hospice, defined as research dealing with formally organized supportive care of terminally ill patients either at home or in an institution; and
• "other palliative care," including any supportive care (e.g., psychological counseling, relief of nausea, or other symptom management) that is not coded as pain or hospice.

In addition to the research grants, $1.7 million was spent in 1999 on training grants related to end-of-life or palliative care (Begg, 2000). While the 1999 NCI expenditure on palliative and hospice care was just over $26 million, or about 0.9 percent of the total 1999 budget of $2.9 billion.

CONCLUSIONS AND RECOMMENDATIONS

People with cancer suffer from an array of symptoms at all stages of the disease (and its treatment), though these are most frequent and severe in advanced stages. Much of the suffering could be alleviated if currently available symptom control measures were used more widely. For symptoms not amenable to relief by current measures, new approaches could be developed and tested, if even modest resources were made available. Both the use of current interventions and the development of new ones are hindered by the barriers discussed earlier (and in the chapters that follow). The National Cancer Policy Board's recommendations are intended to break down or lower the barriers to excellent palliative care for people with cancer today and for those who will develop it in years to come. The recommendations describe a series of initiatives directed largely—though not exclusively—at the federal government, which should be playing a more powerful role than it has done.

The recommendations are not laid out in parallel to the barriers, as earlier in this chapter. They have been consolidated as "packages" for particular organizations and entities, and some address more than one barrier. Recommendation 1, in particular, which focuses on the role of NCI-designated cancer centers, contains elements that address all the barriers.

NCI-designated cancer centers should play a central role as agents of national policy in advancing palliative care research and clinical practice, with initiatives that address many of the barriers identified in this report.

Recommendation 1: NCI should designate certain cancer centers, as well as some community cancer centers, as centers of excellence in symptom control and palliative care for both adults and children. The centers will deliver the best available care, as well as carrying out research, training, and treatment aimed at developing portable model programs that can be adopted by other cancer centers and hospitals. Activities should include, but not be limited to, the following:

   • *formal testing and evaluation of new and existing practice guidelines for palliative and end-of-life care;*
   • *pilot testing "quality indicators" for assessing end-of-life care at the level of the patient and the institution;*
   • *incorporating the best palliative care into NCI-sponsored clinical trials;*
   • *innovating in the delivery of palliative and end-of-life care, including collaboration with local hospice organizations;*
   • *disseminating information about how to improve end-of-life care to other cancer centers and hospitals through a variety of media;*
   • *uncovering the determinants of disparities in access to care by minority populations that should be served by the center and developing specific programs and initiatives to increase access; these might include educational activities for health care providers and the community, setting up outreach programs, and so forth;*
   • *providing clinical and research training fellowships in medical and surgical oncology in end-of-life care for adult and pediatric patients;*
   • *creating faculty development programs in oncology, nursing, and social work; and*

• *providing in-service training for local hospice staff in new palliative care techniques.*

Recommendation 2: NCI should add the requirement of research in palliative care and symptom control for recognition as a "Comprehensive Cancer Center."

Practices and policies that govern payment for palliative care (in both public and private sectors) hinder delivery of the most appropriate mix of services for patients who could benefit from palliative care during the course of their illness and treatments.

Recommendation 3: The Health Care Financing Administration (HCFA) should fund demonstration projects for service delivery and reimbursement that integrate palliative care and potentially life-prolonging treatments throughout the course of disease.

Recommendation 4: Private insurers should provide adequate compensation for end-of-life care. The special circumstances of dying children— particularly the need for extended communication with children and parents, as well as health care team conferences—should be taken into account in setting reimbursement levels and in actually paying claims for these services when providers bill for them.

Information on palliative and end-of-life care is largely absent from materials developed for the public about cancer treatment. In addition, reliable information about survival from different types and stages of cancer is not routinely included with treatment information.

Recommendation 5: Organizations that provide information about cancer treatment (NCI, the American Cancer Society, and other patient-oriented organizations [e.g., disease-specific groups]; health insurers; and pharmaceutical companies) should revise their inventories of patient-oriented material, as appropriate, to provide comprehensive, accurate information about palliative care throughout the course of disease. Patients would also be helped by having reliable information on survival by type and stage of cancer easily accessible. Attention should be paid to cultural relevance and special populations (e.g., children).

Practice guidelines for palliative care and for other end-of-life issues are in comparatively early stages of development, and quality indicators are even more embryonic. Progress toward their further development and implementation requires continued encouragement by professional societies, funding bodies, and payers of care.

Recommendation 6: Best available practice guidelines should dictate the standard of care for both physical and psychosocial symptoms. Care systems, payers, and standard-setting and accreditation bodies should strongly encourage their expedited development, validation, and use. Professional societies, particularly the American Society of Clinical Oncology, the Oncology Nursing Society, and the Society for Social Work Oncology, should encourage their members to facilitate the development and testing of guidelines and their eventual implementation, and should provide leadership and training for nonspecialists, who provide most of the care for cancer patients.

Recommendation 7: The recommendations in the NCPB report Enhancing Data Systems to Improve the Quality of Cancer Care *(see Appendix B) should be applied equally to palliative and end-of-life care as to other aspects of cancer treatment. These recommendations include*

- *developing a core set of cancer care quality measures;*
- *increasing public and private support for cancer registries;*
- *supporting research and demonstration projects to identify new mechanisms to organize and finance the collection of data for cancer care quality studies;*
- *supporting the development of technologies, including computer-based patient record systems and intranet-based communication systems, to improve the availability, quality, and timeliness of clinical data relevant to assessing quality of cancer care;*
- *expanding support for training in health services research and other disciplines needed to measure quality of care;*
- *increasing support for health services research aimed toward improved quality of cancer care measures;*
- *developing models for linkage studies and the release of confidential data for research purposes that protect the confidentiality and privacy of health care information; and*
- *funding demonstration projects to assess the impact of quality monitoring programs within health care systems.*

Research on palliative care for cancer patients has had a low priority at NCI, and as a result, few researchers have been attracted to the field and very few relevant studies have been funded over the past decades. NCI should continue to collaborate on end-of-life research with the National Institute of Nursing Research (the lead NIH institute for this topic) but cannot discharge its major responsibilities in cancer research through that mechanism.

Recommendation 8: NCI should convene a State of the Science Meeting[2] on palliative care and symptom control. It should invite other National Institutes of Health, and government research agencies with shared interests should be invited to collaborate. The meeting should result in a high-profile strategic research agenda that can be pursued by NCI and its research partners over the short and long terms.

Recommendation 9: NCI should establish the most appropriate institutional locus (or more than one) for palliative care, symptom control, and end-of-life research, possibly within the Division of Cancer Treatment and Diagnosis.

Recommendation 10: NCI should review the membership of its advisory bodies to ensure representation of experts in cancer pain, symptom management, and palliative care.

---

[2]In 1999, NCI initiated State of the Science Meetings focused on specific types of cancer "to bring together the Nation's leading multidisciplinary experts, to identify the important research questions for a given disease and help define the scientific research agenda that will assist us in addressing those questions."

REFERENCES

Agency for Healthcare Research and Quality (AHRQ). 2001. *Management of Cancer Pain.* Summary, Evidence Report/Technology Assessment: Number 35. AHRQ Publication No. 01-E033, January 20001. Rockville, MD: Agency for Healthcare Research and Quality. http://www.ahrq.gov/clinic/canpainsum.htm.

American Society of Clinical Oncology (ASCO). Cancer care during the last phase of life. *JCO* 1998;16(5):1986-1996.

Begg L. NCI Cancer Training Branch. Personal communication to Hellen Gelband, June 2000.

Cassel CK, Foley KM. 1999. *Principles for Care of Patients at the End of Life: An Emerging Consensus among the Specialties of Medicine.* New York: Milbank Memorial Fund, 32 pp.

Christ GH, Sormanti M. Advancing social work practice in end-of-life care. *Social Work in Health Care* 1999;30(2):81-99.

Christakis NA, Escarce JJ. Survival of Medicare patients after enrollment in hospice programs. *New England Journal of Medicine* 1996;338:172-178.

Colbert K. National Cancer Institute Budget Office. Personal communication to Hellen Gelband, August 2000.

Donnelly S, Walsh D. The symptoms of advanced cancer. *Semin Oncol* 1995;22:67-72.

Emanuel, EJ. National Cancer Institute. Unpublished data, 2000.

Emanuel EJ, Fairclough D, Clarridge BC, Blum D, Bruera E, Penley WC, Schnipper LE, Mayer RJ. Attitudes and practices of U.S. oncologists regarding euthanasia and physician-assisted suicide. *Ann Intern Med* 2000a Oct 3;133(7):527-532.

Emanuel EJ, Fairclough DL, Slutsman J, Emanuel LL. Understanding economic and other burdens of terminal illness: the experience of patients and their caregivers. *Ann Intern Med* 2000b Mar 21;132(6):451-459.

Ferrell B, Virani R, Grant M, et al. Beyond the Supreme Court decision: nursing perspectives on end-of-life care. *Oncology Nursing Forum* 2000;27(3):445-455.

Freeman HP, Payne R. Racial injustice in health care. *New England Journal of Medicine* 2000;342:1045-1047.

Hilden JM, Emanuel EJ, Fairclough DL, Link MP, Foley KM, Clarridge BC, Schnipper LE, Mayer RJ. Attitudes and practices among pediatric oncologists regarding end-of-life care: results of the 1998 American Society of Clinical Oncology survey. *JCO* 2001;19: 205-212.

Hogan C, Lynn J, Gabel J, Lunney J, O'Mara A, Wilkinson A. 2000 *A statistical profile of decedents in the Medicare program.* Washington, D.C., Medicare Payment Advisory Commission.

Hudgings C. National Institute on Nursing Research, personal communication to Hellen Gelband, 2000.

Institute of Medicine (IOM). 1997. *Approaching Death: Improving Care at the End of Life,* Field MJ, Cassel CK, eds. Washington, D.C.: National Academy Press.

IOM. 1999. *Ensuring Quality Cancer Care,* Hewitt M, Simone JV, eds. Washington, D.C.: National Academy Press.

IOM. 2000. *Enhancing Data Systems to Improve the Quality of Cancer Care,* Hewitt M, Simone JV, eds. Washington, D.C.: National Academy Press.

Joint Commission on Accreditation of Healthcare Organizations. Background on the Development of the Joint Commission Standards on Pain Management, July 31, 2000. JCAHO Web site, http://www.jcaho.org/trkhco_frm.html.

Lagnado L. Rules are rules: hospice's patients beat the odds, so Medicare decides to crack down—terminally ill who don't die within a 6-month period risk losing coverage—Al Ouimet's 9-year survival. *Wall Street Journal* June 5, 2000.

Medicare Payment Advisory Commission (MedPAC). 1999. *Report to the Congress: Selected Medicare Issues.* Washington, D.C.: MedPAC.

MedPAC. 2000. *Medicare Beneficiaries' Costs and Use of Care in the Last Year of Life.* Washington, D.C.: MedPAC.

Morrison RS, Wallenstein S, Natale DK, et al. "We don't carry that"—failure of pharmacies in predominantly nonwhite neighborhoods to stock opioid analgesics. New England Journal of Medicine 2000;342:1023-1026.

NHPCO (National Hospice and Palliative Care Organization). Facts and figures on hospice care in America. NHPCO Web site, January 10, 2001. www.nhpco.org.

Pfeifer MP, et al. The discussion of end-of-life medical care by primary care patients and physicians: a multicenter study using structured qualitative interviews. *Journal of General Internal Medicine;*1994;9(2):82-88.

Phillips RS, Hamel MB, Covinsky KE, Lynn J. Findings from SUPPORT and HELP: an introduction. *Journal of the American Geriatrics Society* 2000;48:S1-S5.

President's Cancer Panel. 1998. *Cancer Care Issues in the United States: Quality of Care, Quality of Life.* NCI Web site, http://deainfo.nci.nih.gov/ADVISORY/pcp/pcp97-98rpt/pcp97-98rpt.htm#letter.

Schroeder SA. The legacy of SUPPORT. *Annals of Internal Medicine* 1999;131(10):780-782.

Singer PA, Martin DK, Kelner M. Quality end of life care—patients' perspectives. *JAMA* 1999;281:163-168.

SUPPORT Principal Investigators. A controlled trial to improve care for seriously ill hospitalized patients. *JAMA* 1995;274(20):1591-1598.

World Health Organization. 1990. *Cancer Pain Relief and Palliative Care.* World Health Organization Technical Report Series 804. Geneva.

APPENDIX 1A

TABLE 1A-1 NCI Funding for Palliative Care Research: Specific Projects, Fiscal Year 1999

Total Project $	Percent[a]	$ Relevant to Palliative Care	Project Title[b]
603,532	100	603,532	Inhibition of Postoperative Gynecological Adhesions
364,549	100	364,549	Intelligent Knowledge Base for Cancer Pain Treatment
367,610	100	367,610	Diana2 Computer-Based Teaching of Elder Care
153,918	100	153,918	Palliative Training for Caregivers of Cancer Patients
133,702	100	133,702	Patterns Care for Cancer Patients at End of Life
103,382	100	103,382	Home Based Moderate Exercise for Breast Cancer Patients
117,792	100	117,792	Stress of Cancer Caregiving—Analysis and Intervention
602,537	100	602,537	Family Home Care for Cancer—A Community Based Model
70,464	100	70,464	Clinical Management of Cancer Pain in US Nursing Homes
500,685	100	500,685	Pain Measurement in Bone Marrow Transplantation
162,671	100	162,671	Method for the Analysis of Pain Clinical Trials

continued on next page

TABLE 1A-1 Continued

Total Project $	Percent[a]	$ Relevant to Palliative Care	Project Title[b]
413,030	100	413,030	Laboratory Studies of Pain Control Methods
292,011	100	292,011	Cost Effectiveness of Lung Cancer Chemotherapy
360,637	100	360,637	Comparison of Psychosocial Intervention in Breast Cancer
498,233	100	498,233	Self Care Intervention to Control Cancer Pain
540,262	100	540,262	Breast Cancer—Preparing for Survivorship
175,615	100	175,615	Recycling of Urea Nitrogen in Cancer Cachexia
203,436	100	203,436	Adjustment to Breast Cancer
248,889	100	248,889	Clinical Investigations in Hodgkin's Disease
588,097	100	588,097	Cancer Pain and Its Management
1,205,625	100	1,205,625	Maximizing the Therapeutic Index of Childhood ALL
1,778,647	100	1,778,647	CCSP in Head and Neck Cancer Rehabilitation
8,747	100	8,747	Feasibility of Physioacoustic Therapy in Cancer Care
405,116	100	405,116	Pain and the Defense Response
79,000	100	79,000	Home Care Training for Younger Breast Cancer Patients
358,290	100	358,290	A Simulator to Teach Therapeutic Communication Skills
412,812	100	412,812	Facilitating Positive Adaptation to Breast Cancer
416,067	100	416,067	Enhancing Recovery from Blood and Marrow Transplantation
451,385	100	451,385	Computerized Pain Report and Nursing Pain Consult Protocol
350,015	100	350,015	Item Banking and Cat for Quality of Life Outcomes
50,000	100	50,000	Menopausal Symptom Relief for Women with Breast Cancer
100,000	100	100,000	Exercise and Quality of Life in Women with Breast Cancer
99,975	100	99,975	Self Advocacy and Empowerment for Cancer Patients
100,000	100	100,000	Apoptosis Inhibitor for Alopecia Due to Cancer Therapy
99,805	100	99,805	Skin Patches for AIDS Patients
12,405	100	12,405	CCG Nursing Workshop—Challenges in CCG Nursing
74,918	100	74,918	Stress Reduction for Women with Breast Cancer

TABLE 1A-1 Continued

Total Project $	Percent[a]	$ Relevant to Palliative Care	Project Title[b]
347,423	100	347,423	Gender Differences in Opioid Analgesia and Side Effects
363,294	100	363,294	Exercise—An Intervention for Fatigue in Cancer Patients
280,410	100	280,410	Cognitive Behavioral Aspects of Cancer Related Fatigue
404,999	100	404,999	Computerized Symptom Report Consult for Cancer Patients
328,624	100	328,624	Endothelin 1 Induced Pain and Metastatic Prostate Cancer
270,936	100	270,936	A Caregiver Intervention to Improve Hospice Outcomes
1,999,999	100	1,999,999	Center for Psycho-oncology Research
249,986	30	74,996	Longitudinal Quality of Life After Marrow Transplant
1,645,030	30	493,509	Epithelial Ovarian Cancer Program Project
2,441,974	30	732,592	Fluorescence Spectroscopy for Cervical Neoplasia
10,000	25	2,500	HIV, Leukemia, and Opportunistic Cancers
584,213	20	116,843	New Approaches to Brain Tumor Therapy CNS Consortium
98,456	20	19,691	New Approaches to Brain Tumor Therapy CNS Consortium
290,809	20	58,162	Synthetic Studies on Tumor Promoters and Inhibitors
14,883	20	2,977	Technical Requirements for Image Guided Spine Procedures
1,578,050	15	236,708	National Black Leadership Initiative on Cancer
250,641	15	37,596	Quality of Life of Gynecologic Cancer Survivors
284,633	15	42,695	Prophylactic Mastectomy in Hereditary Breast Cancer
270,273	5	13,514	Depression, HPA Function and Smoking Abstinence in Women
TOTAL		**$18,331,326**	

NOTE: ALL = acute lymphocytic leukemia; CCG = Cancer Center Grant; CCSP = Cancer Control Science Program; CNS = central nervous system; HPA hypothalamic-pituitary-adrenal.

[a]NCI estimate of percent of total relevant to palliative care
[b]Grant numbers, principal investigators, and specific institutions have not been listed in this table.

SOURCE: Colbert, 2000.

TABLE 1A-2 NCI Funding for Palliative Care Research: Institutional
Grants, Fiscal Year 1999

Total Project $	Percent[a]	$ Relevant to Palliative Care	Project Title[b]
1,427,579	21.20	302,647	Great Lakes Regional Center for AIDS Research
1,682,639	21.20	356,719	Robert H Lurie Cancer Center
1,451,421	18.02	261,546	Cancer Center and Research Institute
554,090	10.63	58,900	University of Texas MD Anderson CCOP Research Base
781,064	10.37	80,996	Cancer Center Support Grant (CCSG)
2,018,050	10.00	201,805	SPORE in Breast Cancer
2,449,134	10.00	244,913	Bay Area Breast Cancer Translational Research Program
947,107	10.00	94,711	Cooperative Core Lab and Clinical Nutrition Research Unit
2,671,424	10.00	267,142	SPORE in Breast Cancer
409,734	8.23	33,721	Comprehensive Cancer Center—Wake Forest University Research Base Grant
1,182,855	6.11	72,272	ECOG CCOP Research Base
271,255	6.07	16,465	Scottsdale Community Clinical Oncology Program
209,774	6.07	12,733	San Juan Minority-Based Community Oncology Program
212,744	6.07	12,914	Cedar Rapids Oncology Project
199,707	6.07	12,122	Geisinger Clinical Oncology Program
262,463	6.07	15,932	Illinois Oncology Research Association CCOP
252,539	6.06	15,304	CCOP
218,728	6.06	13,255	Oklahoma CCOP
881,850	6.06	53,440	Metro Minnesota CCOP
359,450	6.06	21,783	Kalamazoo CCOP
481,448	6.06	29,176	Northern New Jersey Community Oncology Program
108,209	6.05	6,547	University of Michigan CCOP Research Base
455,553	6.05	27,561	CCOP—Colorado Cancer Research Program
269,121	6.05	16,282	Mainline Health CCOP
350,001	6.05	21,175	Toledo CCOP
424,715	6.05	25,695	Marshfield CCOP
483,525	6.05	29,253	Duluth CCOP
563,042	6.05	34,064	Carle Cancer Center CCOP
397,585	6.05	24,054	Meritcare Hospital CCOP
402,567	6.05	24,355	Sioux Community Cancer Consortium
359,785	6.04	21,731	Missouri Valley Cancer Consortium CCOP
399,670	6.04	24,140	Ann Arbor Regional CCOP
393,221	6.04	23,751	Ochsner CCOP
335,086	6.04	20,239	Iowa Oncology Research Association
505,639	6.00	30,338	Clinical Oncology Program
350,433	6.00	21,026	Kansas City CCOP

TABLE 1A-2 Continued

Total Project $	Percent[a]	$ Relevant to Palliative Care	Project Title[b]
273,234	6.00	16,394	University of Illinois Minority Based CCOP
445,098	6.00	26,706	Scott and White CCOP
434,322	6.00	26,059	Greenville, South Carolina CCOP
150,185	6.00	9,011	Gynecologic Oncology Group
296,456	6.00	17,787	Montana Cancer Consortium
185,244	6.00	11,115	Santa Rosa Memorial Hospital Regional CCOP
361,602	6.00	21,696	Hawaii Minority Based CCOP
301,593	6.00	18,096	South Texas Pediatric Minority Based CCOP
184,797	6.00	11,088	Minority Based Clinical Oncology Program
1,035,721	6.00	62,143	Southeast Cancer Control Consortium Inc.
500,180	6.00	30,011	Central Illinois CCOP
451,849	6.00	27,111	Mount Sinai CCOP
304,404	6.00	18,264	Tumor Institute CCOP
847,078	6.00	50,825	CCOP Research Base
165,969	6.00	9,958	CCSG Research Base for CCOP
501,148	6.00	30,069	Pediatric Oncology Group as a CCOP Research Base
510,286	6.00	30,617	Community Clinical Oncology Program
460,201	6.00	27,612	Southern Nevada Cancer Research Foundation CCOP
550,206	6.00	33,012	Northwest CCOP
761,255	6.00	45,675	North Shore CCOP
293,899	6.00	17,634	Greater Phoenix CCOP
462,893	6.00	27,774	Columbus CCOP
286,396	6.00	17,184	CCOP
266,547	6.00	15,993	Florida Pediatric CCOP
551,590	6.00	33,095	Upstate Carolina CCOP
3,877,581	6.00	232,655	CCOP—Biostatistical Center
405,949	6.00	24,357	Louisiana State University Medical Center Minority-Based CCOP
368,614	6.00	22,117	Virginia Commonwealth University Minority-Based CCOP
1,134,032	6.00	68,042	Cancer and Leukemia Group B CCOP Research Base
11,242,692	6.00	674,562	Southwest Oncology Group—CCOP Research Base
519,100	6.00	31,146	CCOP Research Base
1,568,634	6.00	94,118	CCOP
9,772,324	6.00	586,339	CCOP
240,240	6.00	14,414	Baptist Cancer Institute CCOP
406,637	6.00	24,398	Ozarks Regional CCOP
481,158	6.00	28,869	Atlanta Regional CCOP
553,267	6.00	33,196	Christiana Care CCOP

continued on next page

TABLE 1A-2 Continued

Total Project $	Percent[a]	$ Relevant to Palliative Care	Project Title[b]
425,939	6.00	25,556	Syracuse Hematology-Oncology CCOP
509,387	6.00	30,563	Columbia River Oncology Program
260,360	6.00	15,622	St Louis/Cape Girardeau CCOP
187,892	6.00	11,274	Green Mountain Oncology Group
400,043	6.00	24,003	Dayton Clinical Oncology Program
3,660,649	5.71	209,023	CCSG
6,026,463	4.63	279,025	Cancer Center Support (Core) Grant
6,756,815	3.34	225,678	Cancer Center Support
3,092,697	3.32	102,678	Cancer Center Core Support Grant
1,256,873	2.84	35,695	Cancer Center Support Grant
854,004	2.23	19,044	Cancer Center of Wake Forest University
5,818,218	1.37	79,710	CCSG
3,194,572	0.60	19,167	Cancer Center
2,056,974	0.44	9,051	CCSG
2,551,080	0.43	10,970	CCSG
2,220,205	0.41	9,103	Yale Comprehensive Cancer Center
4,876,435	0.30	14,629	Regional Oncology Research Center
3,510,542	0.21	7,372	CCSG
202,113	0.11	222	Genetic Markers for Therapy of Colon Cancer
2,640,213	0.11	2,904	ECOG Statistical Center—Data Management Office
2,329,568	0.11	2,563	ECOG Statistical Office
6,944,062	0.11	7,638	ECOG Operations Office
154,596	0.11	170	ECOG Institution Grant
181,018	0.11	199	ECOG
366,391	0.11	403	ECOG
281,735	0.11	310	ECOG
234,810	0.11	258	ECOG
446,441	0.11	491	ECOG
547,877	0.11	603	ECOG —Wisconsin Studies
393,987	0.11	433	ECOG Clinical Trials
286,855	0.11	316	ECOG
391,656	0.11	431	ECOG
170,319	0.11	187	ECOG
335,704	0.11	369	ECOG Studies
206,311	0.11	227	ECOG
426,499	0.11	469	ECOG
345,144	0.11	380	ECOG
742,780	0.11	817	ECOG Chair's Office
146,456	0.11	161	ECOG
3,001,469	0.05	1,501	University of Michigan Cancer Center
2,865,494	0.02	573	American College of Surgeons Oncology Trials Group

TABLE 1A-2 Continued

Total Project $	Percent[a]	$ Relevant to Palliative Care	Project Title[b]
824,877	0.02	165	Quality Assurance Review Center (QARC)
401,529	0.02	80	EORTC Data Center
735,000	0.02	147	Radiological Physics Center
2,803,329	0.02	561	CCSG
TOTAL		**6,148,591**	

NOTE: CCOP = Community Clinical Oncology Program; CCSG = Cancer Center Support Grant; ECOG = Eastern Cooperative Oncology Group; EORTC = European Organization for Research and Treatment of Cancer; SPORE = Specialized Program of Research Excellence.

[a]NCI estimate of percent of total relevant to palliative care

[b]Grant numbers, principal investigators, and specific institutions have not been listed in this table.

SOURCE: Colbert, 2000.

APPENDIX 1B

Recommendations from *Enhancing Data Systems to Improve the Quality of Cancer Care* (IOM, 2000)

1. Enhance Key Elements of the Data System Infrastructure

Recommendation 1: Develop a core set of cancer care quality measures.

The Secretary of the Department of Health and Human Services (DHHS) should designate a committee made up of representatives of public institutions (e.g., the DHHS Quality of Cancer Care Committee, state cancer registries, academic institutions) and private groups (e.g., consumer organizations, professional associations, purchasers, health insurers and plans) to: 1) identify a single core set of quality measures that span the full spectrum of an individual's care and are based on the best available evidence; 2) advise other national groups (e.g., National Committee for Quality Assurance, Joint Commission for the Accreditation of Healthcare Organizations, Quality Forum) to adopt the recommended core set of measures; and 3) monitor the progress of ongoing efforts to improve standard reporting of cancer stage and comorbidity.

a) Research sponsors (e.g., Agency for Healthcare Research and Quality [AHRQ], National Cancer Institute [NCI], Health Care Financing Administration [HCFA], Department of Veterans Affairs [VA]) should invest in studies to identify evidence-based quality indicators across the continuum of cancer care.

b) Ongoing efforts to standardize reporting of cancer stage and comorbidity should receive a high priority and be fully supported.

c) Efforts to identify quality of cancer care measures should be coordinated with ongoing national efforts regarding quality of care.

Recommendation 2: Congress should increase support to the Centers for Disease Control and Prevention (CDC) for the National Program of Cancer Registries (NPCR) to improve the capacity of states to achieve complete coverage and timely reporting of incident cancer cases. NPCR's primary purpose is cancer surveillance, but NPCR, together with the Surveillance, Epidemiology, and End Results (SEER) Program, has great potential to facilitate national, population-based assessments of the quality of cancer care through linkage studies and by serving as a sample frame for special studies.

Recommendation 3: Private cancer-related organizations should join the American Cancer Society and the American College of Surgeons to provide financial support for the National Cancer Data Base. Expanded support would facilitate efforts underway to report quality benchmarks and performance data to institutions providing cancer care.

Recommendation 4: Federal research agencies (e.g., NCI, CDC, AHRQ, HCFA) should support research and demonstration projects to identify new mechanisms to organize and finance the collection of data for cancer care quality studies. Current data systems tend to be hospital based, while cancer care is shifting to outpatient settings. New models are needed to capture entire episodes of care, irrespective of the setting of care.

Recommendation 5: Federal research agencies (e.g., National Institutes of Health [NIH], Food and Drug Administration [FDA], CDC, and VA) should support public-private partnerships to develop technologies, including computer-based patient record systems and intranet-based communication systems, that will improve the availability, quality, and timeliness of clinical data relevant to assessing quality of cancer care.

Recommendation 6: Federal research agencies (e.g., NCI, AHRQ, VA) should expand support for training in health services research and training of professionals with expertise in the measurement of quality of care and the implementation and evaluation of interventions designed to improve the quality of care.

2. Expand Support for Analyses of Quality of Cancer Care Using Existing Data Systems

Recommendation 7: Federal research agencies (e.g., NCI, AHRQ, VA) should expand support for health services research, especially studies based on the linkage of cancer registry to administrative data and special studies of cases sampled from cancer registries. Resources should also be made available through NPCR and SEER to provide technical assistance to states to help them expand the capability of using cancer registry data for quality improvement initiatives. NPCR should also be supported in its efforts to consolidate state data and link them to national data files.

Recommendation 8: Federal research agencies (e.g., NCI, AHRQ, HCFA) should develop models for the conduct of linkage studies and the release of confidential data for research purposes that protect the confidentiality and privacy of healthcare information.

3. Monitor the Effectiveness of Data Systems to Promote Quality Improvement Within Health Systems.

Recommendation 9: Federal research agencies (e.g., NCI, AHRQ, HCFA, VA) should fund demonstration projects to assess the application of quality monitoring programs within healthcare systems and the impact of data-driven changes in the delivery of services on the quality of health care. Findings from the demonstrations should be disseminated widely to consumers, payers, purchasers, and cancer care providers.

Part 2

2

Reliable, High-Quality, Efficient End-of-Life Care for Cancer Patients: Economic Issues and Barriers

Joanne Lynn, M.D.
RAND Center to Improve Care of the Dying

Ann O'Mara, R.N., Ph.D.
Bethesda, MD

INTRODUCTION

Living with, and eventually dying from, a chronic illness ordinarily runs up substantial costs for the patient, family, and society. Patients are sick, dependent, changing, and needy. Indeed, more than two dollars of every eight spent in Medicare is spent in the last year of life, and one in every eight is spent in the last month (Lubitz and Riley, 1993). Those with cancer have approximately 20 percent higher than average costs (Hogan et al., 2000).

High costs probably would be acceptable to all if patients and families were satisfied with the care provided for those with advanced disease, but few can count on being satisfied. Reports of inadequate symptom relief, uncertain responsibility for patient care across multiple care providers, family disruption and financial distress, inadequate planning ahead for serious disability and death, and other shortcomings are commonplace (IOM, 1997). In short, our society is spending a great deal and not getting what dying cancer patients need.

Many factors contribute to these shortcomings: inadequate attention to the problems, untrained professionals, absent quality standards, and so on. This chapter addresses the contribution to the shortcomings made by the financial arrangements covering care for people with advanced cancer. Changes in financing and coverage will not, on their own, change the standards of care (Vladeck, 1999), but changes in financing and coverage are an essential part of sustainable, comprehensive reform. Engineering a society for better performance requires paying for the essential services at least well enough to allow their providers to make a living. Indeed, financial incentives probably shape professional and public definitions of appropriate care in ways that are hard to trace or to correct. However, understanding these incentives and the distortions they engender is essential when aiming to engineer effective reform.

Briefly, the population of concern is those persons who have advanced malignancy (solid cancers, hematologic malignancies, brain tumors, and others) at such a stage that the patient does not feel well on his or her usual day and the malignancy is not expected to remit substantially before contributing to the patient's death. Not all such patients are given the label of "dying." For example, those who may live many years with an indolent cancer, like the usual prostate cancer, or those with a small chance of remission from ongoing aggressive treatment, might not seem to be dying. Furthermore, not all dying cancer patients actually fit this definition; those with other serious conditions that are likely to cause death before the cancer would might well be dying, though their cancer is only a minor problem (Figure 2-1).

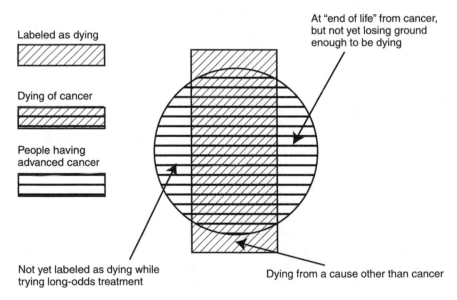

FIGURE 2-1   The population with advanced cancer.

Once, virtually every serious illness, including cancer, spelled a fairly rapid course to death. Malignancies were identified only when large or in a critical location, and most often, no treatments were available that substantially altered the course. The fact that cancer patients often lingered a few months, often with disturbing appearance, odors, and suffering, undoubtedly contributed to cancer's special position of abhorrence in the popular mythology. Now, patients with cancer often live much longer because of better prevention, earlier diagnosis, and treatments that prolong survival, resulting in longer periods of adaptation to cancer as a chronic debilitating disease. However, most still eventually die from the cancer. In fact, mortality from lung, breast, prostate, and colorectal cancers, for example, is not much better than it was 50 years ago (ACS, 2001). Most, too, face discontinuities and other lapses in quality of care at the end of life.

The fact that many will suffer at the end of life from the shortcomings of current care patterns probably arises mostly from our inexperience, as a society, with our new circumstances. As part of our collective inexperience, we have not settled upon language, categories, or methods that serve us well. We persist in talking of "terminal cancer" or "the shift from cure to care" as if these were obvious, natural categories, though they are not. Myriad studies of treatments use prolonged survival as the end point; in contrast, only a handful of studies aim to find ways to improve quality of life, opportunity for life closure, family togetherness, financial well-being, or symptoms.

This chapter describes the following general findings and offers suggestions as to how to improve the experience of end-of-life care for patients with cancer:

- End-of-life care is unavoidably expensive, largely because people are very sick.
- The services most needed are often not covered by Medicare or other insurance, and the services most well-covered may well be overused.
- The transfers that patients endure among care providers might be much more avoidable if continuity were valued.
- The Medicare hospice program could be modified in various ways to improve its usefulness.
- Very little reliable and generalizable information advances the discussion of financing of end-of-life care.

Since we are focused upon those at the end of life, this chapter does not deal with the costs of diagnosis or initial treatment, and since the focus is on cancer care, it does not deal with the effects of comorbidities, although the economics of both earlier care and care of other conditions profoundly affect the economics of cancer care.

CURRENT FINANCING OF ADVANCED CANCER CARE

Private insurance or Medicare covers most of the medical care expenses of people with advanced cancer. Most people with Medicare coverage have expanded benefits (through Medicaid, private pensioners' insurance, or Medigap insurance) that often cover some prescription drugs (Commonwealth Fund, 1998) and also cover most of the deductibles and coinsurance. Since Medicare is the largest and the only nationally uniform coverage plan and the majority of people with cancer are over 65, Medicare will be used as a prototype.

Medicare Coverage and Design

Medicare (in fact, most health insurance) was constructed mainly to make surgery available, and its coverage and financing rules reveal those roots. Although managed care has been introduced and covers a growing portion of the Medicare population, most Medicare payment is currently in the fee-for-service system, in which payment arises as reimbursement for services already given. Medicare fee-for-service provides reasonably well for procedures needed for diagnosis and treatments aimed at disease modification. Coverage extends not only to surgery, radiation treatment, diagnostic testing, and in-patient hospitalization, but also to intravenous medication, skilled nursing for the homebound and those in nursing facilities, oxygen (for those with severely low oxygenation), and durable medical equipment. Medicare also offers hospice; indeed, Medicare pays for 65 percent of all patients receiving hospice care in the United States (National Hospice and Palliative Care Organization, 2001). However, Medicare was originally established for diagnosis and treatment of diseases. The language of the hospice benefit (and the parallel language in the preventive services benefit added later) can be read to imply that assuaging symptoms and supporting the very sick was not part of the original Medicare mandate. Since clinical practice has moved strongly toward incorporating palliative care into routine health care, this interpretation may become irrelevant. However, it may also eventually require modification of the enabling statute.

Medicare (and most insurance) does not generally pay for medications that the patient can take on his or her own, personal care assistance, or disposable supplies. These restrictions are felt all the more keenly with the shift of cancer care to the outpatient setting, greater demands on family caregivers to administer both oral and parenteral medications, and the increasing use of home-delivered chemotherapeutic agents. Furthermore, fee-for-service payments generally have incentives contrary to continuity and do not pay for institutional care outside of hospitals.

A small proportion of Medicare patients and a larger proportion of younger patients are in capitated care systems, in which a provider or insurer receives a set amount of money each month for every member regardless of how much care is provided. In general, these arrangements do not pay the fiscal risk-taking entity better for a patient who is sick, since rates are set "per capita" for a population. (Risk-adjusted payments are being implemented in the Medicare capitated payment system; Iezzoni, 1997). However, capitation also allows much more flexible use of the funding and thus can cover medications, personal care, and other elements not generally covered in Medicare fee for service, if the insurer decides to offer those benefits (to attract enrollees). Capitation undoubtedly creates pressures to reduce services generally, but the one careful study of the effects of provider or payer type on the costs of the last year of life for the frail elderly found no differences between Medicare health maintenance organizations (HMOs), traditional fee for service, and Medicare-Medicaid dual eligibles (in California, in 1990-1993) (Experton et al., 1999).

Innovative approaches that combine elements of these approaches are not hard to find. Some benefits managers are "carving out" care of cancer patients and handling them as a separate capitation to specialists, for example.

Hospice

The most substantial innovation to serve advanced cancer patients is hospice. The Medicare hospice benefit mostly pays the hospice provider organization a daily rate for each patient enrolled and served at home. A small proportion (by law, less than 20 percent) of the days that Medicare pays to hospice providers can cover continuous nursing care, inpatient respite stay, or inpatient symptom management. The services that hospices provide include many elements that are not typically part of Medicare coverage: for example, interdisciplinary team, care planning, personal care nursing, family or patient teaching and support, chaplaincy, medication (with a small copayment), counseling, symptomatic treatment, and bereavement. The attending physician services either are paid within the hospice benefit (if the physician is a hospice employee) or are paid upon a separate billing from the physician to Medicare.

Hospice pioneers did not envision hospice as a part of routine health care, although this is what it has become. More than half of Medicare beneficiaries dying with a cancer diagnosis used at least some hospice care in 1998 (Hogan et al., 2000). However, the ways in which hospice programs are not parallel to (or integrated with) other health care programs are evident. For example, under Medicare, hospice programs may serve only patients enrolled specifically in the hospice benefit (which restricts other types of care they can receive, as discussed below). Even if hospice skills would be useful to other patients, no payment is available, and in some circumstances, the services cannot even be provided for free (since it might amount to an illegal inducement to enroll).

As another example, the interface of hospice services and nursing home care has been quite unsettled. Only a minority of nursing home patients has their stay reimbursed by Medicare (only after a qualifying hospitalization and if requiring skilled services). In general, Medicare reimbursement for skilled nursing home stays is high enough that the few patients who do qualify are not even offered the opportunity to enroll in hospice (only *either* skilled nursing home care or hospice can be in effect at one time). However, most nursing home stays do not qualify as "skilled" and thereby do not qualify for Medicare payment. These patients are often eligible for hospice services if a qualified hospice works out a relationship with the nursing home.

However, two problems complicate the integration of nursing home reimbursement and hospice. First, both the nursing home and the hospice are independently required to establish and implement a plan of care, and it is not clear how conflicts should be resolved. In addition, most such nursing home stays end up being paid by Medicaid. This could offer an opportunity for paying almost double the nursing home rate (by adding the hospice benefit payment to the nursing home payment). Many observers were skeptical that such patients would receive twice as much service, thus raising the possibility of improper profits. While the situation is unstable, the current resolution is that a Medicaid-enrolled patient in a nursing home (who is not using Medicare skilled nursing facility benefits) who is also eligible for hospice can enroll in hospice if the nursing facility and the hospice have a legal agreement as to their responsibilities, the hospice provides certain core services directly, and the hospice accepts the full payments from Medicaid and Medicare and pays the nursing home.

When hospice started in this country, it was a movement that rejected mainstream medicine. The Medicare hospice benefit perpetuated this concept by making hospice quite separate from the rest of health care. Now that hospice is used as mainstream care, unanticipated troubles arise from the many dysfunctional junctures between hospice and the rest of health care, such as the interface with nursing homes or patients still not in hospice care.

Once committed to hospice care, the major problems that affect most patients arise from

- restrictive and varying enrollment criteria,
- substantial variation in service array and financial risk taking across hospices,

- short stays, and
- increasingly costly options for palliative care.

Hospice Enrollment Criteria

Medicare allows hospice enrollment only for patients with a "prognosis of less than six months" who formally consent to forgo curative medical care. These requirements ensure that hospice enrollment is seen as a substantial decision to pursue a death-accepting course. The sense that one is giving up on hopefulness makes some patients resist enrollment.

The hospice requirement of a six-month prognosis has itself been quite troubled. Oddly, the requirement has never been defined. Is the "just barely qualified" patient just "more likely than not" to die within six months, or should that patient be "virtually certain to die"? This may sound like an arcane issue, but the population that includes everyone who is more likely than not to die from a chronic disease within six months is probably two to three orders of magnitude (100 to 1,000 times) larger than the population of persons who can be known to be virtually certain to die. In addition, requiring virtual certainty also engenders eligibility for hospice only within a few days or weeks of death, since our prognosticating ability is simply not precise enough to allow confident prognosis until the patient is visibly failing, bed-bound, and worsening daily (Fox et al., 1999; Lynn et al., 1997).

Fraud investigations for long-stay hospice patients in the past few years have induced an attitude of caution and a reticence to take on patients who might stabilize and live a long time. Until these fraud investigations, when a very sick patient did stabilize and live, most hospices would just keep the patient enrolled, knowing that the illness would eventually worsen again and cut life short. Now, such patients are likely to be discharged from hospice. Their "next-best" service array is often quite limited (as discussed below).

Providers and patients expect much the same services to be available from all programs within each kind of provider. For example, we expect every hospital to have a laboratory and X-ray facilities, operating rooms, inpatient beds, and so on. Indeed, we expect that most hospitals would profess their own competence and scope in just about the same ways as other hospitals. Hospices are different. Right from the start, they were allowed to define their own scope of practice, within broad boundaries. Thus, some hospices will not take patients using feeding tubes, while others not only will take those patients but would also allow tests and medications to keep a patient eligible for transplantation. Some hospices won't take any patient on "chemotherapy," but others will try to accept those with "palliative" treatments (but not those "still aiming at cure"). These terms have become quite difficult to define, but the point here is that, as long as they are honest with patients and others, hospices are free to define their scope of service and enrollment criteria and thereby to limit or expand their financial risks.

This has led to neighboring hospices having quite different practices, populations, and skills. Since they all are paid the same capitation, this also translates to very different foci. Some hospices limit themselves to rather simple medications and limited physician services, for example, and therefore may be more able to provide home health aides. Other hospices are committed to providing whatever treatments the patient and physician think might be helpful. Since the treatments are often costly, these hospices might have much less flexibility to serve psychosocial needs.

In addition, hospices are very different in size. Roughly 30 percent of hospice days are in hospices that are of substantial size—more than 150 patients on the usual day. However, these patients are being served by only about a score of hospice organizations. The other 3,100 hospices mostly serve less than 50 patients on any given day (Stephen Connor, National Hospice and Palliative Care Organization, personal communication, July 13, 2000). Large hospices are more able to take risks and accept patients who might be exceedingly costly. Managers of small hospices realize that one patient with extreme costs would spell financial disaster. These differences are not usually apparent to patients or referring physicians, who may end up seeing differences among hospice programs as simply erratic, unpredictable, and idiosyncratic.

Hospices are bedeviled now with short stays. In 1998, the mean length of stay was 51.3 days and the median length of stay was 25 days (National Hospice and Palliative Care Organization, 2001). In 1990, the mean was nearly 90 days and the median was 36 days (Christakis and Escarce, 1996). Various observers attribute short stays to different causes, including physician and patient reticence to stop active treatment; more treatment options for second-, third-, and fourth-line treatments (e.g., Herceptin, Rituxan, erythropoietin); hospice reticence to enroll patients receiving expensive treatments (even if acknowledged to be palliative); prognosis becoming clear only when death is close (especially in non-cancer diagnoses); and new populations coming into hospice (incompetent persons, very elderly persons, noncancer fatal illnesses, and others). No reliable research has yet sorted out the reasons for increasingly short stays in hospice. However, the financial impact has been substantial. The first day or two in hospice are always costly, as the hospice team gets to know the patient and family, puts needed equipment and medication in the home, and monitors progress with new plans of care. Likewise, the last few days of life are expensive, as the patient and family need more care, more frequent changes in medication, help with declaring death and arranging for the care of the body, and support through at least a year of bereavement. When these days come close together, there are no "stable" days in which costs might often be lower than the daily rate. Thus, short stays threaten the financial viability of hospices.

Hospices are also struggling with a plethora of developments in palliative care. Twenty years ago, it was not much of an exaggeration to claim that the hospice physician could do most everything with little more than cheap opioid medications, steroids, diuretics, and antibiotics. Now, patients are served somewhat better by more technologically advanced interventions, more expensive medications, more use of radiation or surgery, and so on. For example, for some patients, pain could be suppressed with oral or subcutaneous morphine, with the side effect that the patient would be groggy and perhaps sometimes confused. Better alertness and pain control might be possible with an intrathecal pump for morphine, at an initial cost of about $20,000.

Other examples are common. Gemcitabine measurably reduces pain in pancreatic cancer and has been reported to have superior antitumor activity and improved survival over 5-fluorouracil (5-FU; Ulrich-Pur et al., 2000), at a cost of about $500 per week. Many patients with advanced cancer also get pulmonary emboli or thrombosis of the leg veins. Standard treatment with anticoagulants entails certain risks and annoyances that are largely avoided by low-molecular-weight heparin injections. However, the standard treatments cost only a few dollars per day (after initial hospitalization, which is covered by Medicare), while the low-molecular-weight heparin costs about $60-$120 per day it is not covered by Medicare unless a hospice program decides to pay for it from the hospice per diem. Because this is financially unsustainable, medications and interventions that are this costly and are not covered by insurance are largely unavailable. In contrast, if covered by insurance, they are readily available, even if a thoughtful assessment would raise doubts about the merits of investing so heavily in small gains for persons with short life expectancies.

Gap Between Hospice and Home Care

Many patients simply have no Medicare-covered services for a part of their course when they are quite needy but are neither so sure to die within six months that hospice is available (or they are otherwise ineligible for their local hospice) nor so housebound as to qualify for the limited help from Medicare home care (which requires being unable to leave the home except for physician visits). Physicians and nurses are probably fairly customer oriented for this needy group and offer ways to get them some of the services they need (e.g., by short-term certification of homebound status).

The impact of this distortion and the unmet need has not been estimated in the published literature, however.

DESCRIPTION OF COSTS AND COST-EFFECTIVENESS OF TREATMENTS

About half a million patients in the United States die of cancer each year (American Cancer Society, 2001), and on average, about $32,000 per patient is spent in the last year of life for the care of Medicare patients dying of cancers (Hogan et al., 2000). The care of cancer is a major part of the business of health care, and many businesses and provider organizations focus exclusively on cancer care. Most literature on diagnosis, treatment, and cost does not address the entire cancer population, but addresses just one type. Thus, this section reviews descriptive accounts that address costs and cost-effectiveness of treatments offered for particular common cancers and then for symptom management and palliative care more generally.

Advanced Lung Cancer (Non-Small Cell Cancer of the Lung)

In contrast to breast, prostate, and colorectal cancers, very little progress has been made in early diagnosis and long-term remission in lung cancer. Furthermore, as the most common cancer among men and women in the United States, lung cancer accounts for approximately 20 percent of all cancer care costs (Desch et al., 1996). The focus of clinical trials has been to prolong survival and increase the number of one- and two-year survivors. Recently, attention has turned to economic evaluations that compare the cost and benefits of such treatments. In their review of the available economic data, Goodwin and Shepherd (1998) conclude that the costs of combination chemotherapy or combined-modality treatment for locally advanced or metastatic lung cancer are well within the range considered acceptable for interventions used for other diseases.

Smith (Thomas J. Smith, personal communication, 2000) proposed asking about the patient's evaluation of the merits of treatment in this disease in a quite novel and illuminating way. Working with a large regional insurer, Smith generated actuarial estimates of the expenditures from diagnosis of inoperable lung cancer through to death. He proposed to give the patient a choice, after giving the patient a solid understanding of the issues at stake. The patient could choose to have conventional care, with treatments that would probably extend life (for three to four months, on average), or the patient could choose to have hospice care available from the start and also take all of the funds (about $19,000) that would probably have been spent on his or her radiation and chemotherapy. The experiment was terminated after six months, largely because few patients remained outside of managed care plans by the time all of the preliminary arrangements were in place (and the experiment required that patients be in conventional fee for service). However, the mental model is quite illuminating. Would people who had to pay their own bills remain willing to get treatments with small expected gains? Some are quite offended by Dr. Smith's experiment, claiming that it is offensive to consider life in monetary terms. This objection, if widespread, will be difficult to accommodate in policy.

In 1992, the charges for hospitalization in the last year of life for lung cancer patients dying in a hospital in Connecticut averaged $40,000, while those who died at home or in hospice had hospital charges of about $30,000 (Polednak and Shevchenko, 1998). Smith suggests that a fairer comparison would be average total health care costs, rather than limiting it to hospital charges.

Advanced Colorectal Cancer

Evaluating the costs of treating patients with advanced colorectal cancer has been the subject of various research endeavors, most of them outside the United States. Chemotherapy, concomitant medications, surgical procedures, hospitalizations, diagnostic tests, and outpatient visits have been assessed for their economic merit (Cunningham, 1998; Glimelius et al., 1995; Neymark and Adriaenssen, 1999; Recchia et al., 1996; Ron et al., 1996; Ross et al., 1996; Scheidback et al., 1999; Torfs and Pocceschi, 1996). A 1996 U.S. study compared two common protocols (intensive-course 5-FU + low-dose leucovorin versus weekly 5-FU + high-dose leucovorin), including financial cost as an end point (Buroker et al., 1994). Therapeutic efficacy was similar between the two schedules, both groups experienced distinct dose-limiting toxicities, and financial costs were higher for the weekly dose due to increased hospitalizations to manage toxicities. The hospitalization expenses for the weekly protocol ($3,240 per patient) were nearly double those for the intensive-course protocol ($1,781) for 32 weeks of chemotherapy (1994 dollars).

Brown and colleagues (1999) developed an illuminating method for describing costs. They split each patient's course into three parts: initial phase (first 6 months), terminal phase (last 12 months), and continuing care (whatever is left in the middle). They also estimated cancer-related costs and other medical costs by comparing matched control patients. The terminal phase in 1990-1994 had cancer-related costs of $15,000; the overall course had cancer-related costs of $33,700 and about an equal amount for noncancer-related costs.

Advanced Breast Cancer

Recent preliminary reports from several large trials show that the rigorous and costly regimen of high-dose chemotherapy with autologous stem cell rescue for metastatic breast cancer probably offers no survival advantage over standard chemotherapy (Peters et al., 2000). Given the lack of a clear, definitive answer to the question, a number of different chemotherapeutic regimens and doses, as well as the timing of these agents, are continuing to be investigated. Eight years prior to these reports, Hillner and colleagues had shown that autologous bone marrow transplant versus standard chemotherapy in a hypothetical cohort of 45-year old women with metastatic (Stage IV) breast cancer increased life expectancy by six months, using a five-year horizon. However, it came at a considerable cost of $115,800 per year of life gained. They also demonstrated that if the cost of the transplant procedure could be reduced, the cost per life-year gained could be improved to $70,000 (Hillner et al., 2000).

One of the most common metastatic sites in breast cancer is bone, resulting in additional treatment costs for pain management, such as narcotic analgesics or radiation, and surgery to treat bone fractures. On the other hand, many bony lesions are asymptomatic, often found on routine follow-up. Consequently, a balance must be achieved between expending undue resources to find asymptomatic lesions and necessary efforts to prevent or reduce complications. One approach to reducing the risk of complications has focused on the role of bisphosphonates, specifically pamidronate. A post hoc evaluation of the cost-effectiveness of pamidronate revealed that although it was effective in preventing skeletal related events (SREs), the total costs of administering pamidronate far exceeded the cost savings from avoided SREs, which included pathologic fractures, spinal cord compression or collapse, radiation for pain relief, and hypercalcemia. In addition, 80 percent of the projected costs of pamidronate per treatment were due to the drug's costs. The 1998 monthly estimated cost of pamidronate therapy was $775 (Hillner et al., 2000).

Hospital charges for breast cancer patients who died in 1992 in a Connecticut hospital averaged $42,000, while the costs for those who died at home or in hospice care averaged $20,000 (Polednak and Shevchenko, 1998).

Advanced Prostate Cancer

Finding the most effective therapy, both medically and financially, for relieving pain related to metastatic prostate cancer has been a major focus of recent research (Beemstrober et al., 1999; Bennett et al., 1996; McEwan et al., 1994; Shah et al., 1999). Medicare reimbursement policies play a troubling role in physician decisionmaking with regard to new modalities for metastatic prostate cancer. Flutamide, a nonsteroidal antiandrogen, may be effective in prolonging the time to progression of disease, improve overall survival, and have a favorable cost-effectiveness profile (Bennett et al., 1996). Because it is an oral medication, Medicare does not cover it. Findings from physician focus groups indicated that the potential out-of-pocket expenses incurred by patients influenced doctors' prescribing practices and recommendations for or against patient enrollment in flutamide clinical trials (Bennett et al., 1996).

In 1991, the total Medicare payments for prostate cancer care from diagnosis to death (seven years) averaged about $49,000 (Riley et al., 1995). Lifetime lung cancer costs are lower ($29,000), but the longer survival period in prostate cancer ends up costing more in aggregate.

Symptom Management

Pain continues to be the most frequent unrelieved symptom in the advanced cancer patient (Ingham, 1998). As cancer patients approach death, their initial oral analgesic may become inadequate. Although reasonable control could usually be regained with substantial dosage increases, different opioids, routes of administration, and delivery systems often provide more reliable control with fewer side effects. However, advanced pain treatments, such as pamidronate and intrathecal pumps, can greatly increase the cost. Furthermore, Medicare does not generally pay for pain management medications (IOM, 1999). The typical cost for an implanted intrathecal opioid infusion is $23,000, which includes hospitalization and professional fees (G. Fanciullo, personal communication, 2000). This may seem inordinately high, in light of the availability of less expensive modes of pain therapy. Yet, the complexity of the patient's condition might well lead the clinician to choose the implanted intrathecal approach. In their case report, Seamans and colleagues (2000) found it more cost effective to use intrathecal therapy (total estimated cost at three months, $19,645) over a systemic analgesic therapy (total estimated cost at three months, $31,860).

Home management of terminally ill patients could potentially contribute to decreased costs. A retrospective Canadian study compared the cost of managing cancer patients who required narcotic infusions in hospital and at home. Medical costs, in 1991 Canadian dollars, averaged $370 per inpatient-day and $150 per outpatient-day (Ferris et al., 1991). Other symptoms or advanced cancer complications for which health care resources are used include constipation (Agra et al., 1998; Ramesh et al., 1998), dyspnea (Escalante et al., 1996), common bile duct obstructions (Cvetkovski et al., 1999; Kaskarelis et al., 1996), intractable vomiting (Scheidbach et al., 1999), and dehydration (Bruera et al., 1998).

The assortment of clinical trials focused on symptom management and related costs does not accurately reflect the reality of clinically managing terminally ill cancer patients. Aside from the pain management studies that included associated costs, the costs of other frequently occurring debilitating symptoms of dyspnea, diarrhea, constipation, seizures, and terminal delirium have not been assessed adequately. Not only do we know little about how much it costs to treat these symptoms, we know equally little about the costs to society when they are mismanaged, as they often are.

An interesting associated issue arises with the off-label use of therapies that are thought to be helpful to suffering patients. An intriguing example might be erythropoietin alfa (Epo), which is used for cancer-related anemia. Epo is approved by the Food and Drug Administration (FDA) for various indications, but the only cancer indication for Epo is for patients with nonmyeloid malignancies who are concomitantly receiving myelosuppressive chemotherapy. Physician prescribing is not limited to FDA-approved indications, however, and many cancer patients not receiving chemotherapy, or receiving chemotherapy that is not myelosuppressive, are prescribed Epo for anemia. Although lack of FDA approval is not always synonymous with a lack of evidence of effectiveness, in this case, there have been no trials in the general population of cancer patients, so effectiveness has not been demonstrated. Only one active National Cancer Institute (NCI) Phase III clinical trial is exploring the effect of Epo in anemic patients with advanced cancer undergoing platinum-containing chemotherapy. Nonetheless, it is an approved drug that is covered by Medicare, which paid $210 per injection in 1998. In 1998, about 35 million injections were given to about 2 million Medicare patients, at a cost of about $7 billion. If Epo is given in the hospital, it is part of the diagnosis-related group (DRG) payment for each stay, but if it is given in doctor's offices, it is a separate covered expense. Either way, it is free to the patient. It has few side effects, beyond the cost.

METHODOLOGICAL CONSIDERATIONS CONCERNING STUDIES REPORTING COSTS

Assessing Costs and Effectiveness

For a few discrete advanced cancers and their symptoms, we know that certain treatments will *not* provide an improved quantity or quality of life and may be costly as well (Smith, 2001) (Table 2-1). One example of this is second-line chemotherapy for metastatic lung cancer, which entails the use of fairly expensive drugs and a number of toxicities. On the other hand, we know very little about the most efficacious, least costly treatment for the full spectrum of advanced cancers. Indeed, little discussion illuminates the

TABLE 2-1 Targets for Reduction in Resource Use with No Impact on Quantity or Quality of Life

Strategy	Comment
2nd-line chemotherapy for metastatic cancer	For instance, 2nd line chemotherapy with docetaxol improves overall survival and health-related quality of life in nonsmall cell lung cancer. Unclear if 3rd or other lines of chemotherapy have a similar effect. Most cancers have not been studied to see if 2nd or 3rd line chemotherapy is better than supportive care. Current NCCN guidelines call for switch to hospice or palliative care when chemotherapy has been tried and failed, and provide a starting point for "stopping rules." For instance, current NCCN guidelines call for 2 types of chemotherapy in breast cancer, then switch to hospice care. The average patient receives far more types of chemotherapy.
Neoadjuvant chemotherapy and radiotherapy for many solid tumors	Proven modest benefits in resected gastric cancer, head and neck cancer, lung and esophageal cancers. For other cancers, there has been minimal impact on disease, and a marked increase in drug costs and toxicities.
Radiotherapy palliation of bone and other metastasis	1-5 fraction radiotherapy offers pain relief to the majority of patients and reduces the travel and treatment costs.
Radiotherapy palliation of advanced lung cancer	8Gy in 1 fraction or 16 Gy in 2 fraction offers symptom relief to the majority of patients and reduces travel and treatment cost; much higher doses are often used.
Carcinoembryonic Antigens (CEAs), CA 27.29, CA 15.3 blood tests; bone scans, liver ultrasounds, chest X-rays, computerized axial tomography (CATs) and other follow-up tests in breast, lung, and colon cancer	With the exception of the CEA in resected colorectal cancer, these tests offer no advantage in life-years saved, and the cost is prohibitive (for instance, estimates of follow up costs for breast cancer alone are over $1 billion annually). these tests are not recommended by the American Society of Clinical Oncology; for details see the website at www.asco.org and go to the "People Living with Cancer" section.
Discuss "code status" with all patients while they are stable, and document whether resuscitation and ICU stay is medically indicated or desired by the patient and family	The majority of physicians have acted against their conscience in providing aggressively futile care; this costly and tragic waste can be prevented by addressing the issue beforehand.
Consolidation of provider visits, with switch to a primary care provider	Patients may see a radiotherapist, surgeon, medical oncologist, and their primary care physician; only one is necessary, and the primary care provider may be less likely to order low-yield, high-cost diagnostic tests.

Thomas J. Smith, personal communication, 2001.

NCCN = National Comprehensive Cancer Network.

question of how we ought to assess costs, efficacy, or the balance between them. Should oncologists be concerned about the costs of two efficacious treatments that are roughly equal, where one is far more expensive than the other? What about two treatments that have discernible but modest differences in efficacy and substantial differences in costs? As Smith and colleagues have wryly noted, "If oncologists do not work to determine the efficacy and cost effectiveness of cancer treatment, others will do it for them" (Smith et al., 1993). Of course, it may be that oncologists should insist upon others doing this work. Perhaps societal or personal values are what should matter, and oncologists may have no special insight into these matters. Either way, we have no method by which to weigh these issues and to implement any ensuing judgments.

Even defining "cost" turns out to be a difficult endeavor. It cannot be confined to the costs of the particular treatment modality because each treatment has side effects and toxicities and may require different settings for treatment or for living. Yet, to date most research has focused on the cost of medications and insurance-covered medical care.

The many physical, emotional, and financial burdens families take on when caring for loved ones are beginning to be noted in counting costs. The metric for measuring the subjective components of caregiver burdens is quite unsettled. The complexity of human situations seems hard to capture in a single scale that would allow comparisons, for example, of the burdens incurred by an elderly wife caring alone for her aged husband who is dying slowly of metastatic prostate cancer with the burdens felt by a large extended family supporting a younger man dying with very difficult suffering from lung cancer.

Smith and colleagues pose the question of whether palliative cancer care can be cost-effective, at least as that is now operationally defined. For many cancers, palliative therapy may be as expensive as chemotherapy (Smith et al., 1993). However, the end points for palliative therapy, although definable in terms of symptom control and quality of life, are not easily quantified. Hillner and colleagues (2000) believe that the recurring challenge for both cancer and noncancer therapies is to establish the financial value of new medical interventions that are not associated with improved survival.

Paucity of Attention to Costs or Quality of Life in Clinical Trials

Until recently, the gold standards for determining the efficacy of a cancer treatment in a clinical trial have been improved survival, tumor shrinkage, and ultimately, cure. As more costly treatments enter the picture, more attention is being given to the economics of cancer therapies. In addition to the absolute costs of the treatments themselves, increasing numbers of procedures used in cancer therapy and the aging of the population contribute to the overall costs of cancer treatment (Journal of the National Cancer Institute, 1998). While improved survival has resulted for individuals diagnosed with early-stage cancers, eventually succumbing to the disease continues to be a likely outcome for many.

As the scope of clinical trials broadens to include individuals with late-stage disease, improved survival and tumor response remain the primary end points. Clearly, these end points are insufficient for this population. Researchers and clinicians are beginning to identify as end points the distressing symptoms of advanced cancer. The National Cancer Institute provides a comprehensive list of the six different categories of clinical trials— treatment, prevention, diagnostic, genetic, screening, and supportive care —on its Web site (http://cancernet.nci.nih.gov/cgi-bin/srchcgi.exe). A search of the supportive care category revealed 90 ongoing Phase II and III clinical trials. The primary end points were toxicity profiles, side effects, response rate, maximum tolerated dose, dose-limiting toxicities, event-free survival, and pharmacokinetic profile. Only a few studies aimed for other end points. Among the 38 Phase II trials, 7 explored quality of life (QOL) and/or symptom relief as primary or secondary end points in the advanced cancer population. Among the 52 Phase III trials, 13 specifically addressed QOL or symptom management or relief (pain, diarrhea, sleep disturbances, toxicities), in addition to tumor response and survival time.

Irrespective of the physiological or behavioral end point, financial considerations are rarely primary or secondary end points in clinical trials. None of the NCI supportive care clinical trials listed cost as an end point. A MEDLINE search of clinical trials about pain published over the past 10 years in the advanced cancer population yielded 265 trials. However, when cost, cost-effectiveness, health care costs, or economics was entered as a search term, only five remained. An even smaller proportion of advanced lung cancer trials (7 out of 725) listed these financing terms. In both types of studies, financial considerations were most often merely cursory commentaries, not study end points. Given the disturbingly high number of distressing symptoms afflicting the majority of the terminally ill cancer population, much more attention must be given to cost-effective symptom management modalities.

Generalizability

The generalizability of findings from advanced cancer clinical trials is also problematic, particularly with respect to age. Cancer has often been labeled a disease of aging, with estimations of a 10-fold increased likelihood of being diagnosed with cancer for those over 65 than for those under 65. Yet the median age of participants with advanced cancer in clinical trials is almost always many years under 65. For example, the median age of women with metastatic breast cancer participating in two randomized trials that evaluated pamidronate in preventing bone complications was 57 years (Hillner et al., 2000). This is in marked contrast to the 1988-1992 age-adjusted incidence rates of 72.8 per 100,000 for women under 65 and 445.4 per 100,000 for women over 65 (Kosary et al., 2000). The data available for policy are built on a population that is at least a decade younger than the population actually facing these illnesses. This is important because the financial and family resources, physiological reserves, and comorbidities of younger persons are dramatically different than they are in older persons. The burgeoning size of our over-65 population demands that research deal with this target population, especially when the data are used for Medicare policy.

Other considerations make the generalizability of published studies quite problematic. Most studies are carried out in academic centers, which serve populations quite different from random samples. Most require patients who are able to travel and to consent, which eliminates many with cognitive disability or severe poverty. Most also require that the patient have no other serious or life-threatening disease.

Complex Role of the Patient's Setting

As an alternative to aggressive, often futile, expensive therapy requiring repeated hospitalizations, increasing numbers of terminally ill cancer patients are enrolling in hospice or other home care. By opting for hospice or extensive home care, patients commonly remain at home among loved ones, receiving care that is focused on their symptoms, emotions, spiritual concerns, and family.

However, the long-held assumption that hospice care can contain costs at the end of life is being challenged on a number of fronts. These supposed benefits were among the reasons for hospice becoming a benefit in the Medicare program in 1983. Early research appeared to confirm this (Brooks, 1989a, 1989b; Brooks and Smyth-Staruch, 1984; Kidder, 1992; Mor and Masterson-Allen, 1990). Kidder estimated that during the first three years of the hospice benefit program, Medicare saved $1.26 for every dollar spent on Part A expenditures. Mor and colleagues examined data from the National Hospice Study to assess the time in the hospice program that would be the most informative period for which to evaluate associated costs. Enrollment periods of one to three months tend to yield the most savings (Brooks and Smyth-Staruch, 1984; Kidder, 1992). However, when the time period extended six months and beyond, the savings were not substantial. The National Hospice Organization commissioned a study that found that hospice saved $1.52 for every $1 spent by Medicare (Lewin-VH1, 1995).

This study was, however, largely uninterpretable because the key comparison was between cancer patients who had used hospice and those who had not. Even with a multivariable modeling technique, the comparability is uncertain. Furthermore, these data are now outdated, having focused on patients who died in 1992, and much has changed since that time. Since Medicare Part A and B expenditures cover less than 50 percent of medical care costs for patients over 65, examination of Medicare claims alone also limits our full understanding of the potential savings or costs of hospice enrollment.

Recent unadjusted comparisons (Hogan et al., 2000) showed that the total costs of care (from the Current Medicare Beneficiary Survey) were not significantly different, although Medicare's proportion of payment was higher for hospice users. Emanuel addressed the question of whether better care at the end of life would generally reduce costs (Emanuel, 1996). Using his assumptions and estimates, hospice and advance directives might save 25-40 percent of the last month's costs and 10-17 percent over the last six months. A recent analysis for the Medicare Payment Advisory Commission (MedPAC) showed that patients who used hospice tended to be high-cost users before hospice enrollment (at the least, they did not include any very low cost users) and their costs were similar to non-hospice-using cancer patients at the end of life (Hogan et al., 2000).

Pritchard and colleagues reported on regional variation in where patients died and found that the availability of Medicare hospice services affected the likelihood of dying at home (Pritchard et al., 1998). However, the overwhelming predictor was regional hospital bed supply. The amount of regional variation is substantial: between 14 percent and 49 percent of Medicare beneficiaries in different areas use intensive care units (ICUs) in the last six months of life, and the aggregate Medicare costs of that time are between $6,200 and $18,000 (Dartmouth, 1999). Work on regional variation illustrates the complex relationship of location, costs, service supply, and patient preferences. Higher bed supply is almost always a strong predictor of higher costs and more hospitalization, but it is not at all clear whether there is an optimum rate or whether increased availability of other services is necessary to support low rates of hospital supply.

While patients with cancer wish to die at home among familiar surroundings, labeling this as cost-effective (or cost-saving) may be premature, given the complex nature of the disease, technological advances, family resources. Very little research has described the costs to caregivers of terminally ill cancer patients. One study of cancer patients who were undergoing active treatment reported that the average cancer home care costs for a three-month period were not much lower than the costs of nursing home care (Stommel et al., 1993).

Problem of Varying Lengths of Life

Virtually our entire slim database on costs implicitly turns on a problematic assumption that the time to death is not affected by the treatments given or the choices of patients and others. On the few occasions when a researcher aimed to learn whether an intervention could be justified in terms of lengthening life, a rough estimate of cost per year of life might be made. However, if good palliative care extends life by a few months or if nursing home placement shortens life, these effects have not been assessed. Thus, since patients' length of life varies substantially anyway, it would be hard to notice whether interventions or patterns of care altered survival time by a few months. Yet, this effect could be substantial in financial terms. The last few weeks or months characteristically have the highest costs. If some patterns drag out this time and others foreshorten it, analyses that do not take this into account could yield seriously misleading assessments of costs. Once the patient is very sick, the most substantial contributor to lifetime costs is survival time. No method corrects costs per unit time for changes in the numbers of units of time. Indeed, policymakers would reasonably be concerned about whether to focus on lifetime costs or costs for each unit of time.

REFORMS IN FINANCING ARRANGEMENTS TO IMPROVE END-OF-LIFE CARE

End-of-life care is unavoidably expensive, largely because people are very sick, but also because prognoses are ordinarily ambiguous until very close to death. One could certainly aim reforms at using existing funds more cleverly, but one cannot hope to reduce the costs of care substantially for those who are living with serious disability from cancer or for treatments that might still give the patient a chance to live longer or better.

Medicare and other insurers do not often cover the services most needed, and the services best covered may well be overused. While some surgeries or invasive procedures still offer benefits to patients coming to the end of life, the balance of burdens and benefits makes it much less likely that these treatments still offer net benefits. Instead, the kinds of things that ordinarily have few side effects and substantial benefits are prescription medications (such as opioid analgesics), family support, and respite care. These either are not covered at all or are covered only under unusual circumstances. Some services, such as psychosocial support, family and patient education, and advance care planning, are partly covered if provided by a qualified provider and supported by adequate documentation, but the time and effort needed to meet requirements may exceed the reimbursement.

Once a person has advanced cancer, many of the problems that he or she will face can be anticipated, and plans can be put in place to provide thoughtfully designed responses. This anticipation of future possibilities and implementation of customized plans has come to be called "advance care planning," and it functions to avoid emergency responses that no longer serve the patient well, such as resuscitation at the end of life. Advance care planning also functions to implement the patient's and family's perspective on the merits of various courses of care.

Care patterns that routinely transfer patients from one provider of care to another do not generally focus upon advance care planning. Making plans requires envisioning the patient's situation comprehensively, effectively communicating about the situation and its possible treatments with patient and family, and having the capability to implement plans where the patient lives (including home, assisted living, or nursing home). The usual physician in an office or hospital has few incentives to take the time and endure the problems of doing this, since it seems to be enough to implement the recommended treatment protocols or address the patient's current problem.

Indeed, the interfaces between provider types cause many "built-in" disruptions in care. Some physicians who work in hospitals do not even register to write prescriptions for controlled drugs for patients at home. When their patients leave the hospital, they have to get opioid medications from another physician, leading to a delay, which invites recurrence of pain. Often, the physician in the nursing home simply prefers different medications from the physician in the hospital, thus guaranteeing a period of risk from overdosing or underdosing with each transfer. Many provider organizations, as a matter of policy, do not trust the decisions made in other settings to forgo resuscitation, artificial feeding, or other important treatments. Thus, when the patient is transferred, these plans have to be reestablished. If communication is difficult or the situation is deteriorating rapidly, repeating the discussion of plans may not be done in time. Again, the patient's plans end up not being implemented.

In short, continuity matters to the seriously ill and dying, but the payment arrangements do not generally support this good aim. Physicians actually are paid better for having many initial examinations rather than for continuity. Hospices are barred from providing care to patients who are not yet eligible for hospice. Indeed, hospices and home care agencies cannot arrange integrated services with one another, even though such services might insulate patients from the problems of transfers. Once enrolled in hospice (or PACE, the Program of All-Inclusive Care for the Elderly), patients enjoy continuity and comprehensiveness, and these programs have nearly universal advance care planning and the lowest rates of transfer in health care. Transfers in these programs arise almost entirely from patient choice or from the forced discharge of hospice patients who stabilize and cannot be certified as continuing to have less than six months to live. Various options could be made available to rearrange payment and coverage to encourage continuity.

With continuity comes a drive for comprehensiveness. Issues such as family support, bereavement counseling, and housing are unavoidable when care providers stay with the patient through whatever comes up. More continuity and comprehensiveness may well encourage innovations such as paying family caregivers (as much of Europe already does), providing respite care, developing supported housing, and ensuring that medications are available.

Modifications to hospice seem to be an obvious target for improving end-of-life care for patients with cancer (President's Cancer Panel, 1999). Hospice could be made available on the basis of the extent of illness or disability and then be lifelong, rather than requiring a confident prediction of death within six months. Hospice expertise could be made available to patients who are not eligible for direct services by allowing consultation by the hospice team. It makes sense for hospice team members to become known to patients with eventually fatal malignancies during the course of their illness, rather than just at the very end of life. In short, enrollment into hospice should be a less dramatic change and a more expected and integrated transition. Hospice programs could be paid somewhat more for the first day or two and the last day or two (and perhaps less for longer-term stays). Payments for costly treatments should be considered on their own merits. If evidence shows that the costs are worth it in the community's judgment, then those interventions that cannot generally be provided within the hospice capitation should be paid separately for small programs or should be folded into the overall capitation rate for large programs.

How could society move to make these reforms? We need an era of innovation and evaluation, aiming to learn how to engineer our care system to provide reliably competent, comprehensive services from the time of onset of serious illness through to death.

In doing this, society will need more reliable data on the relevant populations. The available research has usually measured costs in a referral clinic serving a population that is more than a decade younger than the average of those who face the problem. Policymakers need data about the effects and costs of various treatment strategies and approaches to organizing care delivery, in samples that represent the entire population at risk. This information requires developing new methods and substantial commitments.

Until now, society has focused mainly on premature deaths and disability. Having won many of these battles, most people now get the opportunity to live long and die of degenerative conditions such as cancer. As a society, we need to learn new framing, new approaches, and new ways of paying for the care that people need at the end of life. It can be done, and done within just a few years, if we set about the job now.

POSSIBLE STRATEGIES TO IMPROVE FINANCING FOR CARE OF PATIENTS COMING TO THE END OF LIFE WITH CANCER

Reshaping the financing of end-of-life care for those with cancer requires attention to three elements: serviceable methods, adequate description and monitoring, and innovation with evaluation. Many organizations bear responsibility for addressing these needs, some of which are noted (in parentheses) in the discussion that follows.

Methods Development Priorities

- Metrics for costs and effects (Agency for Healthcare Research and Quality [AHRQ], Health Care Financing Administration [HCFA], National Center for Health Statistics [NCHS], MedPAC, Department of Veterans Affairs [VA])
- Benchmarks—what quality can real systems yield? (AHRQ, Health Resources and Services Administration [HRSA], HCFA, VA)
- Developing models to correct for nongeneralizable populations (AHRQ, HCFA)
- Efficient methods to monitor population experience with end-of-life care in cancer, measuring outcomes and processes (Centers for Disease Control and Prevention [CDC], AHRQ).
- Efficient reporting and analysis of costs, in aggregate and to various payers (HCFA, MedPAC, AHRQ)
- Exploration of the relationship between costs and life span, and development of language and methods to correct for varying life span in assessment of cost (National Institutes of Health [NIH], AHRQ, VA)

Descriptive Data Priorities

- Developing surveillance methods to monitor trends and comparisons among populations by age, race, diagnosis, and geographic locality (CDC, states)
- Describing service use (including hospice) by outcomes, variations, and comparisons across geographical areas (HCFA, AHRQ)
- Assessing the costs and benefits of interventions in generalizable populations (NIH, AHRQ)

Innovation and Evaluation

We urgently need a period of innovation, with thoughtful evaluation and learning, in order to shape the care system and payment arrangements so they will better serve cancer patients coming to the end of life. Here, a list of possibilities is provided. Many agencies and programs should take part, but it seems likely that NCI, AHRQ, HRSA, HCFA, and the VA should be in the lead. In each case, an innovation is listed, but it is essential that each innovation be evaluated and that insights be gained from the trial. These examples are meant to be illustrative, not comprehensive or sufficient. The important conclusion is that innovations such as these should be tried out, in substantial numbers, and soon.

PRESCRIPTION DRUG COVERAGE

• If Medicare covers medications, examine effects on end-of-life care.
• If there is a formulary or purchasing cooperative, evaluate comprehensiveness and efficiency of symptom treatments.
• If Medicare does not cover medications generally, experiment with coverage for symptoms only.

HOSPICE

• Change enrollment criterion from prognosis to severity (or extent) of illness and allow continuous enrollment from onset of a certain severity to the end of life.
• Pay more for the first day or two and the last day or two.
• Carve out certain high-cost treatments or "pay down" their cost to the program to a reasonable cost share.
• Allow the hospice team to consult on nonhospice patients.
• Increase the daily rate, tailored to specific diagnoses.
• Encourage "bridge" and "graduate" programs, with funding beyond home care.
• Require coverage of hospice in Medicaid.
• Reward physicians (e.g., with better administrative arrangements) for signing up patients on hospice.

NURSING FACILITY OR LONG-TERM CARE

• Integrate hospice care and nursing home care at a fair rate of pay.
• Develop regional guidelines on management of common symptoms and advance care planning to ease transfers.
• Make key consultations for difficult symptoms readily available on-site.
• Provide incentives so that most residents can live to the end of life in their residence.

- Evaluate high rates of hospital transfer as evidence of potentially avoidable adverse events.

HOME CARE

- Modify home care eligibility to ease the homebound requirement.
- Ensure quick availability of key consultations for difficult symptoms arising in a home care patient.
- Establish rate and enrollment criteria encouraging "bridge programs" that are integrated with hospice.
- Try out integrated home-hospice-institutional care programs (PACE, MediCaring).
- Encourage geographic concentration by programs.

CAPITATED PLANS

- In PACE, the payment rate for Medicare is set at the nursing home rate and Medicaid makes up the rest. The Medicare rate is almost certainly too low for cancer patients, forcing Medicaid to make up more of the overall rate and thereby making PACE care of cancer patients unattractive for the states. PACE's Medicare payments could mirror the risk adjustment rates, once those are set.
- Make risk adjustment plans cover end-of-life care (e.g., for patients not likely to live into next year; for patients cared for mainly out of hospital).
- Purchase on quality of end-of-life care.
- Adjust the risk adjustment plan to improve end-of-life care.

FEE FOR SERVICE

- Reduce the differential between procedure and counseling payments.
- Designate palliative care specialization, to avoid problems with concurrent care.
- Provide incentives for advance planning before repeat hospitalization.
- Provide incentives for coordinated care before repeat hospitalizations.
- Provide incentives for services in centers of proven quality in end-of-life care.

FOR FAMILY CAREGIVERS

- Pay family caregivers a discounted rate for their services (e.g., half the going rate for paid services).
- Provide health insurance for full-time family caregivers who have no other source of insurance.
- Provide payment for respite help, either in-home or in-facility.

- Provide more paid help at home, including in PACE and hospice.

FOR HIGH-COST PALLIATIVE CARE

- Require accounting of the aggregate costs and benefits of costly interventions in realistically representative populations.
- Develop a regional or national review process that can limit coverage for particular interventions to particular kinds of patients or can keep a particular treatment from being covered at all.
- Monitor effects of high-cost interventions, especially effects on availability of aide care and psychosocial services.

FOR CAPACITY BUILDING AND QUALITY IMPROVEMENT

- Involve HRSA in addressing the concerns of the population needing end-of-life care, including cancer. This would bring to bear the skills and attention of professional educators, manpower experts, health services delivery managers, and innovators and evaluators.
- Tie Medicare payments to quality (e.g., the upcoming effort to tie managed care payments to heart failure performance standards).
- Build culture of quality improvement; pay for the work.
- Consider the role of routine autopsy.

CONCLUSION

The quality, reliability, and comprehensiveness of end-of-life care are important to cancer patients and their families. Some of the current shortcomings arise from financing and regulations; others, from habit patterns. Enduring reforms must be guided by descriptive and evaluative data, which are not available. This shortcoming should be corrected quickly. We need a decade of vigorous innovation and evaluation, learning how to improve policies. As we settle upon desirable changes, we will also need to forge the political will for reform.

REFERENCES

Agra Y, Sacristan A, Gonzalez M, Ferrari M, Portugues A, Calvo MJ. Efficacy of senna versus lactulose in terminal cancer patients treated with opioids. *Journal of Pain Symptom Management* 1998;15:1-7.

American Cancer Society. 2000. http://www.cancer.org/statistics/index.html

Beemstrober PM, de Koning HJ, Birnie E, et al. Advanced prostate cancer: course, care and cost complications. *Prostate* 1999;40:97-104.

Bennett CL, Matchar D, McCrory D, McLeod DG, Crawford ED, Hillner BE. Cost-effective models for flutamide for prostate carcinoma patients: are they helpful to policy makers? *Cancer* 1996;77:1854-1861.

Brooks CH. A comparative analysis of Medicare home care cost savings for the terminally ill. *Home Health Care Services Quarterly* 1989a; 10:79-96.

Brooks CH. Cost differences between hospice and nonhospice care. A comparison of insurer payments and provider charges. *Eval Health Prof* 1989b;12:159-178.

Brooks CH, Smyth-Staruch K. Hospice home care cost savings to third-party insurers. *Medical Care* 1984;22:691-703.

Brown ML, Riley GF, Potosky AL, Etzioni RD. Obtaining long-term disease specific costs of care: application to Medicare enrollees diagnosed with colorectal cancer. *Medical Care* 1999;37:1249-1259.

Bruera E, Pruvost M, Schoeller T, Montejo G, Watanabe S. Proctoclysis for hydration of terminally ill cancer patients. *Journal of Pain Symptom Management* 1998;15:216-219.

Buroker TR, O'Connell MJ, Wieand HS, Krook JE, Gerstner JB, Mailliard JA, et al. Randomized comparison of two schedules of fluorouracil and leucovorin in the treatment of advanced colorectal cancer [see comments]. *Journal of Clinical Oncology* 1994;12:14-20.

Christakis NA, Escarce JJ. Survival of Medicare patients after enrollment in hospice programs. *New England Journal of Medicine* 1996;338:172-178.

Commonwealth Fund. 1998. *Improving Coverage for Low-Income Medicare Beneficiaries.* New York: Commonwealth Fund.

Cunningham D. Mature results from three large controlled studies with raltitrexed ('Tomudex'). *British Journal of Cancer* 1998;77 (Suppl) 2:15-21.

Cvetkovski B, Gerdes H, Kurtz RC. Outpatient therapeutic ERCP with endobiliary stent placement for malignant common bile duct obstruction. *Gastrointestinal Endoscopy* 1999;50:63-66.

Dartmouth Medical School, Center for the Evaluative Clinical Sciences. 1999. *The Quality of Medical Care in the United States: A Report on the Medicare Program. The Dartmouth Atlas of Health Care in the United States, 1999,* Wennberg JE, Cooper MM., eds. Chicago: AHA Press.

Desch CE, Hillner BE, Smith TJ. Economic considerations in the care of lung cancer patients. *Current Opinion in Oncology* 1996;8:126-132.

Emanuel EJ. Cost savings at the end of life. What do the data show? [see comments]. *Journal of the American Medical Association* 1996;275:1907-1914.

Escalante CP, Martin CG, Elting LS, Cantor SB, Harle TS, Price KJ, et al. Dyspnea in cancer patients. Etiology, resource utilization, and survival-implications in a managed care world. *Cancer* 1996;1978:1314-1319.

Experton B, Ozminkowski RJ, Pearlman DN. How does managed care manage the frail elderly? The case of hospital readmissions in fee-for-service versus HMO systems. *American Journal of Preventive Medicine* 1999;16(3):163-172.

Ferris FD, Wodinsky HB, Kerr IG, Sone M, Hume S, Coons C. A cost-minimization study of cancer patients requiring a narcotic infusion in hospital and at home. *Journal of Clinical Epidemiology* 1991;44:313-327.

Fox E, Landrum McNiff, Zhong Z, et al. Evaluation of prognostic criteria for determining hospice eligibility in patients with advanced lung, heart, or liver disease. SUPPORT Investigators. Study to Understand Prognoses and Preferences for Outcomes and Risks of Treatment. *Journal of the American Medical Association* 1999;282(17):1638-1645.

Glimelius B, Hoffman K, Graf W, Haglund U, Nyren O, Pahlman L, et al. Cost-effectiveness of palliative chemotherapy in advanced gastrointestinal cancer [see comments]. *Annals of Oncology* 1995;6:267-274.

Goodwin PJ, Shepherd FA. Economic issues in lung cancer: a review. *Journal of Clinical Oncology* 1998;16:3900-3912.

Hillner BE, Weeks JC, Desch CE, Smith TJ. Pamidronate in prevention of bone complications in metastatic breast cancer: a cost-effectiveness analysis. *Journal of Clinical Oncology* 2000;18:72-79.

Hogan C, Lynn J, Gabel J, Lunney J, O'Mara A, Wilkinson A. 2000. *A Statistical Profile of Decedents in the Medicare Program.* Washington, D.C.: Medicare Payment Advisory Commission.

Iezzoni LI. The risk of adjustment. *Journal of the American Medical Association* 1997; 278(19):1600-1607.

Ingham JM. 1998. The epidemiology of cancer at the end stage of life. In *Principles and Practice of Supportive Oncology,* Berger A, Portenoy R, Weissman DE, eds. Philadelphia: Lippincott-Raven.

IOM (Institute of Medicine). 1997. *Approaching Death: Improving Care at the End of Life.* Field MJ, Cassel CK, eds. Washington, D.C.: National Academy Press.

IOM. 1999. *Ensuring Quality Cancer Care.* Hewitt M, Simone JV, eds. Washington, D.C.: National Academy Press.

Journal of the National Cancer Institute. Integrating economic analysis into cancer clinical trials: the National Cancer Institute-American Society of Clinical Oncology Economics Workbook. *Journal of the National Cancer Institute Monograph* 1998;1924:1-28.

Kaskarelis IS, Minardos IA, Abatzis PP, Malagari KS, Vrachliotis TG, Natsika MK, et al. Percutaneous metallic self-expandable endoprostheses in biliary obstruction caused by metastatic cancer. *Hepatogastroenterology* 1996;43:785-791.

Kidder D. The effects of hospice coverage on Medicare expenditures. *Health Services Research* 1992;27:195-217.

Kosary C L, Ries LAG, Miller BA, Hankey BF, Harras A, Edwards BK. 2000. SEER Cancer Statistics Review, 1973-1992: Tables and graphs, NIH Pub. No. 96-2789. Bethesda, MD: National Cancer Institute.

Lewin-VHI, Inc. 1995. An Analysis of the Cost Savings of the Medicare Hospice Benefit. Commissioned by the National Hospice and Palliative Care Organization.

Lubitz JD, Riley GF. Trends in Medicare payments in the last year of life. *New England Journal of Medicine* 1993;328:1092-1096.

Lynn J, Harrell F, Cohn F, et al. Prognoses of seriously ill hospitalized patients on the days before death: implications for patient care and public policy. *New Horizons* 1997;5(1): 56-61.

McEwan AJ, Amyotte GA, McGowan DG, MacGillivray JA, Porter AT. A retrospective analysis of the cost effectiveness of treatment with Metastron (89Sr-chloride) in patients with prostate cancer metastatic to bone. *Nucl Med Commun* 1994;15:499-504.

Mor V, Masterson-Allen S. A comparison of hospice vs conventional care of the terminally ill cancer patient. *Oncology* 1990;4:85-91.

National Hospice and Palliative Care Organization. 2001. http://www.NHPCO.org/facts.htm

Neymark N, Adriaenssen I. The costs of managing patients with advanced colorectal cancer in 10 different European centres. *European Journal of Cancer* 1999;35:1789-1795.

Peters WR, Dansey RD, Klein JL, Baynes RD. High-dose chemotherapy and peripheral blood progenitor cell transplantation in the treatment of breast cancer. *Oncologist* 2000;5:1-13.

Polednak Ap, Shevchenko Ip. Hospital charges for terminal care of cancer patients dying before age 65. *Journal of Health Care Finance* 1998;25(1)26-34.

President's Cancer Panel. 1998. *Cancer Care Issues in the United States: Quality of Care, Quality of Life.* Bethesda, MD: National Cancer Institute, 1999. (http://deainfo.nci.nih.gov/ADVISORY/pcp/reports/index.htm)

Pritchard RS, Fisher ES, Teno JM, et al. Influence of patient preferences and local health system characteristics on the place of death. SUPPORT Investigators. Study to Understand Prognoses and Preferences for Risks and Outcomes of Treatment. *Journal of the American Geriatrics Society* 1998;46(10): 1242-1250.

Ramesh PR, Kumar KS, Rajagopal MR, Balachandran P, Warrier PK. Managing morphine-induced constipation: a controlled comparison of an Ayurvedic formulation and senna. *Journal of Pain, Symptom Management* 1998;16:240-244.

Recchia F, Nuzzo A, Lalli A, Lombardo M, Di Lullo L, Fabiani F, et al. Randomized trial of 5-fluorouracil and high-dose folinic acid with or without alpha-2B interferon in advanced colorectal cancer. *American Journal of Clinical Oncology* 1996;19:301-304.

Riley GF, Potosky AL, Lubitz JD, et al. Medicare payments from diagnosis to death for elderly cancer patients by stage at diagnosis. *Medical Care* 1995;33(8):828-841.

Ron IG, Lotan A, Inbar MJ, Chaitchik S. Advanced colorectal carcinoma: redefining the role of oral ftorafur. *Anticancer Drugs* 1996;7:649-654.

Ross P, Heron J, Cunningham D. Cost of treating advanced colorectal cancer: a retrospective comparison of treatment regimens [see comments]. *European Journl of Cancer* 1996;32A (Suppl)5:S13-S17.

Scheidbach H, Horbach T, Groitl H, Hohenberger W. Percutaneous endoscopic gastrostomy/jejunostomy (PEG/PEJ) for decompression in the upper gastrointestinal tract. Initial experience with palliative treatment of gastrointestinal obstruction in terminally ill patients with advanced carcinomas. *Surgical Endoscopy* 1999;13:1103-1105.

Seamans DP, Wong GY, Wilson JL. Interventional pain therapy for intractable abdominal cancer pain. *Journal of Clinical Oncology* 2000;18:1598-1600.

Shah Syed GM, Maken RN, Muzzaffar N, Shah MA, Rana F. Effective and economical option for pain palliation in prostate cancer with skeletal metastases: 32P therapy revisited. *NuclMedCommun* 1999;20:697-702.

Smith TJ, Hillner BE, Desch CE. Efficacy and cost-effectiveness of cancer treatment: rational allocation of resources based on decision analysis [see comments]. *Journal of the National Cancer Institute* 1993;85:1460-1474.

Stommel M, Given CW, Given BA. The cost of cancer home care to families. *Cancer* 1993;71:1867-1874.

Torfs K, Pocceschi S. A retrospective study of resource utilisation in the treatment of advanced colorectal cancer in Europe. *European Journal of Cancer* 1996;32A (Suppl)5:S28-31.

Ulrich-Pur H, Kornek GV, Raderer M, Haider K, Kwasny W, Depisch D, Greul R, Schneeweiss B, Krauss G, Funovics J, Scheithauer W. A phase II trial of biweekly high dose gemcitabine for patients with metastatic pancreatic adenocarcinoma. *Cancer* 2000;88(11):2505-2511.

Vladeck BC. The problem isn't payment: Medicare and the reform of end-of-life care. *Generations* 1999;21:52-57.

3

Quality of Care and Quality Indicators for End-of-Life Cancer Care: Hope for the Best, Yet Prepare for the Worst

Joan M. Teno, M.D., M.S.
Brown University School of Medicine
and Department of Community Health

INTRODUCTION

Cancer is a life-defining illness. Half of those who get cancer die from it. Decades of research have resulted in cures for some forms of cancer, and for others, it is now a chronic, progressive, but still fatal illness. For those who die, quickly or after a long period of illness, health care providers must guide a patient through a disease trajectory where one must hope for the best, but prepare for the possibility of the worst. The management of this transition from hope for a cure to focus solely on comfort is key to quality end-of-life care. Important to this transition is medical care that is consistent with professional knowledge and that is based on informed patient preferences, to the extent the patient desires involvement in decisionmaking. The National Cancer Policy Board (NCPB) in its report *Ensuring Quality Cancer Care* (IOM, 1999) outlined a vision for the development of quality indicators to cover the spectrum of cancer care, including the dying process.

We are not close to meeting this NCPB mandate for care at the end of life, either for cancer or for other conditions. Research and demonstration programs will be needed before a preliminary set of satisfactory indicators can be developed. Ideally, such efforts should entail the collaboration of the National Cancer Institute (NCI), the Agency for Healthcare Research and Quality (AHRQ), the National Institute for Nursing Research (NINR), and the National Institute on Aging (NIA). The focus of early work will be on the development and validation of measurement tools based on administrative data, medical records, and interviews with patients, family members, and health care providers. These instruments must be developed and adapted for different cultures and ethnicities.

Measurement tools should be consistent with professional guidelines and the best available research. For many cancers, there is a strong evidence base to inform treatment decisions. However, research on the risks and benefits of cancer treatment, especially in those cases where chemotherapy, radiation treatment, and other treatment modalities are labeled palliative, is sorely lacking.

Ongoing national data collection efforts include little information to describe the quality of care of dying persons and their families. An occasional survey, the U.S. National Mortality Followback Survey (NMFBS), has collected information on access to care and functional status but not on important domains that are central to the quality of care of the dying. A redesigned NMFBS could collect information on key domains to describe the quality of care for cancer patients who died based on the perspective of the bereaved family member. Currently, there are no plans for further iterations of the NMFBS, however.

Quality indicators are needed for two main purposes: accountability (external use by regulators, health care purchasers, or consumers) and quality improvement (internal use for the purpose of monitoring or continuous quality improvement). The same types of indicators may serve both purposes, but the indicators may also be different. At this early stage in development, there is a strong evidence base to support the development of quality indicators for pain management for the purpose of accountability. However, demonstration programs will be needed before pain management indicators can be implemented nationally, and more basic research is needed to develop indicators for managing other common symptoms (e.g., emotional distress and depression, fatigue, gastrointestinal symptoms). An important aspect of demonstration and validation is monitoring for potential unintended consequences (e.g., patients are sedated contrary to their preferences to improve accountability statistics).

Besides the domain of symptom management, four other domains should be considered for early development and implementation of accountability measures: (1) patient satisfaction, (2) shared decisionmaking, (3) coordination, and (4) continuity of care. In each of these domains, indicators must validly represent the perceptions of the dying person and family members. This means investing in new survey methods that are patient centered and include questions that get at unmet needs, which has not always been the norm.

Shared decisionmaking has been increasingly recognized as a key aspect throughout the continuum of care. While the focus of research has been on resuscitation decisions, the most important decision for the majority of cancer patients is the one to stop active treatment, but there is little research examining this decision.

There is strong support for the domains of pain (and other symptoms), shared decisionmaking, satisfaction, coordination, and continuity of care, but there is debate about which other domains are important in the care of the dying. Various conceptual models have been proposed to examine the quality of end-of-life care, emphasizing different domains. Research is now needed to examine the correlations among structures of the health care system, processes of care, and important outcomes to identify the most fruitful areas for developing new quality measures.

Two national data collection systems warrant consideration for the development of quality indicators: Medicare claims files and the Minimum Data Set (MDS). NCPB has recommended that hospice enrollment and length of stay be examined as quality indicators (IOM, 1999) From a national perspective, the only data set with that information is Medicare claims data. Other indicators based on administrative data have also been proposed (Wennberg, 1998). Work to develop and validate these indicators using claims data is still to be done.

The second national data collection effort is the MDS, which routinely collects extensive information on every nursing home resident in the United States. Nursing homes increasingly are providing end-of-life care for frail and older Americans (Teno, 2000a). In 1998, an estimated 10 percent of cancer patients died in a nursing home. The Health Care Financing Agency (HCFA) is now embarking on a national program of examining nursing home quality performance. There are important lessons to be learned from the MDS, including concerns about the institutional response burden in implementing data collection and the potential for unintended consequences. In the nursing home setting, the main concern is with applying quality indicators developed for populations where the goals of care are on restoring function to those who are dying. For example, the rates of dehydration and weight loss are now among the core quality indicators for nursing homes (HCFA, 2000). With increased scrutiny of these indicators, there is concern that unintended consequences for the dying include increased use of feeding tubes, which could be contrary to patient preferences.

At this time, health care providers usually apply the term "dying" to individuals in the last days of life, allowing little time for preparation or life closure. Given the inherent imprecision of predicting the day of death, we need to move back on the continuum and identify people with "life-limiting illness" or "serious, progressive illness," which would imply a median survival of less than one year.

"Hope for the best, prepare for the worst" is not something we say to people dying of cancer. In one sense, it forces us to admit failure to a disease that is the second leading cause of death in the United States. While it is the disease that we are "fighting," our ultimate obligation is to provide the best-quality care to each individual patient, and we must recognize that individual preferences are central to defining the quality of medical care. Health care providers must not only provide the best available clinical care, as desired by patients, but must become adept at helping patients and families make choices about transitions in goals of care. The goal of quality indicators is to measure the extent to which the health care system is succeeding in this at the end of life.

QUALITY OF END-OF-LIFE CANCER CARE

Few, if any, would argue seriously against the current emphasis on prevention and cure in cancer research and treatment. Yet this emphasis should not be allowed to result in inadequate care of the half-million people who die from cancer each year in the United States, whose final needs are for treating symptoms as they approach death. The National Cancer Policy Board, in *Ensuring Quality Cancer Care* (IOM, 1999), noted the wide disparity between the "ideal" cancer care system and the reality that confronts people with cancer today. The gaps are nowhere as large as they are in the realm of care for the dying.

A central premise of this chapter is that patient expectations and preferences are fundamental to defining the quality of medical care for people with chronic, progressive, and eventually fatal illnesses. Fundamental to any discussion of quality of care, however, are measures of quality that are valid and reliable. This chapter focuses on the status of "quality indicators" for assessing the care of dying individuals, particularly those dying from cancer.

Dying is unlike any other time in a person's life. A 41-year-old with his first heart attack will most likely value the same health outcomes as others with the same diagnosis: a focus on minimizing the extent of damage to the heart, preserving cardiac function, and reducing the risk of another heart attack. Those dying from chronic, progressive, and eventually fatal illnesses, however, may choose very different courses. The goals of care for a dying person cannot reasonably be anticipated, as they can in the case of a heart attack patient. To care well for a dying person, health care providers must understand that person, his or her needs and expectations, and the disease trajectory itself.

Care of the dying is distinct from other aspects of health care in that it is delivered not just to the patient, but in the context of a "family" (in its most inclusive definition, not restricted to the legal definition of "family") (WHO, 1990). Ideally, care is "patient focused," which is defined as care that promotes informed patient involvement in decisionmaking and attends to physical comfort and emotional support.

In the past century, the United States has seen a striking transformation in how people die. In contrast to the late 1800s, people now die of chronic, progressive, and eventually fatal illness such as cancer, which they may live with for years or decades. Faced with caring for an older and chronically ill population, public policy and research efforts have focused on examining not only survival but also quality of life and health care costs.

In a *New England Journal of Medicine* editorial, accountability was identified as the "third revolution in medical care," following on the heels of health care expansion and cost containment (Relman, 1988). Yet, to date, little attention has been given to how best we can measure the quality of end-of-life care. Despite the universality of death, few generalizable research studies (Addington Hall and McCarthy, 1995; Emanuel et al., 2000; Greer et al., 1986; Lynn et al., 1997; Seale et al., 1997; Wolfe et al., 2000) have examined the experiences of dying persons. At this early stage, cancer represents an ideal disease trajectory on which to initiate work measuring quality of care of the dying for the purposes of accountability (i.e., external release of data to the purchaser, regulator, or consumer in order to compare and contrast quality between health care institutions), quality improvement, and research.

Cancer, in contrast to other leading causes of death (e.g., congestive heart failure, chronic obstructive lung disease, stroke), has a more predictable functional trajectory prior to death with less uncertainty in prognosis (Fox et al., 1999; Teno et al., 2001). Some cancers have an authoritative scientific evidence base to guide treatment decisions. Health care providers now have access to evidence-based treatment algorithms, including some for palliative treatment (ASCO, 1997). For these reasons, cancer is a good place to start designing and implementing a national system to measure the quality of end-of-life care.

What Is an Ideal System for Monitoring Quality of Care for Cancer?

The NCPB has outlined the characteristics of an ideal system for measuring quality of care for cancer patients. In order to meet these goals, we will need appropriate measurement tools for research to develop the scientific evidence base, for quality improvement, and for public accountability (Table 3-1), all of which may be different.

The areas of emphasis and desired characteristics vary for measurement tools intended for different purposes (Table 3-2). For example, the intended audience for quality improvement (QI) measures is the institutional and QI staff, whereas the intended audience for public accountability is the health care purchaser and consumer. Given the intended audiences and implica-

TABLE 3-1 Purposes of Quality Measures

Purpose	Description
Quality improvement	Measures to provide information for health care institutions to reform or shape how care is provided
Clinical assessment	Measures to guide individual patient management
Research	Measures that assess the phenomenon of interest
Accountability	Measures that allow comparison of quality of care for the purposes of quality assurance or for consumer choice between health care institutions or practitioners

SOURCE: Teno et al., 1999.

TABLE 3-2 Areas of Emphasis Based on the Purpose of Quality Measure

	Purpose of Measure			
	Clinical Assessment	Research	Improvement	Accountability
Audience	Clinical staff	Science community	QI team and clinical staff	Payers, public
Focus of measurement	Status of patient	Knowledge	Understand care process	Comparison
Confidentiality	Very high	Very high	Very high	Low
Evidence base to justify use of measure	Important; measure should have face validity from a clinical standpoint	Builds on existing evidence to generate new knowledge	Important	Extremely important in that proposed domain ought to be under control of the institution
Importance of psychometric properties	Important to individual provider	Extremely important to the research effort	Important within specific setting	Valid and responsive across multiple settings

SOURCE: Adapted from Solberg et al. (1997) and Teno et al. (1999).

tions of the use of measurement tools, more stringent psychometric properties than are now employed must be put into measures that will be used for public accountability. In addition, there must be either normative or empirical research substantiating a claim that the construct being measured for public accountability is under the control of the health care institution.

It seems easy to conceptualize quality measures for various purposes, but in practice, we are at an early stage in measuring the quality of end-of-life care. Substantial normative and empirical research is still needed to develop and validate a conceptual model of quality end-of-life care, to develop and test the psychometric properties of proposed measurement tools, and to demonstrate the tools' effectiveness in multisite studies before they can be used nationally. This chapter describes what is known and what still needs to be done to develop widely applicable quality indicators for end-of-life care for cancer patients. The following questions guide the discussion:

1. What is currently known about the quality of care for dying cancer patients?
2. What are the proposed definitions and conceptual models for quality of care of dying persons and their family?
3. What can we currently measure with existing nationally collected data?
4. What do we want to be able to say in the future?
5. What research is needed?

What Is Currently Known About
Quality of Care of the Dying Cancer Patient?

Few studies have characterized the experience for dying cancer patients and their families. From a national perspective, only one ongoing data collection effort routinely characterizes dying from cancer, and a second occasional survey was carried out six times between the early 1960s and 1993. The National Center for Health Statistics (NCHS) compiles data from all death certificates nationwide and publishes annual summaries that include cause of death, place of death, and other demographic information.

The other survey that has characterized aspects of dying is the NMFBS, last carried out in 1993. The 1993 survey represents a 1 percent sample of all deaths at age 15 and older. Unlike the mortality followback surveys in the United Kingdom (Addington Hall and McCarthy, 1995a, 1995b), the NMFBS does not characterize the quality of the dying experience (e.g., pain management, satisfaction). Rather, the U.S. survey collects information on socio-demographics, use of alcohol and medications, lifestyle, health care resource utilization, and difficulties with functioning (Lentzner et al., 1992; NCHS, 1998).

What can be learned from the available data? In 1998, 538,947 people died of cancer in the United States. Five types of cancer account for 70 percent of those deaths (Figure 3-1; NCHS Web site). Over the past decade, there has been a trend toward more cancer patients dying at home (Figure

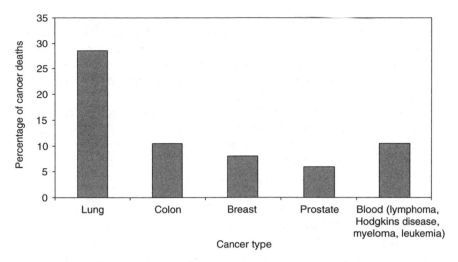

FIGURE 3-1   Leading causes of cancer death, 1998.

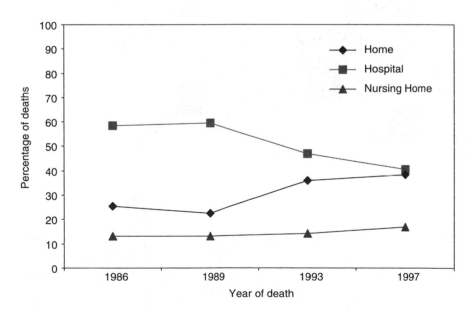

FIGURE 3-2   Site of cancer deaths, 1986-1997 (selected years).

3-2; mortality files and NMFBS). There is, however, substantial geographic variation in the site of death (Figure 3-3) (Pritchard et al., 1998; Wennberg, 1998). For example, Oregon has experienced a dramatic increase in the proportion of people dying at home (probably due to a number of factors, including closing of hospital beds and a vigorous public debate about physician aid in dying) (Tolle et al., 1999).

Based on the 1993 NMFBS, cancer patients are less likely to be functionally impaired in the last year of life and experience a more precipitous functional decline in the last five months of life than those dying from other causes (Figure 3-4), as measured by difficulty with activities of daily living (ADL: bathing, dressing, eating, transferring from a bed or chair, and using the toilet). In that year, nearly half of these deaths occurred in an acute care hospital, and 36 percent, at home. Only 19.7 percent of those who died from cancer in 1993 used hospice care. The functional trajectory measured as the number of ADL impairments in the last five months of life was associated with dying at home and with hospice involvement (Teno et al., 2001).

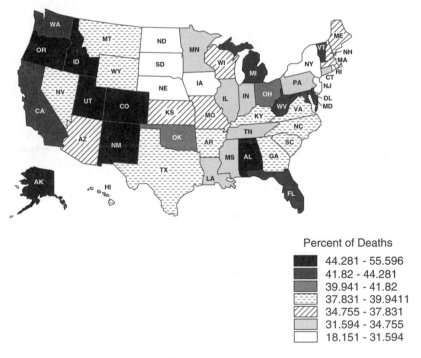

Percent of Deaths

- 44.281 - 55.596
- 41.82 - 44.281
- 39.941 - 41.82
- 37.831 - 39.9411
- 34.755 - 37.831
- 31.594 - 34.755
- 18.151 - 31.594

FIGURE 3-3   Proportion of cancer home deaths in 1997.
Copyright, Center for Gerontology and Health Care Research, used by permission.

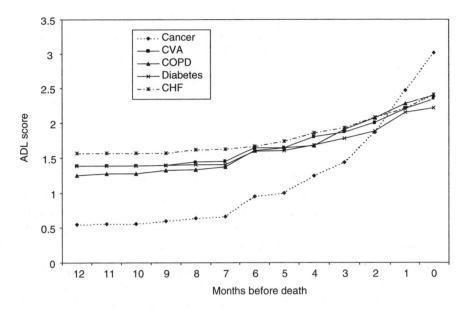

FIGURE 3-4   Age-adjusted ADL scores by time before death.
NOTE: ADL = activities of daily living; CHF = congestive heart failure, COPD = chronic obstructive pulmonary disease; CVA = cardiovascular accident (stroke).

In *Ensuring Quality Cancer Care* (IOM, 1999), the NCPB recommended ensuring timely referral of dying cancer patients to palliative and hospice care. Currently, the only data that can shed light on the timing of these referrals are from Medicare claims files, and these do not tell the story of whether referrals are "timely." However, they do demonstrate a dramatic reduction in the median length of hospice stay during the late 1990s and substantial geographic variation in length of stay. In 1990, reported median length of stay was 36 days (Christakis and Escarce, 1996). According to the National Hospice Organization (NHO), this had declined to 25 days by 1998. There has been some speculation that the decline is due, in part, to efforts to avoid charges of Medicare fraud, which may cause practitioners and hospice providers to delay enrolling patients until they are very close to death.

Information on access to medical care was collected in the 1986 and 1993 NMFBS. In 1993, the question asked was, Were there any times during the last year of life that ... needed health care, but didn't get it? Eleven percent of respondents stated that they had difficulty obtaining needed care, which seems relatively small. However, this question should be repeated in future surveys, because access to care is continually changing.

While the NMFBS has provided some information about the dying experience, health care providers cannot answer the important question, What will my dying be like? Information about the bereaved family member's perspective on the quality of care, concerns about pain management, or whether medical care was in accord with the patient's informed preferences is not included. To address these issues, we must rely on less generalizable studies.

Future Directions:

Funding a seventh wave of the National Mortality Followback Survey should be considered. If carried out, it should include data collection to document a surrogate perspective on quality of care with a focus on issues that proxies are known to report accurately—access to care, decisionmaking, advance care planning, coordination of care, and the financial impact on dying persons and families.

Additional research should be conducted to improve the quality of followback reporting (e.g., to examine the best timing of interviews within the constraints of current reporting of death data). Research is also needed to examine the types of people best able to serve as proxies, what they are able to validly report on, the impact of bereavement, and the validity of interviews with family members.

Pain

Pain is common among people dying from cancer. Severe pain may signify that death is not far off (Conill et al., 1997; Foley, 1979; Portenoy et al., 1994a; Turner et al., 1996). Cancer pain, itself, can lead to anxiety, depression, and even suicide (Spiegel et al., 1994; Strang, 1992). One study found that requests for physician aid in dying were withdrawn once the patient was appropriately treated for pain (Foley, 1991). The general public is fearful that the discomfort associated with cancer will be "extremely painful" (Levin et al., 1985). Nearly 70 percent of people believe cancer pain can be so severe that a patient considers suicide. Are such concerns warranted?

Multicenter studies in hospitals (Desbiens et al., 1996; SUPPORT Principal Investigators, 1996), outpatient settings (Cleeland et al., 1994), and nursing homes attest to important public health concern with pain assessment and management (Bernabei et al., 1998). In the Study to Understand Prognosis and Preferences for Outcomes and Risks of Treatments (SUPPORT), 22.7 percent of patients reported moderately or extremely severe pain at least half the time during their first week of hospitalization. Bereaved family members reported that more than 40 percent of those who died of colon or lung cancer had severe pain in the last three days of life. Despite this level of pain, family members reported satisfaction with pain control, which seems to reflect relatively low expectations.

Among 54 outpatient clinics participating in the Eastern Cooperative Oncology Group (ECOG), about one-third of patients with metastatic cancer had pain that limited their function. Of the two-thirds of patients with pain, 42 percent reported that their pain was not adequately treated (Cleeland et al., 1994). Supporting these patient reports, 86 percent of ECOG physicians stated that pain was undermedicated. In a study of nursing homes in five states, 40 percent of patients discharged with a diagnosis of cancer had daily pain (Bernabei et al., 1998). Of even greater concern, one in four of these patients was not receiving any pain medication—not even a World Health Organization (WHO) step 1 drug, such as acetaminophen.

Even in a hospice or palliative care setting, pain remains an important concern (Higginson and McCarthy, 1989; Hockley et al., 1988; Morris, Mor et al., 1986; Turner et al., 1996; Vainio and Auvinen, 1996). Although pain may always be ameliorated by sedation with barbiturates as a last resort (Truog et al., 1992), significant controversy exists over the rate at which a dying cancer patient's suffering requires deep sedation. Ventafridda and colleagues found that more than half of the dying people treated through a home care program in Italy could achieve palliation of suffering only by sedation (Ventafridda et al., 1986; 1989). Must they sleep before they die? asked an editorial, questioning whether this represents overtreatment (Roy, 1990). A study of dying patients in a palliative care unit in Canada found that only 16 percent of patients required sedation for symptom relief (Fainsinger et al., 1991).

In summary, there is strong evidence that pain is prevalent and too often untreated, despite clear, appropriate guidelines. If guidelines were followed, pain could be ameliorated for up to 90 percent of patients. Because of the high prevalence of pain and because it can be alleviated with proper treatment, pain and its control should be an outcome measure used to judge the quality of end-of-life care for purposes of public accountability.

Future Directions:

The NCI, AHRQ, Department of Defense, and Department of Veterans Affairs could consider research and demonstration efforts to implement accountability measures for pain management. In these efforts, the potential unintended consequences of measuring pain management (e.g., more persons being sedated without informed discussion) should be monitored. If warranted by the results, HCFA could require monitoring of pain management as part on ongoing quality reporting from health care institutions that participate in Medicare.

Dyspnea and Other Symptoms

Patients, family members, and health care providers report that dyspnea is one of the most burdensome and difficult symptoms to treat in the last days of life (Dudgeon and Rosenthal, 1996; Farncombe, 1997; Hockley et al., 1988; Kuebler, 1996; Nelson and Walsh, 1991; Ripamonti and Bruera, 1997; van der Molen, 1995). Between 21 percent and 89 percent of dying people report directly (Donnelly and Walsh, 1995; Dudgeon et al., 1995; Hay et al., 1996; Hopwood and Stephens, 1995; Portenoy et al., 1994; Roberts et al., 1993; Vainio and Auvinen, 1996) or are observed to have difficulty breathing in the final phase of life (Addington Hall and McCarthy, 1995b; Coyle et al., 1990; Desbiens et al., 1997; Edmonds et al., 2000; Fainsinger et al., 1991; Goodlin et al., 1998; Higginson and McCarthy, 1989; Hockley et al., 1988; Lynn et al., 1997; Marin et al., 1987; Muers and Round, 1993; Reuben and Mor, 1986; Robinson et al., 1997. Similar to worsening pain, increasing dyspnea implies a shorter survival time. Half of all lung cancer patients presenting to an emergency room with dyspnea die in the following month (Escalante et al., 1996).

Research has shown that unlike pain, dyspnea persists as a troublesome symptom even in patients receiving palliative care. Both pharmacological and nonpharmacological interventions are limited (Higginson and McCarthy, 1989; Ripamonti, 1999) (although a recent trial suggests an important role of nonpharmacological interventions using relaxation techniques; Breitbart et al., 1995). This is not unexpected, because for many cancer patients, lung tissue is replaced with nonfunctional tumor tissue such that the patient follows the clinical course of a person with restrictive lung disease.

In addition to the distressing symptoms of pain and dyspnea, cancer patients often endure a constellation of other symptoms. More than 90 percent of people with advanced cancer who are close to death have more than three distressing symptoms (Donnelly and Walsh, 1995). Weakness afflicts between 51 percent and 88 percent of dying cancer patients, and at least one-quarter have one or more gastrointestinal symptom, including nausea, vomiting, and anorexia (Conill et al., 1997; Donnelly and Walsh, 1995; Hockley et al., 1988; Portenoy et al., 1994b; Turner et al., 1996; Vainio and Auvinen, 1996). Confusion, which is often devastating to family members, is found in between 8 percent and 85 percent of dying cancer patients (Breitbart et al., 1995; Conill et al., 1997; Donnelly and Walsh, 1995; Hockley et al., 1988; Turner et al., 1996; Vainio and Auvinen, 1996).

With the exception of pain, interventions for managing these symptoms are not well characterized and the tools themselves are probably inadequate. In addition, there are disagreements among professionals about appropriate treatment. The use of intravenous fluids, for example, is often viewed as not the "hospice way" to care for actively dying patients. The argument is that it is a natural part of the dying process for persons to decrease their intake of fluids and that symptoms attributable to dehydration can be managed by ice chips and aggressive mouth care (McCann et al., 1994). However, others suggest that hydration through subcutaneous saline injection can ameliorate or reverse agitation in dying persons (Fainsinger and Bruera, 1997).

Despite reports of striking levels of patient distress, reliable and valid tools to measure symptoms are often lacking. For example, many dying persons are unable to report either their pain or discomfort from dyspnea. It will be difficult to document progress unless the necessary tools are developed.

Future Directions:

The scientific evidence base of, and current measurement tools for physical symptoms other than pain need further refinement prior to their use for public accountability. For physical symptoms other than pain, existing measures have to be refined, new measurement tools must be developed, research on treatment effectiveness has to be conducted, and guidelines must be formulated. NCI, in collaboration with other federal research agencies, could take the lead in developing this scientific evidence base for the palliation of physical symptoms of persons dying from cancer.

Emotional Distress

Emotional distress greatly diminishes the quality of life of dying patients and their families. Depression and anxiety inhibit the patient's ability to experience pleasure and to focus on the conclusion of significant relationships (Block, 2000) and may impair the ability to make critical decisions. From a clinical standpoint, health care workers should recognize and treat emotional distress to enable the patient and family to participate fully in end-of-life decisionmaking and attain a sense of closure in the time remaining before death.

Depression and anxiety, as well as an increased risk of suicide, among patients with cancer and other terminal illnesses have been documented for two decades, but the reported prevalences vary widely, depending on diagnostic criteria and study design (DeFlorio and Massie, 1995). Using a self-report measure of common symptoms, 65 percent of patients with breast, colon, prostate, or ovarian cancer reported feeling sad, and 61 percent reported feeling nervous (Portenoy et al., 1994a). In a study limited to those with advanced cancer, 21 percent of patients reported moderate or severe depression, and 13 percent of women and 9 percent of men reported moderate or severe anxiety (Donnelly et al., 1995). Using the Diagnostic and Statistic Manual of Mental Disorders, Third Revised Edition (DSM-IIIR) diagnostic criteria adapted for terminally ill patients, 26 percent of terminally ill cancer patients met the criteria for depression (Power et al., 1993).

Thoughts of suicide among terminally ill patients are relatively common (Block, 2000). In a sample of patients with terminal cancer in palliative care hospital units for example, 44.5 percent acknowledged occasional desires for death (Chochinov et al., 1995). Even though the majority of suicidal thoughts among patients with terminal illnesses are transient, the reported suicide rate among patients with cancer is twice that of the general population, with the greatest risk during advanced illness. Moreover, the actual suicide rate among cancer patients may be underestimated since some family members may be unwilling to report that a terminally ill cancer patient died as a result of suicide (Chochinov et al., 1998). Despite the wide variation in reported rates of emotional distress and the difficulty of assessing the true suicide risk among patients with cancer, it is clear that depression, anxiety, and suicidal ideation affect a large enough portion of cancer patients to warrant further research regarding their measurement and the efficacy of both pharmacological and nonpharmacological treatments (e.g., individual or group therapy) that can help patients come to terms with impending death (Block, 2000; Spiegel et al., 1994).

Although there is no consensus regarding the best or most useful tool for diagnosing emotional distress among terminally ill cancer patients, two broad categories of assessment tools have been employed: self-report questionnaires and clinical interview diagnostic criteria. Researchers have used many self-report questionnaires measuring psychological well-being to assess emotional distress among cancer patients; however, only the Memorial Symptom Assessment Scale (Portenoy, et al., 1994b) was designed specifically to measure symptoms common to cancer. Similarly, although standard clinical diagnostic criteria (e.g., the DSM series) are widely used in the general population, versions modified for people with medical illness have to be validated (Kathol et al., 1990), and tools geared toward palliative care that are sensitive to cultural and ethnic differences must be developed (Breitbart et al., 1995; Lewis-Fernandez and Kleinman, 1995).

Future Directions:

NCI could fund development of measures, descriptive studies, and research on treatment for anxiety and depression among cancer patients diagnosed as having a life-limiting condition.

Shared Decisionmaking

With the development of more effective treatments, cancer has become curable for some, and for others, a chronic, progressive illness that people live with and, with their health care providers, manage over time. One consequence of this change is that physicians and patients must communicate with each other in ways that previously were unimportant. Communication research has focused largely on decisionmaking at the end of life, in particular, on the single issue of a "do-not-resuscitate" (DNR) decision. As important as that is, even more important for many patients is a decision to stop chemotherapy or other active treatment, but this decision has yet to be fully studied.

Patient preferences have an important role in shared medical decisionmaking. Published guidelines regarding end-of-life care strongly endorse a patient's right to participate in health care decisions (Teno et al., 2001a). For example, the American Society of Clinical Oncology (ASCO) calls for physicians to speak truthfully to cancer patients and families about prognosis, treatment options, and advance care planning (ASCO, 1998). Despite widespread endorsement by professional guidelines, the Patient Self-Determination Act, and court rulings, there is still significant concern about whether patients' preferences are honored along with persistent claims that they are "trumped" by physicians. The evidence to support this claim is scant and derives in large part from misinterpretations of SUPPORT results and studies that asked for the perceptions of nurses and physicians in training (e.g., a report that one in two health care providers believe they had provided overly aggressive medical care to a dying person) (Solomon et al., 1993).

The SUPPORT results were widely reported and have had a lasting impact that does not necessarily represent their most accurate interpretation. *US News and World Report* headlines were, "Doctors Don't Listen" and "...Doctors Don't Talk About Bad News"—the implication being that physicians were ignoring individuals' informed preferences. Half of the patients in SUPPORT with colon cancer who voiced a preference to avoid resuscitation did not have a DNR order (Haidet et al., 1998), but even so, these patients were not resuscitated against their preferences (Hakim et al.,1996). Similarly, a review of those deaths with an advance directive found only one case in which an advance directive was trumped at the request of the family (not by a physician) (Teno et al., 1998). Whether it was ethically defensible to delay the death of this unconscious patient so that his daughter could come to grips with the decision can be debated.

The larger area of concern is not that patient preferences are being ignored but rather questions regarding the timing of communication and interpretation of the intended meaning of "hopelessly ill." In a qualitative study of advance directives in SUPPORT, Teno and colleagues (1998) found that advance directives were invoked and often played a role in decision making. However, directives were invoked only when the patient was "hopelessly ill."

Moving this decision upstream from a point when treatment is judged almost certainly futile will take a fundamental change in the dialogue that occurs between patients, families, and physicians. Discussion of prognosis at an earlier stage must be accomplished in such a way that it does not shatter hope, yet allows a dying person to make realistic choices about medical care. Cancer, unlike other leading causes of death, does have a relatively predictable disease trajectory that would allow for such dialogues to be developed and implemented.

The lack of impact of the SUPPORT intervention (which provided physicians with information on patient preferences and prognoses but did not result in increased physician understanding of patient preferences, timing of DNR orders, reduction in days spent in undesirable outcome states, and reduction in resource utilization) has been taken by some as a rationale for endorsing "glide paths" (i.e., "default pathways"), rather than finding better ways to communicate and, ultimately, implement patient self-determination. A careful review of the SUPPORT findings, however, suggests that the intervention itself was inadequate to improve communication, not that improved communication is impossible.

Given the existing research, the only firm conclusion that can be drawn is that communication is lacking between physicians and patients (Haidet et al., 1998; SUPPORT Principal Investigators, 1996) and that physicians often misunderstand patient preferences (Teno et al., 1995). Research in communication and decisionmaking has focused largely on the last days of life. The more sentinel decisions, though, may be stopping active treatment or choosing palliative chemotherapy, radiation therapy, or surgical treatment earlier in the course of illness. The evidence base to support guidelines for these decisions is preliminary at best. Research on how best to communicate this information to patients has only begun.

Future Directions:

NCI and AHRQ could fund research to develop the evidence base for palliative chemotherapy, radiation, and other treatment modalities. Such research should consider the treatment's meaning to patients and families, toxicity, and impact on quality of life.

Cooperative Oncology Groups could standardize measures and schedules to examine both treatment toxicity and quality of life. This would facilitate meta-analyses to develop the evidence base for palliative chemotherapy, radiation, and surgical treatments.

NCI could sponsor research with the NIA and AHRQ to study communication of information about risks and burdens of chemotherapy in making treatment decisions with persons whose cancer is expected to be fatal. Consideration could be given to funding a center of excellence in communication regarding end-of-life care. Such a center would address issues such as stopping active cancer treatment and the use of chemotherapy, radiation, and other modalities for palliative intent only.

ASCO and other professional organizations could develop clinical guidelines regarding the point at which physicians should discuss the burdens and benefits of continued chemotherapy, including the presentation of information about hospice and/or palliative care.

Decisions regarding treatment approaches in cancer require consideration of the trade-offs of quality versus quantity of life. With increasing use of capitation, the incentive may be to provide less care. Measurement tools that examine whether treatment decisions reflect informed patient preferences should be developed and validated. Such measures, if validated, could be incorporated into HCFA's ongoing effort to monitor the quality of managed care.

Proposed Definitions and Conceptual Models of Quality of Care

Dying is a time unlike any other, and more than at any other time, patients' preferences are central to defining the quality of care. While one patient may choose an experimental chemotherapeutic trial and even continued intravenous (IV) hydration in an inpatient hospice unit, another patient with the same diagnosis may choose aggressive treatment with IV opiates for distress from dyspnea but no chemotherapy. Essential to the quality of care for a cancer patient is meeting the patient's needs and expectations within society's imposed constraints.

A previous Institute of Medicine (IOM) report defined quality of care as the "degree to which health services for individuals and populations increased the likelihood of desired health outcomes and are consistent with professional knowledge" (IOM, 1990). This definition implies that conceptual models for quality of care (as well as instruments measuring quality) must be based on both professional knowledge (based on scientific evidence) and informed patient preferences. Most conceptual models have been built either around expert opinion (Emanuel and Emanuel, 1998; IOM, 1997; Lynn, 1997; NHO, 1997; Stewart et al., 1999) or on qualitative data from patients, families, or health care providers Singer et al., 1999; Steinhauser et al., 2000; Teno et al., in preparation). Only one proposed model incorporates both the expert and the consumer perspectives (Table 3-3).

TABLE 3-3   Comparison of Domains of Experts, Patients, Family
Members, Health Care Providers, and New Proposed Model

Expert Opinion			Consumer Opinion
Emanuel and Emanuel (1998)	IOM (1990)	NHO Pathway (1997)	Patients with HIV, Renal Failure on Dialysis, and Nursing Home Residents (Seale et al., 1997)
Physical symptoms	Overall quality of life	Safe and comfortable dying	Receiving adequate pain and symptom management
Psychological and cognitive symptoms	Physical well-being and functioning	Self-determined life closure	Avoiding inappropriate prolongation of the dying
Social relationships and support	Psychosocial well-being and functioning	Effective grieving	Achieving sense of control
Economic demands and caregiving demands	Family well-being and perceptions		Relieving burdens
Hopes and expectations			Strengthening relationships
Spiritual and existential beliefs			

SOURCE: Based on Teno et al., 2001.

Experts and consumers agree in many ways about what is important to
end-of-life care—physical comfort, emotional support, and autonomy—but
they have significant areas of disagreement, as well (e.g., on unmet needs;
Table 3-3). Family members want more information on what to expect and
how they can help their dying loved ones. Patients and families emphasize
the importance of closure at the end of life, including issues of personal
relationships. Families often speak of frustration with the lack of coordination of medical care. It often isn't clear who was in charge, different health

	Combined Model	
Patients, Families, and Health Care Providers	Bereaved Family Members from the Current Study	New Proposed Conceptual Model of Patient-Focused, Family-Centered Medical Care
Pain and symptom management	Providing desired physical comfort	Provide desired level of physical comfort and emotional support
Clear decisionmaking	Achieving control over health care decisions and everyday decisions	Promote shared decisionmaking
Preparation for death	Burden of advocating for quality medical care	Focus on the individual. This includes closure, respect, and patient dignity.
Completion	Educating on what to expect, and increasing confidence in providing care	Attend to the needs of the family for information, increasing their confidence in helping with patient care and providing emotional support prior to and after the patient's death.
Contributing to others	Emotional support prior to and after the patient's death	Coordination and continuity of care
Affirmation of the whole person		Informing and educating

care providers provide conflicting information, and transitions can be fraught with confusion.

Teno and colleagues' (2001) model of patient-focused, family-centered medical care (Table 3-3) is based on a review of existing professional guidelines and focus groups conducted with family members. For the seriously ill patient, institutions and care providers striving to achieve patient-focused, family-centered medical care should

- provide the desired level of physical comfort and emotional support;
- promote shared decisionmaking, including advance care planning;
- focus on the individual patient by facilitating situations in which patients achieve their desired level of control, staff members treat patients with respect and dignity, and patients are aided in achieving their desired levels of closure; and
- attend to the needs of caregivers for information and skills in providing care for the patient, and provide emotional support to the family before and after the patient's death.

In the ideal quality-monitoring system for cancer, guidelines and proposed quality indicators should be strongly linked. Guidelines should be based on both normative and empirical research. A quality indicator can measure information about the structure of the health care institution (e.g., availability of certain services, existence of policies), processes (i.e., interactions of health care providers, patients, and family), and outcomes (i.e., effectiveness of treatment). Currently, most quality indicators measure either structure or processes of care. Outcome measures are intuitively more attractive, but they are more difficult to apply because of our limited ability to adjust for differences in patient characteristics and the relatively small numbers of people with a particular condition treated at institutions each year (Brook et al., 1996). One argument in favor of process data is that they are a more sensitive measure of quality because adverse outcomes do not occur every time there is an error in the provision of medical care (Brook et al., 1996). Also, important outcomes—both positive and negative—often appear months or even years after care has been given. Quality indicators based on measures of structure or process, however, are only as good as their predictiveness for outcomes of importance.

Future Directions:

NCI and AHRQ could fund research to elucidate the interrelations of structure, process, and outcomes of care, in order to develop valid quality indicators.

Surveys and chart abstraction tools have been designed to examine the quality of care of the dying for purposes of quality improvement and research. SUPPORT used both chart abstraction tools (examining reported patient involvement in decisions and the point at which a decision was made) and interviews with patients and family members. Other tools have been developed that examine the documentation regarding pain management (Weissman et al., 2000).

SUPPORT demonstrated that a majority of seriously ill patients cannot be interviewed (Wenger et al., 1994). As a result, the research choice becomes either to eliminate those cases or to rely on information given by a surrogate, usually a family member. The tools developed for SUPPORT reflect survey methodologies of the early 1980s, which had important limitations—including lowered patient expectations and subsequent high satisfaction with the quality of care. For example, Desbiens and colleagues (1996) reported that persons were satisfied with pain management despite reporting severe pain more than one-half the time.

Responding to the need to develop tools to measure quality of life and quality of care at the end of life, the Brown University Center for Gerontology and Health Care Research and the IOM have convened a series of multidisciplinary conferences (Teno et al., 1999). The result has been a series of recommendations for a "Toolkit of Instruments to Measure End of Life Care," with the initial target of developing tools that measure the perspectives of the dying person and the family for the purposes of research and quality improvement.

Since medical decisions increasingly are based on quality of life and quality of life is a subjective concept, cancer patients must be allowed their desired role in decisionmaking. Medical records can document treatments received and whether physicians state that they discussed treatment decisions with patients and/or their families. Even though this can be useful information, a consumer perspective on communication, decisionmaking, coordination, and other domains is important when assessing the quality of care of the dying. Ultimately, it is not documentation of the event, but whether the information was provided in a way that the cancer patient could understand and use in making decisions that should be the ultimate judge of the quality of care.

Typically, "satisfaction measures" have been relied on for the consumer perspective on the quality of health care (Table 3-4). In these cases, consumers are asked to rate the quality of care using scales ranging from either "excellent" to "poor" or "very satisfied" to "very dissatisfied." Typically, respondents must go through a cognitive process in which they first ask whether a particular event occurred, formulate their expectations regarding that event, and then rate that event using the provided response scale. Unfortunately, expectations are usually low, causing respondents to express high satisfaction with care that is less than optimal.

Newer methods have begun using either "patient-centered reports" (Cleary and McNeil, 1988) or "preference-based questions" (i.e., unmet needs) to capture consumer perspectives. These methodologies, unlike typical satisfaction questions that rely on ratings, provide information that can guide improvement of the quality of care. For example, knowing that 85 percent of patients believe a health care provider is "very good" does not supply that provider with information on how to improve. On the other hand, knowing that 20 percent of patients did not understand a provider's directions for taking pain medications does provide an important target for improving and enhancing the quality of care. Moreover, patient-centered reports and preference-based questions have strong face validity with health care providers. In the future, surveys have to rely on all three methodologies to capture the consumer perspective on quality of care at the end of life. (See Figure 3-5 for examples of questions from a bereaved family member survey to examine the quality of care for dying persons and their families.)

TABLE 3-4   Status of Quality Indicator Development for End-of-Life Care

Domain	Proposed Indicators	Readiness
Pain	Frequency and severity of pain from Minimum Data Set	Proposed indicators require validation, but can be measured for all hospitalized cancer patients
		Major limitation: captures only health care provider perspective
	Patient and family perspective on pain management	Instruments available (e.g., from American Pain Society or Toolkit of Instruments to Measure End-of-Life Care)
Satisfaction	Measures of patient satisfaction, based on patient or surrogate responses	New instruments have undergone reliability and validity testing. Additional questions are specific for cancer (e.g., whether patients are informed of recommended treatments, access to high-quality clinical trials) and incorporation into ongoing data collection efforts
	New instruments include some questions relevant to people dying from cancer	
Shared Decisionmaking	Questions from Toolkit of Instruments to Measure End-of-Life Care	Reliability and validity testing completed
		Examination of responsiveness not complete
Coordination and Continuity of Care	No indicators yet available	

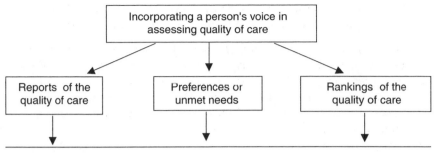

Reports of specific events
Did your doctor talk to you about other treatment approaches for your condition?

Unmet Needs

In the last X days while (he/she) was at [LAST PLACE], did [PATIENT] receive too much, too little, or just the right amount of medication for (his/her) pain?

Rankings of specific aspects of care
Now we would like you to rate some aspects of the care [PATIENT] received at [LAST PLACE]. For the following questions, please rate the care at [LAST PLACE] on a scale of 0 to 10, where 0 means care was as bad as possible and 10 means care was as good as possible.

(In the last X days of (his/her) life) how well did those taking care of [PATIENT] at [LAST PLACE] make sure (his/her) symptoms were controlled to a degree that was acceptable to (him/her)?

Reports of specific events conditioned on respondent assessment
Were you told the purpose of your pain medication in a way that you could understand?

Preferences and discrepancy
Would you like someone to spend more time helping you eat?

FIGURE 3-5 Proposed scheme for measuring patient and family voice about quality of medical care.
SOURCE: Author.

What Can We Measure with Current Nationally Collected Data? What Do We Want to Be Able to Measure in the Future?

The ultimate goal is a national system that measures the quality of care for people with cancer, from diagnosis through cure, long-term survival, or death. Good care (1) is based on scientifically sound evidence, (2) incorporates informed patients' preferences, (3) provides access to appropriate services including high-quality clinical trials, (4) coordinates services across multiple segments of the health care "system," and (5) is compassionate, attending to both the physical and the psychological needs of the patient and family.

Reliable indicators of quality can be powerful motivators for health care providers at all levels to improve the quality of their care. The development of quality indicators for end-of-life care remains at an early stage. At this point, there are two relevant questions: (1) for which domains is there either empirical or normative evidence to support quality indicators for the purpose of accountability; and (2) are there reliable and valid measures in existing data sets?

There is both normative and empirical evidence of the importance of pain management, something that is entirely under the control of health care systems. While the evidence is not as strong as for pain management, satisfaction also could be measured for purposes of public accountability. The evidence that health care institutions can improve satisfaction with hospice interventions is very strong (Greer and Mor, 1986; Hanson et al., 1997; Kane et al., 1984).

There is strong normative evidence based on both guidelines and court rulings that attest to the importance of shared decisionmaking (i.e., decisions regarding treatment choices that are based on informed patient preferences if the patient desires a role in decisionmaking). One last domain for which measures could be developed is coordination and continuity of medical care. Recurrent concerns in focus groups are that medical care is fragmented, that a physician often is not in charge, and that health care providers give conflicting information about treatment plans. Unlike pain and satisfaction, the conceptual framework and measurement tools for coordination and continuity of care are in need of further development.

Future Directions:

Measures of pain management, shared decisionmaking, coordination and continuity of care, and patient or family perspectives of the quality of care (i.e., satisfaction) must be developed, validated, and benchmarked. These measures have to be tested for validity and responsiveness in demonstration programs to assess the quality of care for persons dying from cancer.

Some of these domains can be examined in part with two national databases: the Minimum Data Set of Nursing Home Residents and Medicare claims files. The MDS is federally mandated and reports data from the Resident Assessment Instrument, which collects information on the presence, severity, and frequency of pain for nursing home residents at admissions, quarterly, and with changes in health status (Hawes et al., 1995; Morris et al., 1990). With computerized drug data, quality indicators can be formulated to examine the frequency and severity of pain and the degree to which pain is treated. Based on an examination of the MDS database available from five states, nearly one in four cancer patients with daily pain was not prescribed any analgesic (Bernabei et al., 1998). Although only about 10 percent of cancer patients die in a nursing home, they are often the most frail and vulnerable patients.

The MDS is a potentially useful tool for public accountability, but it has limitations. For one thing, the data are recorded by staff members, not by the patient, so reports of pain and other symptoms depend on the accuracy of proxy staff reporting. An indication that reporting may not be accurate, or at least not uniform, is the range of values found in nursing homes from 10 different states, which Teno and colleagues found to vary between 8 and 49 percent of patients reported as having daily pain (Teno, 2000b). This variation could reflect inadequate pain assessment, inconsistent pain management, or the different types of people cared for by a facility. A likely explanation is inadequate assessment, given the challenges of evaluating pain in this frail population, more than half of whom have moderate to extensive cognitive impairment.

Since July 1999, HCFA has identified a series of performance indicators that are examined based on the MDS. Experience with the use of the MDS indicators has yet to be evaluated, but there are important concerns. Specifically, the experience of nursing homes is increasingly revealing the importance of unintended consequences of applying quality indicators to populations in which they are not applicable.

For example, two of the proposed nursing home indicators focus on dehydration and weight loss. A quality indicator is composed of a numerator (e.g., those persons with pain) and a denominator (e.g., conscious persons in that nursing facility). For the dehydration and weight loss indicators, the denominator is everyone in the health care facility, including those who are dying. The potential unintended consequence is that nursing homes will increase the use of nasogastric tube feeding, IV hydration, and hospitalizations of dying individuals. The obvious and simplistic solution is to eliminate the dying patients from the denominator. However, identifying patients who are dying—particularly those dying from illnesses other than cancer—can be quite difficult given the limitations of prognostication and knowing that the functional trajectory is relatively flat for noncancer patients (Teno and Coppola, 1999).

For Medicare beneficiaries enrolled in fee-for-service plans (but not in Health Maintenance Organizations), Medicare claims files collect information on charges, reimbursement, hospitalizations, hospice enrollment, Current Procedural Terminology (CPT) codes, and *International Classification of Diseases, Ninth Edition* (ICD-9) codes. Researchers have used these records for a variety of purposes. Pritchard and colleagues (1998) examined the national pattern of proportion of deaths in hospitals. Wennberg and colleagues have examined records for the last six months of life to determine whether patients spent time in an intensive care unit (ICU), the number of physician visits, and whether 10 or more physicians were involved in the decedent's care, all of which are potentially useful indicators of aspects of quality. The importance of this work is the striking variation around the country in each of these statistics (which was also found in two studies based on SUPPORT data, after adjustment for disease severity and patient preferences) (Pritchard et al., 1998; Teno et al., 2001e). However, Medicare claims data alone cannot be used as appropriate quality indicators because they lack information on disease severity and patient preferences. One way around this is to link a measure of severity (site and stage of cancer) from NCI's Surveillance, Epidemiology and End Results (SEER) database to Medicare claims. Data linkages such as this are becoming easier but still require considerable development before they can be used routinely.

Future Directions:

HCFA, AHRQ, or NCI could sponsor research to develop and validate the use of quality indicators based on data from Medicare claims files.

None of the existing databases captures the patient perspective on the quality of care. The only federally sponsored effort that has attempted this is the Consumer Assessment of Health Plans Survey (CAHPS; http://www.ahrq.gov/qual/cahpfact.htm). This five-year research effort has developed, validated, and used new surveys tools to capture the patient experience with managed care. The goal of CAHPS is to develop information to be used by consumers and health care purchasers in choosing managed care plans. CAHPS consists of core questions and modules addressed to specific populations (e.g., Medicaid managed care enrollees) and covering specific content areas (e.g., well-child care, prescription medicines). There is a CAHPS chronic disease module, but it is not specific enough to assess the quality of care for advanced cancer, and it would be difficult to construct a module that could do so within CAHPS.

The discussion thus far has focused on indicators to be used for public accountability. Equally important are indicators for "quality improvement," which takes in a range of purposes from institutional audits to identify opportunities to improve care, to indicators designed to examine the impact of small interventions tested through multiple "Plan, Do, Study, and Act" cycles. The measures used for different purposes differ, but are related, and fall along a continuum. Measures developed for quality improvement with the correct psychometric properties may evolve into accountability measures.

There are currently no quality indicators in national use that deal specifically with palliative care or other end-of-life issues. However, the degree to which indicators may be in use for QI or other institutional purposes is not known. The author contacted six NCI-designated Comprehensive Cancer Centers with strong palliative care interests to determine the extent of their current systematic efforts to examine quality of care of the dying. Only one of the centers is collecting any such information, using the NHO family satisfaction survey for people who died in an affiliated hospice program and ongoing satisfaction surveys to examine the quality of care for dying patients discharged home from its hospital. Two other centers did monitor symptoms as a "fifth vital sign."

Future Directions:

Comprehensive Cancer Centers should set the benchmarks for excellence in cancer care, and this includes validating and reporting on quality indicators.

What Research Is Needed?

In *Ensuring Quality Cancer Care* (IOM, 1999), the National Cancer Policy Board recommended development of a core set of quality measures for the continuum of cancer care, including care at the end of life. The elements of quality care identified were an "agreed upon care plan that outlines the goals of care, policies to ensure full disclosure of information with appropriate treatment options, a mechanism to coordinate services, psychosocial support services, and compassionate care." There are gaps all along the continuum of care, but nowhere more severe than for end-of-life care, for which the following are needed: the development of new measurement tools; research to both validate measurement tools and examine their real-world application in terms of responsiveness and burden; and if these measurement tools are to be used for accountability, a consensus-building process between the public, the government, and the health care industry.

The importance of guidelines has also been recognized by the NCPB and is especially true for examining quality of end-of-life care. A key question for advance care planning to formulate end-of-life contingency plans consistent with patient preferences is, When? Guidelines that recognize different needs at different points along the disease trajectory are necessary, especially those that are of particular importance when a person accepts that he or she is dying, such as spirituality and transcendence.

Patient preferences and satisfaction are important at every stage of treatment, but they take on added significance at the end of life. The measurement tools now available are based on review of medical records or administrative data. New measures are needed that incorporate the extent to which a patient's care is based on informed preferences, that measure whether patients receive psychological support if needed and wanted, and that they assess whether care is both coordinated and compassionate. The perceptions of the dying patient and family provide an important perspective on each of these aspects of medical care. These surveys should be developed according to a conceptual model that is based on guidelines and the concerns voiced by dying persons and their families.

Some work has been started toward surveys of bereaved family members. One effort (Teno et al., 2001a; Teno, et al., 2001b) uses current guidelines and results of focus groups from around the country to develop questions on unmet needs and on the family's perspective of the quality of care delivered to the dying person and to themselves. A second survey (Patrick and Curtis, 2001) focuses on the quality of dying. As these and other tools are developed, some questions will be applicable to all dying persons, but there will also be a need for disease-specific questions (e.g., management of toxicity from chemotherapeutic agents is a very important concern, and the specifics of management are different for cancer patients than for those dying from other causes).

The initial work has focused on retrospective surveys of surviving family members largely because the denominator is easily defined (based on cancer registry or death certificate data) and family members are often the only ones able to be interviewed in the last month of a patient's life. Surveys that directly capture the patients' perspective are needed, as well, however. The design of such surveys could be linked to sentinel events or triggers (e.g., admission to palliative care or hospice program, reaching a certain disease stage), with consideration give to which domains are included and the point (or points) along the patient's disease trajectory at which questions should be asked.

An important tension that the developers of surveys will face is between respondent's burden and the desire to be comprehensive. The eventual goal is to minimize the respondent burden, but initially a larger number of items will be tested and a winnowing process used to arrived at a parsimonious set of questions.

The mode of survey administration is another important research question: can valid information be gathered through a self-administered questionnaire (by either the patient or a proxy respondent), or should it be professionally administered? Self-administered surveys cost less, but their validity must be demonstrated for these sensitive areas. At a later stage, it will be necessary to examine the correlation of different quality indicators based on administrative data, chart reviews, and surveys.

The constraints imposed by feasibility and cost must guide the development of quality indicators. A key consideration is to minimize the institutional burdens and maximize the value in achieving the goals of quality care for dying persons and their families. It will be important from the outset to involve health care administrators who would have to implement data collection in partnership with the development of measurement tools.

Future Directions:

Guidelines are needed that outline the triggers for when a cancer is to be considered life limiting (an implied prognosis of less than one year) and normative behaviors (such as advance care planning, discussion of prognosis and options of hospice) are expected. Such triggers should be linked to prospective surveys to measure the quality of medical care. Research to develop population-based prognostic models will be needed to help inform the selection of such triggers.

CONCLUSION

The development of quality indicators for the care of the dying person is at an early stage of development. Basic descriptions of the dying experience and the care given to people who are dying are still lacking. Clinical guidelines, important for synthesizing the available evidence and reaching consensus on what defines quality medical care, have been developed only for certain aspects of palliative and end-of-life care. These need further development within a system that allows regular incorporation of new knowledge. Such guidelines can help in defining who should be counted among the "dying." Quality indicators based on guidelines and the consumer perspective must be developed, validated, and applied in health care settings. Such indicators must examine the structure, processes, and outcomes of health care systems. Research is needed to examine the interrelationships of structure, process, and outcome as well as the correlation of indicators using different data sources. Ultimately, we need indicators that are feasible and cost-effective, that recognize what the best medical care consists of, and that reflect the perspectives of the dying and their families.

REFERENCES

Addington Hall J, McCarthy M. Regional Study of Care for the Dying: methods and sample characteristics. *Palliat Med* 1995a;9(1):27-35.

Addington Hall J, McCarthy M. Dying from cancer: results of a national population-based investigation. *Palliat Med* 1995b;9(4):295-305.

American Pain Society. Quality improvement guidelines for the treatment of acute pain and cancer pain. American Pain Society Quality of Care Committee [see comments]. *JAMA* 1995;274(23):1874-1880.

ASCO (American Society of Clinical Oncology). Clinical practice guidelines for the treatment of unresectable non-small-cell lung cancer. Adopted on May 16, 1997 by the American Society of Clinical Oncology. *J Clin Oncol* 1997;15(8):2996-3018.

ASCO (American Society of Clinical Oncology). ASCO Special Article: Cancer care during the last phase of life. J Clin Oncol 1998;16(5):1986-1996.

Bernabei R, Gambassi G, Lapane K et al. Management of pain in elderly patients with cancer. SAGE Study Group. Systematic Assessment of Geriatric Drug Use via Epidemiology [see comments] [published erratum appears in *JAMA* 1999 Jan 13;281(2):136]. *JAMA* 1998; 279(23):1877-1882.

Block SD. Assessing and managing depression in the terminally ill patient. ACP-ASIM End-of-Life Care Consensus Panel. American College of Physicians - American Society of Internal Medicine. *Ann Intern Med* 2000;132(3):209-218.

Bredin M, Corner J, Krishnasamy M, Plant H, Bailey C, A'Hern R. Multicentre randomised controlled trial of nursing intervention for breathlessness in patients with lung cancer. *BMJ* 1999;318(7188):901-904.

Breitbart W, Bruera E, Chochinov H, Lynch M. Neuropsychiatric syndromes and psychological symptoms in patients with advanced cancer. *J Pain Symptom Manage* 1995; 10(2):131-141.

Brock DB, Foley DJ. Demography and epidemiology of dying in the U.S. with emphasis on deaths of older persons. *Hosp J* 1998;13(1-2):49-60.

Brook RH, McGlynn EA, Cleary PD. Quality of health care. Part 2: measuring quality of care [editorial] [see comments]. *N Engl J Med* 1996;335(13):966-970.

Chochinov HM, Wilson KG, Enns M, et al. Desire for death in the terminally ill. *Am J Psychiatry* 1995;152(8):1185-1191.

Chochinov HM, Wilson KG, Enns M, Lander S. Depression, Hopelessness, and suicidal ideation in the terminally ill. *Psychosomatics* 1998;39(4):366-370.

Christakis NA, Escarce JJ. Survival of Medicare patients after enrollment in hospice programs [see comments]. *N Engl J Med* 1996;335(3):172-178.

Cleary PD, McNeil BJ. Patient satisfaction as an indicator of quality care. *Inquiry* 1988; 25(1):25-36.

Cleeland CS, Gonin R, Hatfield AK et al. Pain and its treatment in outpatients with metastatic cancer [see comments]. *N Engl J Med* 1994;330(9):592-596.

Conill C, Verger E, Henriquez I et al. Symptom prevalence in the last week of life. *J Pain Symptom Manage* 1997;14(6):328-331.

Coyle N, Adelhardt J, Foley KM, Portenoy RK. Character of terminal illness in the advanced cancer patient: pain and other symptoms during the last four weeks of life [see comments]. *J Pain Symptom Manage* 1990;5(2):83-93.

De Florio ML, Massie MJ. Review of depression in cancer: gender differences. *Depression* 1995;3:66-80.

Desbiens NA, Mueller Rizner N, Connors AF, Wenger NS. The relationship of nausea and dyspnea to pain in seriously ill patients. *Pain* 1997;71(2):149-156.

Desbiens NA, Wu AW, Broste SK et al. Pain and satisfaction with pain control in seriously ill hospitalized adults: findings from the SUPPORT research investigations. For the SUPPORT investigators. Study to Understand Prognoses and Preferences for Outcomes and Risks of Treatment [see comments]. *Crit Care Med* 1996;24(12):1953-61.

Donnelly S, Walsh D. The symptoms of advanced cancer. *Semin Oncol* 1995;22(2 Suppl 3):67-72.

Donnelly S, Walsh D, Rybicki L. The symptoms of advanced cancer: identification of clinical and research priorities by assessment of prevalence and severity. *J Palliat Care* 1995; 11(1):27-32.

Dudgeon DJ, Raubertas RF, Doerner K, O'Connor T, Tobin M, Rosenthal SN. When does palliative care begin? A needs assessment of cancer patients with recurrent disease [see comments]. *J Palliat Care* 1995;11(1):5-9.

Dudgeon DJ, Rosenthal S. Management of dyspnea and cough in patients with cancer. *Hematol Oncol Clin North Am* 1996;10(1):157-171.

Edmonds P, Higginson I, Altmann D, Sen Gupta G, McDonnell M. Is the presence of dyspnea a risk factor for morbidity in cancer patients? *J Pain Symptom Manage* 2000;19(1):15-22.

Emanuel EJ, Emanuel LL. The promise of a good death. *Lancet* 1998;351 Suppl 2:SII21-29.

Emanuel EJ, Fairclough DL, Slutsman J, Emanuel LL. Understanding economic and other burdens of terminal illness: the experience of patients and their caregivers. *Ann Intern Med* 2000;132(6):451-459.

Escalante CP, Martin CG, Elting LS et al. Dyspnea in cancer patients. Etiology, resource utilization, and survival—implications in a managed care world. *Cancer* 1996;78(6): 1314-1319.

Fainsinger RL, Bruera E. When to treat dehydration in a terminally ill patient? Support Care Cancer 1997;5(3):205-211.

Fainsinger R, Miller MJ, Bruera E, Hanson J, Maceachern T. Symptom control during the last week of life on a palliative care unit. *J Palliat Care* 1991;7(1):5-11.

Farncombe M. Dyspnea: assessment and treatment [see comments]. *Support Care Cancer* 1997;5(2):94-99.

Foley KM. 1979. *Management of Pain of Malignant Origin.* Boston: Houghton Mifflin.

Foley KM. The relationship of pain and symptom management to patient requests for physician-assisted suicide. *J Pain Symptom Manage* 1991;6(5):289-297.

Fox E, Landrum McNiff K, Zhong Z, Dawson NV, Wu AW, Lynn J. Evaluation of prognostic criteria for determining hospice eligibility in patients with advanced lung, heart, or liver disease. SUPPORT Investigators. Study to Understand Prognoses and Preferences for Outcomes and Risks of Treatments [see comments]. *JAMA* 1999;282(17):1638-1645.

Glaser B, Strauss A. 1968. *Time for Dying.* Chicago: Aldine Publishing Company.

Goodlin SJ, Winzelberg GS, Teno JM, Whedon M, Lynn J. Death in the hospital. *Arch Intern Med* 1998;158(14):1570-1572.

Greer DS, Mor V. An overview of National Hospice Study findings. *J Chronic Dis* 1986;39:5-7.

Greer DS, Mor V, Morris JN, Sherwood S, Kidder D, Birnbaum H. An alternative in terminal care: results of the National Hospice Study. *J Chronic Dis* 1986;39(1):9-26.

Haidet P, Hamel MB, Davis RB, et al. Outcomes, preferences for resuscitation, and physician-patient communication among patients with metastatic colorectal cancer. SUPPORT Investigators. Study to Understand Prognoses and Preferences for Outcomes and Risks of Treatments. *Am J Med* 1998;105(3):222-229.

Hakim RB, Teno JM, Harrell FE Jr, et al. Factors associated with do-not-resuscitate orders: patients' preferences, prognoses, and physicians' judgments. SUPPORT Investigators. Study to Understand Prognoses and Preferences for Outcomes and Risks of Treatment. *Ann Intern Med* 1996;125(4):284-293.

Hanson LC, Danis M, Garrett J. What is wrong with end-of-life care? Opinions of bereaved family members. *J Am Geriatr Soc* 1997;45(11):1339-1344.

Hawes C, Morris JN, Phillips CD, Mor V, Fries BE, Nonemaker S. Reliability estimates for the Minimum Data Set for nursing home resident assessment and care screening (MDS). *Gerontologist* 1995;35(2):172-178.

Hay L, Farncombe M, McKee P. Patient, nurse and physician views of dyspnea. *Can Nurse* 1996;92(10):26-29.

Health Care Financing Administration (HCFA). Nursing Home Compare, 2000. http://www.medicare.gov/NHCompare/Home.asp.

Higginson I, McCarthy M. Measuring symptoms in terminal cancer: are pain and dyspnoea controlled? *J R Soc Med* 1989;82(5):264-267.

Hockley JM, Dunlop R, Davies RJ. Survey of distressing symptoms in dying patients and their families in hospital and the response to a symptom control team. *Br Med J Clin Res Ed* 1988;296(6638):1715-1717.

Hopwood P, Stephens RJ. Symptoms at presentation for treatment in patients with lung cancer: implications for the evaluation of palliative treatment. The Medical Research Council (MRC) Lung Cancer Working Party. *Br J Cancer* 1995;71(3):633-636.

Institute of Medicine. 1990. *Medicare: A Strategy for Quality Assurance.* Washington, D.C.: National Academy Press.

Institute of Medicine. 1997. *Approaching Death: Improving Care at the End of Life.* Field MJ, Cassel CK (eds.) Washington, D.C.: National Academy Press.

Institute of Medicine. 1999. *Ensuring Quality Cancer Care.* Hewitt M, Simone JV (eds.) Washington, D.C.: National Academy Press.

Kane RL, Wales J, Bernstein L, Leibowitz A, Kaplan S. A randomised controlled trial of hospice care. *Lancet* 1984;1(8382):890-894.

Kathol RG, Noyes R Jr, Williams J, Mutgi A, Carroll B, Perry P. Diagnosing depression in patients with medical illness. *Psychosomatics* 1990;31(4):434-440.

Kuebler KK. Hospice and palliative care clinical practice protocol: dyspnea. *Hosp Nurse Assoc* 1996;1-28.

Lawton MP, Moss M, Glicksman A. The quality of the last year of life of older persons. *Milbank Q* 1990;68(1):1-28.

Lentzner HR, Pamuk ER, Rhodenhiser EP, Rothenberg R, Powell Griner E. The quality of life in the year before death. *Am J Public Health* 1992;82(8):1093-1098.

Levin DN, Cleeland CS, Dar R. Public attitudes toward cancer pain. *Cancer* 1985;56(9):2337-2339.

Lewis-Fernandez R, Kleinman A. Cultural psychiatry. Theoretical, clinical, and research issues. *Psychiatr Clin North Am* 1995;18(3):433-448.

Lynn J. Measuring quality of care at the end of life: a statement of principles [see comments]. *J Am Geriatr Soc* 1997;45(4):526-527.

Lynn J, Teno JM, Phillips RS et al. Perceptions by family members of the dying experience of older and seriously ill patients. SUPPORT Investigators. Study to Understand Prognoses and Preferences for Outcomes and Risks of Treatments [see comments]. *Ann Intern Med* 1997;126(2):97-106.

Marin I, Andrieu JM, Chretien J. [Bronchopulmonary cancers: medical approach of the last weeks of life. Study of 191 patients.] *Ann Med Interne Paris* 1987;138(2):90-95.

McCann RM, Hall WJ, Groth Juncker A. Comfort care for terminally ill patients. The appropriate use of nutrition and hydration [see comments]. *JAMA* 1994;272(16):1263-1266.

Morris JN, Hawes C, Fries BE et al. Designing the national resident assessment instrument for nursing homes. *Gerontologist* 1990;30(3):293-307.

Morris JN, Mor V, Goldberg RJ, Sherwood S, Greer DS, Hiris J. The effect of treatment setting and patient characteristics on pain in terminal cancer patients: a report from the National Hospice Study. *J Chronic Dis* 1986a;39(1):27-35.

Morris JN, Suissa S, Sherwood S, Wright SM, Greer D. Last days: a study of the quality of life of terminally ill cancer patients. *J Chronic Dis* 1986b;39(1):47-62.

Muers MF, Round CE. Palliation of symptoms in non-small cell lung cancer: a study by the Yorkshire Regional Cancer Organisation Thoracic Group. *Thorax* 1993;48(4):339-343.

NCHS (National Center for Health Statistics). Fast Stats A to Z. http://www.cdc.gov/nchs/fastats/deaths.htm.

NCHS. 1998. The National Mortality Followback Survey—Provisional Data, 1993. Public User Data File Documentation. Hyattsville, MD: Centers for Disease Control and Prevention.

National Hospice Organization. 1997. *A Pathway for Patients and Families Facing Terminal Illness: Self-Determined Life Closure, Safe Comfortable Dying and Effective Grieving.* Arlington, VA: National Hospice Organization.

Nelson K, Walsh D. Management of dyspnea in advanced cancer. *Cancer Bull* 1991;43(5): 423-426.

Patrick DL, Curtis JR. Evaluating the quality of dying and death. Manuscript under review, 2001.

Portenoy RK, Kornblith AB, Wong G, et al. Pain in ovarian cancer patients. Prevalence, characteristics, and associated symptoms. *Cancer* 1994a;74(3):907-915.

Portenoy RK, Thaler HT, Kornblith AB, et al. Symptom prevalence, characteristics and distress in a cancer population. *Qual Life Res* 1994b;3(3):183-189.

Portenoy RK, Thaler HT, Kornblith AB, et al. The Memorial Symptom Assessment Scale: an instrument for the evaluation of symptom prevalence, characteristics and distress. *Eur J Cancer* 1994c;30A(9):1326-1336.

Power D, Kelly S, Gilsenan J et al. Suitable screening tests for cognitive impairment and depression in the terminally ill—a prospective prevalence study. *Palliat Med* 1993;(3): 213-218.

Pritchard RS, Fisher ES, Teno JM, et al. Influence of patient preferences and local health system characteristics on the place of death. SUPPORT Investigators. Study to Understand Prognoses and Preferences for Risks and Outcomes of Treatment [see comments]. *J Am Geriatr Soc* 1998;46(10):1242-1250.

Relman AS. Assessment and accountability: the third revolution in medical care [editorial]. *N Engl J Med* 1988;319(18):1220-1222.

Reuben DB, Mor V. Dyspnea in terminally ill cancer patients. *Chest* 1986;89(2):234-236.

Ripamonti C. Management of dyspnea in advanced cancer patients [see comments]. *Support Care Cancer* 1999;7(4):233-243.

Ripamonti C, Bruera E. Dyspnea: pathophysiology and assessment. *J Pain Symptom Manage* 1997;13(4):220-232.

Roberts DK, Thorne SE, Pearson C. The experience of dyspnea in late-stage cancer. Patients' and nurses' perspectives. *Cancer Nurs* 1993;16(4):310-320.

Robinson WM, Ravilly S, Berde C, Wohl ME. End-of-life care in cystic fibrosis [see comments]. *Pediatrics* 1997;100(2 Pt 1):205-209.

Roy DJ. Need they sleep before they die? [editorial] [see comments]. *J Palliat Care* 1990;6(3):3-4.

Seale C, Addington Hall J, McCarthy M. Awareness of dying: prevalence, causes and consequences. *Soc Sci Med* 1997;45(3):477-484.

Singer PA, Martin DK, Kelner M. Quality end-of-life care: patients' perspectives [see comments]. *JAMA* 1999;281(2):163-168.

Solberg LI, Mosser G, McDonald S. The three faces of performance measurement: improvement, accountability, and research. *Jt Comm J Qual Improv* 1997;23(3):135-147.

Solomon MZ, O'Donnell L, Jennings B, et al. Decisions near the end of life: professional views on life-sustaining treatments [see comments]. *Am J Public Health* 1993;83(1):14-23.

Spiegel D, Sands S, Koopman C. Pain and depression in patients with cancer. *Cancer* 1994; 74(9):2570-2578.

Steinhauser KE, Clipp EC, McNeilly M, Christakis NA, McIntyre LM, Tulsky JA. In search of a good death: observations of patients, families, and providers. *Annals of Internal Medicine* 2000;132(10):825-832.

Stewart AL, Teno J, Patrick DL, Lynn J. The concept of quality of life of dying persons in the context of health care. *J Pain Symptom Manage* 1999;17(2):93-108.

Strang P. Emotional and social aspects of cancer pain. *Acta Oncol* 1992;31(3):323-326.

SUPPORT Principal Investigators. A controlled trial to improve care for seriously ill hospitalized patients. The Study to Understand Prognoses and Preferences for Outcomes and Risks of Treatments (SUPPORT). [published erratum appears in *JAMA* 1996 Apr 24; 275(16):1232]. *JAMA* 1995;274(20):1591-1598.

Teno, J. Toolkit of Instruments to Measure End of Life Care, 1999: http://chcr.brown.edu/pcoc/toolkit.htm.

Teno, J. Facts on Dying: Brown Atlas Site of Death 1989-1997, 2000a; http://www.chcr.brown.edu/dying/factsondying.htm.

Teno, J. Rhode Island Partnership to Improve End-of-Life Care: Improving the Quality of Care for Our Most Vulnerable Population. 2000b; http://www.chcr.brown.edu/commstate/homepagewithframes.htm.

Teno JM, Byock I, Field MJ. Research agenda for developing measures to examine quality of care and quality of life of patients diagnosed with life-limiting illness. *J Pain Symptom Manage* 1999;17(2):75-82.

Teno JM, Casey VA, Welch L, Edgman-Levitan S. Patient focused, family centered end-of-life medical care: views of the guidelines and bereaved family members. Manuscript Under Review 2001a.

Teno JM, Casey V, Edgman-Levitan S. Defining patient focused, family centered medical care. *Ann Intern Med* (in preparation) .

Teno JM, Clarridge B, Casey V, Fowler J. Toolkit of instruments to measure end of life care bereaved family member interview—psychometric properties. Manuscript under review. 2001b.

Teno JM, Coppola KM. For every numerator, you need a denominator: a simple statement but key to measuring the quality of care of the "dying." *J Pain Symptom Manage* 1999;17(2):109-113.

Teno JM, Hakim RB, Knaus WA, et al. Preferences for cardiopulmonary resuscitation: physician-patient agreement and hospital resource use. The SUPPORT Investigators. *J Gen Intern Med* 1995;10(4):179-186.

Teno JM, Stevens M, Fisher E. Variation in ICU utilizations: insights from qualitative and quantitative data. Manuscript under review. 2001e

Teno JM, Stevens M, Spernak S, Lynn J. Role of written advance directives in decision making: insights from qualitative and quantitative data. *J Gen Intern Med* 1998; 13(7):439-446.

Teno JM, Weitzen S, Fennell M, Mor V. Dying trajectory in the last year of life: does cancer trajectory fit other diseases? *J Palliat Med.* In press 2001d.

Tolle SW, Rosenfeld AG, Tilden VP, Park Y. Oregon's low in-hospital death rates: what determines where people die and satisfaction with decisions on place of death? *Ann Intern Med* 1999;130(8):681-685.

Truog RD, Berde CB, Mitchell C, Grier HE. Barbiturates in the care of the terminally ill [see comments]. *N Engl J Med* 1992;327(23):1678-1682.

Turner K, Chye R, Aggarwal G, Philip J, Skeels A, Lickiss JN. Dignity in dying: a preliminary study of patients in the last three days of life. *J Palliat Care* 1996;12(2):7-13.

Vainio A, Auvinen A. Prevalence of symptoms among patients with advanced cancer: an international collaborative study. Symptom Prevalence Group. *J Pain Symptom Manage* 1996;12(1):3-10.

van der Molen B. Dyspnoea: a study of measurement instruments for the assessment of dyspnoea and their application for patients with advanced cancer. *J Adv Nurs* 1995; 22(5):948-956.

Ventafridda V, Ripamonti C, Bianchi M, Sbanotto A, De Conno F. A randomized study on oral administration of morphine and methadone in the treatment of cancer pain. *J Pain Symptom Manage* 1986;1(4):203-207.

Ventafridda V, Ripamonti C, De Conno F, Tamburini M, Cassileth BR. Symptom prevalence and control during cancer patients' last days of life [see comments]. *J Palliat Care* 1990;6(3):7-11.

Ventafridda V, Saita L, Barletta L, Sbanotto A, De Conno F. Clinical observations on controlled-release morphine in cancer pain. *J Pain Symptom Manage* 1989;4(3):124-129.

Weissman DE, Griffie J, Muchka S, Matson S. Building an institutional commitment to pain management in long-term care facilities. *J Pain Symptom Manage* 2000;20(1):35-43.

Wenger NS, Oye RK, Bellamy PE, et al. Prior capacity of patients lacking decision making ability early in hospitalization: implications for advance directive administration. The SUPPORT Investigators. Study to Understand Prognoses and Preferences for Outcomes and Risks of Treatments. *J Gen Intern Med* 1994;9(10):539-543.

Wennberg JE (ed.). 1998. *The Dartmouth Atlas of Health Care 1998*. Dartmouth, N.H.: American Hospital Association.

Wolfe J, Grier HE, Klar N, et al. Symptoms and suffering at the end of life in children with cancer [see comments]. *N Engl J Med* 2000;342(5):326-333.

World Health Organization. 1990. *Cancer Pain Relief and Palliative Care: Report of a WHO Expert Committee*. Technical Report Series No. 804. Geneva: World Health Organization.

4

The Current State of Patient and Family Information About End-of-Life Care

Aaron S. Kesselheim
University of Pennsylvania

INTRODUCTION

When faced with a diagnosis of cancer, many people respond by gathering information about the cause of their ailment, their treatment options, and advances in medical research. They hope to become better educated about their disease, wanting to know what to expect and better ways to fight it. Patients can cull this information from any number of sources, including personal discussions with health professionals, family, friends, and religious leaders; printed materials in libraries or physician offices; telephone hotlines; mail order; and increasingly, the World Wide Web. The question is, How well does this information address patients' full range of options during the continuum of their cancer care, from diagnosis and treatment to survivorship or end-of-life concerns? Unfortunately, these materials emphasize curative treatment and living as a cancer survivor to the relative exclusion of palliative care and end-of-life issues, two significant aspects of cancer care.

The National Cancer Policy Board has placed a high priority on improving the care received by cancer patients as they enter the terminal phase of their disease. One highly relevant factor in ensuring such quality care is the availability, nature, and delivery of information about end-of-life issues. People with cancer confront very different issues in their end-of-life care than they faced during the primarily curative phases of their cancer treatment. In addition to an emphasis on symptom management and quality of death, novel practical and psychosocial matters emerge. For example, eight clinical symptoms are frequently associated with advanced cancer and the stages approaching death—pain, nausea and vomiting, fatigue, anorexia, confusion or delirium, anxiety, depression, and insomnia (Portenoy et al., 1994)—so their alleviation grows in importance for patients at this stage. Moreover, the approach of persistent disability or death requires decision-making on matters not purely medical, including advanced directives and home care options, sources of psychosocial support, burial arrangements, estate planning, and preparations for loved ones' grief and bereavement. Handling these issues with appropriate, honest discussions in anticipation of their arrival—not based on unfounded assumptions or after the fact— can help ensure that they are managed as smoothly as possible and in accordance with the patient's wishes. To accomplish this goal, patients and their family members must be well informed and well educated about the experience of dying and the end-of-life care options open to them.

This chapter surveys the sources of information available to cancer patients and investigates the extent to which these sources adequately address the concerns faced by cancer patients whose survival is limited. It then identifies the barriers to dissemination of information and patient education about end-of-life issues and makes recommendations for future initiatives to resolve the information gap between cancer cure and cancer death.

ACQUIRING END-OF-LIFE INFORMATION FROM HEALTH CARE PROVIDERS

Health Professional Resources

Patients first learn of their cancer diagnosis from their physicians, and then depend on them to monitor the progression of the disease and efficacy of treatment. It is natural, therefore, that the physician stands as the primary outlet for questions relating to symptoms, therapeutic options, and outcomes of cancer. Oncologists are involved in the care of most cancer patients at some point, but primary care physicians and other specialists provide a great deal of their care at various points during the illness, during recovery, and throughout survivorship (IOM, 1999). Nurses, social workers, and spiritual leaders are among the other health professionals who also deal directly and frequently with cancer patients about end-of-life care.

The dynamics of these patient-provider interactions depend on where they take place. In community physicians' offices, patients are likely to spend more time talking directly to their personal physician or to a limited number of nursing specialists. In larger institutions such as those that the National Cancer Institute (NCI) officially designates as cancer centers, patient care is usually managed by health care teams of physicians in different specialties, as well as nurses, social workers, and students. An informal survey of a dozen cancer centers reveals that most discussion of end-of-life issues occurs in face-to-face conversations between the patient and the patient's social worker. At Johns Hopkins University, for example, a social worker is assigned to a particular patient at his or her first visit and maintains this contact over the course of the patient's illness (Nye, 1999). The two most significant end-of-life matters that lie outside the realm of social services at these centers are spiritual concerns, which are handled by the chaplain service or the person's own religious leader, and specific medical questions, which are addressed either by the patient's physician or by the appropriate specialist. Most institutions have a "pain team" of physicians and nurses with special expertise in pain control, and some centers go beyond that—in addition to its Pain Management Center, the Jonsson Comprehensive Cancer Center at the University of California, Los Angeles (UCLA) offers a Non-Pain Symptom Management Center focused on fatigue, nausea, depression, and other symptoms (Abe, 1999).

To complement the personal interactions between patients and their health providers at large centers, the NCI has instructed all designated cancer centers to name one of their staff members as the official "patient educator" (Crosson, 1999). The NCI Office for Cancer Information, Communication, and Education (OCICE) has formulated a set of guidelines, *Guidelines for Establishing Comprehensive Cancer Patient Education Services* (NCI, 1999, 36 pp.), to guide these educators in developing local resources for cancer patient education. In addition, the OCICE distributes a resource list to all these educators listing available learning tools, and it convenes annual meetings to discuss advances in patient education (Crosson, 1999). At institutions such as Fox Chase Cancer Center, these educators are active in keeping patients informed about such matters as hospice and burial arrangements (Herman, 1999).

Shortcomings

Despite the presence of multiple outlets for discussions with trained health professionals about end-of-life concerns, patients and their families remain undereducated about hospice care, symptom management, and psychosocial realities. Reports indicate that patients' experiences with cancer are often characterized by uncertainty and ambiguity (Yates and Stetz, 1999). Why are patients not receiving this information?

One explanation is that they are not asking for it. Physicians report that it falls on them to initiate discussions about terminal care, indicating that patients are reluctant to bring up the topics of death and dying in face-to-face conversations (Pfeifer et al., 1994). This reluctance is partly attributable to the general cultural attitude that rejects death as an option, leading to strong feelings of denial or, at the very least, making discussions about death and dying uncomfortable for patients and their families. In addition, patients' personal views of their health and medical prognosis influence their avoidance of such discussion. A paper from the Study to Understand Prognoses and Preferences for Outcomes and Risks of Treatment (SUPPORT) indicates that patients' estimates of their prognoses influence their personal treatment preferences and that patients generally overestimate their chances for survival (Weeks et al., 1998). If patients and their family members do not realize that death is approaching, they cannot be expected to be active participants in such discussions with their health care providers. A thin line exists in the minds of patients and health professionals between genuine hope and pragmatic acceptance of death and disability.

Recent studies indicate that even when patients and their family members are fully educated about their end-of-life options, they can misunderstand the information they are given (Smith and Swisher, 1998; Tattersall et al., 1994). For example, even after much publicity and laws mandating the discussion of advanced directives with hospital patients, studies have indicated that many patients do not know what advanced directives are and why they matter in end-of-life situations (IOM, 1997). Some factors contributing to this misunderstanding have already been identified, including the stress and anxiety surrounding the communication of information about death, patients' denial of their health status, and health providers' tendency to use technical jargon without further explanation (Tattersall, 1994). At the other extreme, patients can feel confused or overwhelmed if they receive information from too many sources, for example, lectures and informational materials from the physician, the nurse, the social worker, and the patient educator. It is important for health care professionals not only to communicate end-of-life issues, but also to ensure that the people on the receiving end of the discussion can digest what is being said.

A second major reason for the failure of these health provider resources to inform patients about end-of-life issues is the inadequate general implementation of many of these patient education initiatives. For example, the NCI patient educator program does not provide additional funds to the cancer centers for the program (Crosson, 1999). As such, the proficiency and level of involvement of these educators can vary widely; personal interviews with people at these institutions suggest that the directors of some cancer centers do not even know patient educators exist. Another illustration of this deficiency can be found in the execution of advanced directives, mandated by law in some states and by hospital policy in some institutions. Many physicians and nurses will admit that these forms are often handed to newly admitted patients among a large stack of paperwork with little explanation. In this milieu, it is no wonder that these patients, even after signing an advanced directive, might still claim no knowledge of what one is.

Finally, even though many NCI-designated cancer centers might advertise themselves as extremely effective sources of patient education and information, the number of people who have access to these institutions is limited. The NCI reports that 80 percent of terminal cancer patients are cared for in community hospital settings (Crosson, 1999). Also, the 58 NCI-designated centers are not uniformly distributed throughout the nation, representing only 29 states and the District of Columbia. Therefore, the great majority of dying cancer patients cannot or do not have access to their resources. Calling or mailing these centers is not an option: an informal telephone survey of the centers indicated that the great majority of them are currently reluctant (or unable) to provide information to outsiders who are not, or have not been, patients at their institution.

The current deficiencies in communication between patients and their physicians about end-of-life issues have many other origins. Poor provider communication skills and knowledge of end-of-life issues, and a health care market that discourages referrals to hospice and rewards medical procedures and treatments over cognitive therapy, are also sad, but true, reasons that keep patients out of terminal care. These issues lie outside the scope of this chapter, however.

Future Directions

One important way to resolve these deficiencies in patient-provider communication is for patients to become better information consumers. We must work to raise expectations about the education patients should receive when their cancer is no longer curable. If the public is aware of palliative care and end-of-life benefits and, as a result, expects to learn about issues such as pain control or advanced directives, then patients and their family members will solicit this information from their health care provider. They will not only engage in discussions they might not have otherwise, but they will also try to overcome ambiguities or misunderstandings that currently can prevent the execution of superior end-of-life cancer care.

Accomplishing this educational effort will be complex, but some prototypical initiatives are already under way. The Robert Wood Johnson Foundation (RWJF), through its "Last Acts" program, is funding projects aimed at consumer empowerment. Among other programs, Last Acts is currently supporting a consultant to help plan public engagement initiatives in end-of-life care, the development of a public television series on end of life, and a public education effort to promote a long-term care system to "allow aging with dignity" (RWJF, 1999). Another methodology is found in the Conquering Pain Act of 1999, a proposed amendment to the Public Health Service Act, which would ensure that all materials distributed on pain management include language, where relevant, to inform people that they should "expect" to have their pain managed (U.S. Congress, 1999a). Working through these and other proposed methodologics, we can begin to impart the need for terminal or disabled cancer patients to seek out proper education on end-of-life issues.

In addition, the NCI and the 58 cancer centers could expand their educational resources. The NCI and many centers have the institutional resources to become focal points of vigorous patient education efforts. The NCI is already taking some steps in this direction. The OCICE is currently beginning work with the Association of Community Cancer Centers to expand the reach of its educational initiatives (Crosson, 1999). Yet more needs to be done. The NCI and the centers should better integrate and support the patient educator program, so that it can serve as an effective information-gathering tool at more institutions. They also could make their educational and informational resources more widely available, for example, to hospice patients not associated with their systems or to patients or family members who contact them over the phone or by e-mail. One way to do this would be for the NCI to make the development of these high-quality educational programs essential to a cancer center's NCI sponsorship. This type of "top-down" policy initiative has worked before in this arena. In 1997, the Veterans Health Administration (VHA) commenced a quality performance measure mandating comprehensive palliative care planning for patients diagnosed as terminally ill, which encompassed six different factors, from advanced directives to pain and symptom management. As a result, the hospitals in the network individually took measures to improve their performance, and an external chart review analysis of VHA patients showed an increase in compliance with the national end-of-life care plan from 52 percent in late 1996 to 94 percent by mid-1999 (Ryan, 1999). Creating model patient education programs at these centers will place institutional pressure on the smaller hospitals to improve their facilities as well.

Finally, the deficiencies in patient-provider interactions about end-of-life care must be further explored. Studies have already indicated that if patients and their family members are provided educational information by their physicians, it helps support the patient, reinforce treatment goals, and assist in managing the side effects of therapy and disease (Ferrell et al., 1995). Yet more must be learned about the preferences and attitudes of terminal cancer patients regarding the discussion of death and dying, such as when in the course of their treatment these issues are best broached, how the information can be imparted most clearly, and whether they really understand what they are being told. It is also important to analyze ethnic and cultural diversity in the way people are most comfortable receiving this information and how these differences influence the effectiveness of educational efforts.

Armed with this information, cancer centers, professional organizations, and patient educators can begin to bridge the communication gap between health professionals and patients. Physicians and researchers are already making advances in this field. The NCI and RWJF are supporting various studies, including ones to research Americans' values regarding end-of-life care and to survey the educational needs of patients and their family caregivers regarding pain management (Ferrell et al., 1999). Some enterprising oncologists and hospital staffs are developing new communication tools, such as videotapes or personalized audiotapes, to make patients more aware of end-of-life issues and their health status in general (Ryan, 1999; Tattersall et al., 1994). The NCI, RWJF, and other institutions that fund research initiatives should place more emphasis on investigating patient preferences for learning about terminal and palliative care and novel techniques for improving the flow of information.

ACQUIRING END-OF-LIFE INFORMATION FROM THE NCI AND ACS

Resources Available

Terminal cancer patients or their family members who want more specialized, in-depth, or hands-on information about certain aspects of their illness, their future expectations, and their end-of-life care look to sources outside the immediate interactions with their health care providers. The materials they obtain reinforce their personal discussions, educate family members who might not be able to meet face-to-face with the providers, and provide needed psychological comfort to patients overwhelmed with their terminal prognosis. The NCI and the American Cancer Society (ACS) write the majority of the supplementary educational materials for cancer patients in the form of booklets, pamphlets, and fact sheets. These products can be obtained at no cost by direct solicitation, in waiting rooms, in the patient resource rooms that exist at some large cancer centers (such as the Dana Farber Cancer Institute and Fox Chase Cancer Center), and from some other more grassroots or specialized cancer groups. The preponderance of these materials deals with cancer prevention, basic background descriptions of various cancers and their treatments, clinical trials, and survivorship concerns. Only recently have the NCI and ACS begun publishing materials related to end-of-life issues.

The NCI's primary patient-oriented document dealing with terminal cancer is *Advanced Cancer: Living Each Day* (NCI, 1998, 46 pp.). This booklet is divided into four sections: living each day, the personal reaction of cancer patients to their terminal prognosis, the reactions of their friends and family, and choices for care. The first three sections succinctly describe many of the psychosocial concerns of end-of-life care, while the final section tackles more practical issues such as introducing patients to hospice care, advanced directives, family planning, and the Patients' Self-Determination Act. The booklet concludes with a list of supplementary resources and personal checklist and inventory sheets for the patient to use. The NCI publishes other booklets for some of the classic end-of-life concerns: *Eating Hints for Cancer Patients* (NCI, 1999, 60 pp.), *Get Relief From Cancer Pain* (NCI, 1994), *Understanding Cancer Pain* (NCI, 2000), and *Pain Control* (NCI, 2000, 57 pp.), published in conjunction with the ACS.

NCI also offers patients and their family members collections of photocopied pages—to be received by mail or at a fax machine—from NCI's Physician Data Query (PDQ) database and its collection of "Cancer Facts" sheets about various types of cancers and aspects of disease. One section of the PDQ database deals with "Supportive Care Topics" and covers all eight of the Memorial Symptom Assessment Scale end-of-life-related symptoms. In addition, Cancer Facts information sheets exist about hospice care and national and local cancer support organizations.

Finally, the NCI oversees the Cancer Information Service (CIS), a group of 19 resource centers across the country that patients and/or their family members can reach either locally or by calling 1-800-4-CANCER. These centers are independent but can be associated with major cancer centers (e.g., the center in Buffalo is attached to the Roswell Park Cancer Institute). CIS telephone representatives mail patients NCI-produced booklets, PDQ printouts, or Cancer Facts sheets, as well as any other information deemed appropriate to the individual patient's situation (e.g., chapters from textbooks, ACS resources).

In addition to distributing NCI material, the ACS offers its own booklets, including one directed at end-of-life care, called *Caring for the Patient with Cancer at Home* (ACS, 1998; 121 pp.). This booklet focuses on helping loved ones and patients themselves manage the symptoms associated with end-stage cancer. Other chapters explain the function and significance of health insurance, hospice care, and certain signs of approaching death. The book is written in simple language with one explanatory section for each topic, followed by points of what to do and what not to do. The ACS also offers source packs of information tailored for individual educational needs by counselors assigned to those who contact the ACS (either by calling 1-800-ACS-2345 or e-mailing ACS from its Web site). These packets can include chapters from its booklets, as well as more extensive notes on "Hospice Concept" and "Coping with Grief and Loss."

Shortcomings

Despite the NCI's and ACS' recent efforts, these organizations still inadequately address the range of terminal cancer patients' end-of-life concerns. One significant issue is the sheer lack of resources devoted to a topic that, even with modern advances in medical sciences, half of all cancer patients will face. *Advanced Cancer*, the one NCI-sponsored booklet on end-of-life concerns, can be contrasted with the 24 booklets the NCI produces on different types of cancer. The notion that one treatise can satisfy educational needs for the varied types of death and issues related to death is as incongruous as producing a booklet called *Solid Tumors* to provide background information on cancers of the breast, gastrointestinal (GI) tract, lung, and so forth. In addition, although the NCI reprints some of its booklets in Spanish, nearly all of these end-of-life materials are currently available only in English. This puts an increased burden on patients of Hispanic, Asian, or Russian descent, et cetera, who must face these issues and either do not speak English or use it as a second language.

Of greater concern is the lack of end-of-life content found in books not designed specifically for terminal disease. For example, the NCI booklet, *What You Need to Know About Ovarian Cancer* (NCI, 1993; 30 pp.) mentions nothing about the possibility that a patient might die of an ovarian tumor. The issue of death is introduced only with suggestions to "talk with the doctor about [your] chance of recovery" and a warning that "the disease can return." For a type of cancer often diagnosed at its late, terminal stages, this disregard for terminal or palliative care is disconcerting. ACS materials tend to be somewhat more realistic. The ACS document on lung cancer relays the generally low overall survival rates from lung cancer and, in its discussion of the treatment options for lung cancer, breaks down the five-year survival percentages at each stage. Significantly, the ACS suggests "supportive care" as a viable choice for patients diagnosed as Stage IV non-small cell lung cancer and mentions the importance of treating pain and weight loss. Still, for another cancer that is most often diagnosed at its later stages, these paragraphs are given less space than highly investigational treatments such as "immunotherapy" and "gene therapy" and thus underemphasize the importance of end-of-life care. The supplementary materials that the NCI and ACS offer to deal with other end-of-life symptoms (e.g., pain and loss of appetite) also mention little about death and dying. The 1997 booklet *When Cancer Recurs: Meeting the Challenge Again* discusses pain control during treatment, but mentions nothing about palliative care more generally.

The NCI and ACS materials are also filled with troubling "symbolic language." The title of the NCI book on terminal care, *Advanced Cancer: Living Each Day*, is just one illustration of how the NCI and ACS use oft-misunderstood euphemisms when discussing death and palliative care. Although this inclination in part reflects the feelings of patients and society in general, by evading straightforward discussions of these topics, the NCI inadvertently helps propagate an ignorance of the real issues. Another aspect of this symbolic treatment of death can be seen in the NCI's and ACS' separation of their cancer information books into books about the disease and its treatment and those about death and palliative care. By separating cancer care in the eyes of patients into treating the disease, on one hand, and dying from it, on the other, these documents can subvert the notion of continuity of care—quality treatment by trained professionals from diagnosis to conclusion, no matter what that outcome may be. Any model of care should include all potential outcomes of their disease, so that patients understand they will not be abandoned if their curative treatment is unsuccessful, and this should be emphasized in the literature they read.

Finally, materials produced by NCI, ACS, and other organizations about end-of-life care are useful only if they find their way into the hands of patients and their families. Of the 235,000 calls that NCI's CIS received in 1998 from patients and their family or friends, only 6,065 (2.5 percent) of these concerned metastatic cancer and only 798 callers (0.34 percent) callers specifically inquired about hospice (Thomsen, 1999). Moreover, it appears that patients facing death or disability may not receive palliative care and end-of-life materials unless they explicitly ask for them. A caller contacted both the NCI and the ACS hotlines to acquire information on treatment options and expectations on behalf of an 85-year-old family member just diagnosed with inoperable non-small cell lung cancer. Neither organization sent its designated palliative care or end-of-life materials. A subsequent call was made regarding a 78-year-old family member with inoperable non-small cell lung cancer, whose disease was "progressing" after three months of chemotherapy and radiation and who was experiencing a lot of pain. A similar information request was made. Although the organizations now sent their resources on pain management, neither organization sent its specific end-of-life materials. Both of these situations present strong indications that death may be approaching and certainly suggest the possibility of treatment with palliative intent. Yet, in these instances, NCI and ACS cancer specialists are put in a difficult and delicate situation because they cannot determine how callers who do not explicitly ask for end-of-life care materials will respond to being sent such information unsolicited. Still, the end result is that necessary information is not communicated.

Future Directions

The NCI and ACS are currently working to improve their end-of-life materials; the NCI is revising *Advanced Cancer* (Ades, 1999; Crosson, 1999). However, these organizations could spearhead a more comprehensive evaluation of their extant materials, analyzing the amount and quality of information relayed to patients, as well as the more sweeping notions of symbolic language and continuity of care. The results should be incorporated into a list of specific concerns and recommendations regarding the adequacy of the end-of-life and palliative care content and the symbolic language of the NCI and ACS materials. Through this effort, NCI and ACS should be inspired to develop more realistic and culturally relevant information booklets—translated, if there is sufficient demand, into Spanish and other languages—that are more responsive to the needs of cancer patients.

The NCI and ACS must subsequently intensify their efforts to distribute these supplementary materials so more patients get them. By targeting community oncology offices, hospitals, and support groups, in addition to the larger NCI-sponsored cancer centers, these organizations can use their considerable resources and influence to support the dissemination to patients of materials that address end-of-life and palliative care. As indicated in the previous section, this information may represent the first time some patients or their family members hear about hospice, advanced directives, and other topics and might therefore help stimulate discussion between cancer patients and their health care providers.

Improving the quality of communication about end-of-life issues from the NCI and ACS hotlines is one important way to support this information distribution effort, because records show that hundreds of thousands of people and patients call these hotlines each month (Ades, 1999; Thomsen, 1999). Members of the NCI and ACS support staff need to recognize better when palliative care or end-of-life information is appropriate and should perhaps be given methodologies by which to start discussions with callers on these issues. The NCI and ACS should develop more specific guidelines for these specialists and counselors that address the need for education about death and dying, in addition to diagnosis and treatment concerns.

ACQUIRING END-OF-LIFE INFORMATION FROM OTHER ORGANIZATIONAL RESOURCES

Resources Available

Numerous other organizations supplement and complement the NCI and ACS in their efforts to educate cancer patients and their family members. All of these groups issue their own educational materials (and may distribute NCI and ACS booklets as well), and some are also designed to set up patients with "peer counselors," other non-health professionals who have survived the patients' particular cancer diagnosis. Among their many topics, they handle end-of-life care issues.

General cancer organizations have grown out of grassroots advocacy efforts by citizens and private institutions, and these organizations devote some resources to end-of-life care issues. Cancer Care, Inc., in New York, for example, offers written materials, personal support from trained social workers, and telephone educational programs and conferences on such topics as coping strategies, pain, and cancer fatigue. Cancer Care distributes four "Cancer Care Briefs"—three- to five-page pamphlets on issues in cancer treatment, prevention, and resources—to address different concerns of people with advanced cancer and a number of others specifically directed at symptom management. Cancer Care can also disburse information from a rich library of practical, psychosocial, and medical information produced by its specialists, or acquired from other institutions, about palliative care and end-of-life issues.

Many groups also exist to inform and advocate on behalf of patients with a particular type of cancer (e.g., the National Association of Breast Cancer Organizations [NABCO], the Alliance for Lung Cancer Advocacy, Support, and Education [ALCASE], and the National Kidney Cancer Association [NKCA]). Some also offer resources to terminal patients with a particular cancer. NABCO, for one, compiles a list of manuscripts that deal with "recurrence and metastatic breast cancer" and will give inquiring callers directions on how to obtain these materials. ALCASE has published a 12-chapter *Lung Cancer Manual* (200 pp.) that integrates palliative care and end-of-life issues into all aspects of its discussions. NKCA's *We Have Kidney Cancer* (1991, 52 pp.) provides background information on kidney cancer cause and treatment and includes a chapter on dealing with death. In addition, NKCA publishes *Reflections* (1997, 62 pp.), a physician-written guide to end-of-life issues for patients and their families, which it will also freely include in mailings to interested parties.

Relatively few organizations dedicate themselves specifically to end-of-life concerns in cancer care. One major institution, the National Hospice Organization (NHO), produces informational pamphlets on hospice care for patients or their loved ones who contact the NHO with questions. The American Pain Society, Wisconsin Cancer Pain Initiative, and City of Hope Pain/Palliative Care Resource Center are among the groups that advocate for the relief of pain and thus serve as important informational resources for terminal cancer patients. They offer support, advice, and a few supplementary publications on pain control (though most of their written materials are directed at health care professionals). Some initiatives are under way to create more such resource centers that specifically focus on end-of-life care. For example, the proposed Advance Planning and Compassionate Care Act of 1999 would establish an information clearinghouse and telephone hotline for end-of-life decisionmaking under the auspices of the Department of Health and Human Services (U.S. Congress, 1999b).

Pharmaceutical companies who manufacture drugs used in terminal care have also developed educational materials. Ortho Biotech, which distributes the cancer fatigue agent Procrit (erythropoietin), has developed a document for patients on psychological and practical tips to help overcome cancer fatigue (one of the eight primary end-of-life symptoms). Roxane

Laboratories—makers of morphine, oxycodone, and clonidine anti-pain medications—runs an on-line Pain Institute to answer patient questions about pain control. Janssen Pharmaceutica (which makes Duragesic, another alternative for pain management) also offers articles on recent advances in pain control and tips for people with chronic pain on its Web site.

Shortcomings

The major drawback to the effectiveness of these organizations is that not enough cancer patients use them. A 1992 study of cancer survivors revealed that only 11 percent contacted cancer organizations (including the higher-profile NCI and ACS) after their diagnosis for information or support (Hewitt et al., 1999). Potentially fewer patients use them for questions specifically relating to end-of-life care. The NABCO information services reveal that although they get anywhere from 20 to 100 calls a day, at most one or two callers a month request hospice or end-of-life care information (McClure, 1999). The NKCA reports that the majority of its contacts are with newly diagnosed renal cell carcinoma patients and that most requests for its *Reflections* booklet come from the medical community (Dison, 1999). There are numerous explanations for these findings. Many of these organizations are small, not-for-profit entities, and so cannot take the steps needed to increase their national exposure. Moreover, patients and their family members might not think to contact these organizations because they believe—justifiably or not—that their personal physician or social worker has provided them with all the relevant information about their disease, treatment options, and what to expect in the future. Furthermore, patients may be in denial or feel self-conscious about their health status and not want to share information they consider private outside the provider-patient relationship. It is hard to reach out for new information when overwhelmed with recent bad news.

Another significant problem is that these organizations vary widely in how well they address end-of-life issues. As indicated above, Cancer Care, Inc., NABCO, ALCASE, and NKCA proficiently integrate palliative care information into all their materials. On the other hand, the National Brain Tumor Association (NBTA) publishes *A Primer of Brain Tumors: A Patient's Reference Manual* (1998, 140 pp.), which never mentions palliative care or the potential for disability and death – not even in the final five page section on "Comfort and Coping." The National Ovarian Cancer Coalition (NOCC), an organization dedicated to "providing complete and accurate information regarding ovarian cancer," sends inquiring patients a large packet of materials on ovarian cancer. However, end-of-life issues are addressed either obliquely, such as by including an Ortho Biotech pamphlet on cancer fatigue, or not at all, as in the NOCC publication *Myths and*

Facts About Ovarian Cancer: What You Need to Know (1997, 64 pp.), which does not discuss palliative care.

In addition, these organizations have limited abilities to adapt the information they distribute to the individual needs of patients. An informal survey indicated that most patients who call, no matter how advanced their condition is, receive the same introductory packet and pamphlets (or a small variation thereof). As a result, while brochures offering hope and goals for living with cancer are appropriate to patients with early-stage disease, these same "educational" materials are being sent to patients with advanced, recurrent, or terminal cancer. This is indicative of a more general inability of some of these organizations to deal with the informational needs of dying or disabled patients.

Perhaps partly as a result of the inadequate information emerging from these sources, pharmaceutical companies that dispense palliative care drugs have started developing their own educational materials. However, letting companies that have a financial stake in end-of-life care be a primary source of education and background information about these concerns can be problematic. For example, the nature of the information produced will inherently be biased and focused, because a pharmaceutical firm that produces an antiemetic has little economic reason to alert people to cancer fatigue, and vice versa. As a result, patients get exposed only to a very piecemeal approach to palliative care education.

Future Directions

Many of these groups should consider increasing their exposure if they are going to be helpful in informing patients and their families about end-of-life care. If more terminal cancer patients contacted Cancer Care, Inc., for example, they could use its many useful resources—both written and verbal—to learn about the parameters of their palliative and end-of-life care. This goal can be pursued on many different fronts. Research on cancer patient preferences and information-gathering behavior should be undertaken, with an emphasis on surveying patients for their views of these organizations and trying to learn how to increase patients' use of them. In addition, supporting joint educational initiatives among these various grassroots, or cancer-specific, organizations and the NCI can plug these groups into a wider range of financial and institutional assets. For example, the NCI's CIS and Cancer Care, Inc., have developed a referral partnership, where NCI cancer information specialists refer patients who need support for psychosocial issues to a Cancer Care social worker, while the Cancer Care staff refers calls requiring technical information to the NCI (Thomsen, 1999). Steps must also be taken to teach health providers, community hospitals, and cancer centers of the existence and availability of these groups, as well as ways in which they can help educate patients about the various aspects of their disease, including end-of-life care.

Equally as important as raising popular consciousness about these organizations is helping them create comprehensive materials that address palliative care and end-of-life issues and integrating materials into their current cancer diagnosis and curative treatment resources. This can be accomplished in different ways. The RWJF is currently supporting a project to create a multimedia curriculum on end-of-life issues for grassroots organizations (RWJF, 1999). Also, these organizations can be encouraged to work with specialists in terminal disease when developing resources. Producing these materials will also give these groups a degree of latitude in the informational material they make available to patients or their family members who call. In this way, the young patient newly diagnosed with a potentially incurable brain tumor will not be inappropriately inundated with end-of-life care materials when calling the NBTA, but an older patient who is more likely to face a terminal diagnosis can be properly educated about his or her treatment options and expectations.

One final objective is increased interorganizational communication. Sharing knowledge and information among the organizations—for example, such as about new methods of increasing exposure, educational tools, and untapped funding resources—will help each group individually pursue its goals of patient education and advocacy. This is especially true with respect to terminal care and the promotion of patient and family education about end-of-life issues. For, while not every type of cancer is treated the same or results in similar psychosocial concerns, every organization that deals with cancer patients will have a certain percentage of patrons facing the prospect of disability and death. Encouraging these groups to work together to educate terminal cancer patients about these issues will stimulate further progress in this developing field.

ACQUIRING END-OF-LIFE INFORMATION FROM THE WORLD WIDE WEB

Resources Available

The Internet, and in particular the graphical World Wide Web, is emerging as a major source of information because it is a powerful archival medium with fast search capabilities. Cancer patients and their family members can instantaneously receive voluminous amounts of materials from sources all over the world, while conveniently (and anonymously) exploring on-line from home, work, or their local library. In addition, the interactive nature of the Web allows people to communicate with personal counselors or support groups, watch or listen to audiovisual clips, and sift quickly through extraneous materials to find the information that fills their particular needs. As a result, many organizations and institutions have started utilizing this medium to distribute information on end-of-life cancer care issues.

Health care providers have thus far made only limited forays into cyberspace. Most independent physician offices do not integrate Web technology into their private practices. However, those physicians who are currently comfortable interacting on-line report that this communication tool allows their patients more time to ask questions and get answers about many topics, including end-of-life concerns (Davis and Miller, 1999). All of the NCI-designated cancer centers support their own Web sites, in which they detail the resources they offer and provide some basic information about end-of-life care. The Johns Hopkins Oncology Center Web site, for example, has a "Guide to Cancer Services" page, which discusses pain control expectations patients should have and the types of support services offered by the center (Johns Hopkins Medicine, 1999).

Nearly all of the cancer organizations that patients and their family members have traditionally contacted by phone or letter have now constructed Web pages to disseminate their informational resources. Some, like Cancer Care, Inc. (http://www.cancercareinc.org) and ALCASE (http://www.alcase.org), offer free on-line reprints of their publications. Others, like the National Coalition for Cancer Survivorship (NCCS) (http://www.cansearch.org), allow visitors convenient ways to order materials. Cancer Care, Inc., also provides on-line support groups. Many organizations, in addition to listing their own information on their sites, supply detailed lists of other on-line resources and hyperlinks to those Web pages, to help patients and health professionals navigate more intelligently around cyberspace and find the information they need. This hyperlink network also promotes less publicized organizations and sites that novice Web users might not find on their own. The NCCS resource database, for example, offers brief descriptions and links to organizations more specifically able to provide psychosocial support to cancer patients and those that can help deal with pain. Through this dense network, patients or their family members who reach one site can begin to broaden their expectations about the various facets of proper end-of-life care (NCCS, 1999).

For additional support, entirely Web-based sources of patient education and information have emerged. On-line clinics have emerged that offer the services of physicians to answer medical questions, as well as diagnose patients or issue prescriptions. One of them, CyberDocs (http://www.cyberdocs.com), records nearly 100,000 visitors per month, indicating its growing popularity (Melton, 1999). Among the articles on its site, to which the on-line support staff can refer inquiring visitors, are those describing hospice care and advanced directives. Other sites, such as the

University of Pennsylvania Cancer Center's Oncolink (http://www.oncolink.com) or DrKoop.com (http://www.drkoop.com), do not offer interactive services, but instead provide the latest information and hyperlinks for cancer patients. A search for "end-of-life issues" on the Oncolink page, for example, led to on-line book reviews of palliative care handbooks, hospice information sites, video downloads with such titles as "Focus on the Final Months," and numerous related articles and hyperlinks.

Shortcomings

The biggest hurdle to effective use of the Web to educate patients and their family members about end-of-life issues is access. Surfing the Internet requires a computer, a modem, and a Web browser, which can be too expensive for some people. Also, the Web has its own distinct technique and language, which is less familiar to older people, who may be uncomfortable in cyberspace (though this will undoubtedly change with the aging of those growing up with access to cyberspace). In 1998, only about 15 percent of Americans using the Internet were older than 50 (Lewis, 1998). Yet this is currently the age group most likely to be diagnosed with cancer and to face difficult end-of-life issues. Still more vexing are the statistics showing most Internet users to be Caucasian and male, indicating that Web-based resources are not reaching entire groups of people—no matter what their wealth or age. Unless these racial, gender, and age-related barriers can be overcome, it may be inappropriate to allocate time and resources to developing Internet end-of-life tools at the expense of the further development of traditional materials. At the least, these Internet-based efforts must be complemented by outreach to populations underserved by the Web.

In addition to access, a major problem is the quality of the information—when and whether to trust the information one finds. The Internet does not provide an automatic check for financial or ideological self-interest. Since there are no restrictions or protections about what information is placed on-line, people can call themselves "experts" and post information, with impunity, that may be out-of-date, misleading, or just plain false. In fact, a recent study of medical HTML (hypertext markup language) pages concluded, "The bulk of information ... is of low applicability and poor quality for answering clinical questions" (Hersh et al., 1998). This limitation is exacerbated by the currently fragmented state of end-of-life information on the Web. Materials on death and dying are scattered diffusely across many different sites purporting to help inform terminal cancer patients about their options. In this milieu, it is difficult for terminal cancer patients or their family members using Internet technology to decipher which advice about end-of-life issues is accurate and evidence based, and which is not.

Future Directions

At this point, with the Web and Internet technology still early in their overall development, increased research should be the main objective regarding the use of this medium to help promote quality end-of-life cancer care. More work needs to be done to identify whether terminal cancer patients and their family members utilize Web-based resources to gather information and, if so, how they can best acquire the necessary education on-line. Research-funding agencies should solicit projects that use the Web to manage end-of-life issues, while addressing pitfalls such as access, reliability of information, and security and confidentiality of discussions. Some inroads have already been made in this area—for example, the American Medical Informatics Association promulgated its "Guidelines for the Clinical Use of Electronic Mail with Patients" (Kane and Sands, 1998)—but more study of patient preferences and attitudes is necessary.

In conjunction with this research, new and innovative ways to use the Web to educate patients needing palliative and end-of-life care have to be developed. One of the primary promises of Internet technology is its ability to go beyond the traditional written materials, or telephone support, in the provision of information. For example, an Internet interactive problem-solving package for people with pain is currently under construction. This Internet modality allows patients and their family members to seek information, while concurrently getting feedback on ways to solve their palliative care problems, so that the users can learn to be problem solvers and not have to rely solely on health professionals (Loscalzo, 1999). We should not be satisfied simply with encouraging the development of Web resources to reprint current written materials and need to support similar ground-breaking ways to disseminate information on palliative and terminal cancer care.

CONCLUSION

The current state of patient and family informational resources about end-of-life cancer care offers many opportunities for terminal cancer patients to obtain the education they need about the medical, practical, and psychosocial concerns that accompany disability and death. Numerous avenues for contact with health professionals exist, as well as a growing library of supplementary resources available from a range of organizations and through various media. However, the fact that many dying and disabled cancer patients remain undereducated about such topics as pain management and palliative care, hospice, and advanced directives indicates that this information is not effectively reaching patients. The reasons for this failure are manifold and relate not only to the poor quality of some of the information and its dissemination, but also to the behaviors of the patients themselves.

To promote the overall quality of palliative and terminal cancer care, the extant information about end-of-life care and its delivery from health care providers, supplementary organizations, and Internet resources must be improved. Some initial suggestions to accomplish this are summarized below.

HEALTH PROFESSIONAL RESOURCES

• Make patients better health consumers and raise their expectations for end-of-life care.
• Develop the 58 NCI-sponsored cancer centers into models of patient education and information delivery.
• Study patients' preferences regarding the delivery of effective end-of-life care information, with an eye toward ethnic and cultural diversity in attitudes.

NCI AND ACS

• Evaluate and subsequently improve extant materials on terminal and palliative care, with emphasis on cultural relevance, symbolic language, and the continuity of care.
• Distribute these materials more universally.
• Improve communication of end-of-life and palliative care information through the popular information hotlines.

OTHER ORGANIZATIONAL RESOURCES

• Increase national exposure of these organizations as sources of patient and family information.
• Evaluate and subsequently improve their educational materials to make these resources more sensitive to patients' end-of-life concerns.
• Increase interorganizational communication and association to address more effectively the concerns of all terminal and disabled cancer patients.
• Point out to pharmaceutical companies the pitfalls of piecemeal, vested-interest approaches to end-of-life care education and encourage them to refocus their informational materials.

THE WORLD WIDE WEB

• Study the ways in which Internet informational resources can most effectively be made available to terminal cancer patients and their families.

• Develop innovative uses of Internet technology to impart information about end-of-life concerns.

REFERENCES

Abe CA. Director of Social Work, Jonsson Comprehensive Cancer Center, University of California at Los Angeles, personal communication, June 14, 1999.

Ades T. Nurse, American Cancer Society, personal communication, August 1, 1999.

Crosson K. Director, Office of Cancer Information, Communication, and Education, National Cancer Institute, personal communication, July 7, 1999.

Davis R and Miller L. Net empowering patients. *USA Today* July 14, 1999, 1A.

Dison C. President and Executive Director, National Kidney Cancer Association. Personal communication, July 27, 1999.

Ferrell BR, et al. The impact of cancer pain education on family caregivers of elderly patients. *Oncology Nursing Forum* 1995;22(8):1211-1218.

Ferrell BR, et al. Family caregiving in cancer pain management. *Journal of Palliative Medicine* 1999;2(2):185-195.

Herman L. Director of Social Work, Fox Chase Cancer Center. Personal communication, June 15, 1999.

Hersh WR et al. Applicability and quality of information for answering clinical questions on the Web. *Journal of the American Medical Association* 1998;280(15):1307-1308.

Hewitt M et al. Cancer prevalence and survivorship issues: analyses of the 1992 National Health Interview Survey. *Journal of the National Cancer Institute* 1999 In press.

Institute of Medicine (IOM). 1997. *Approaching Death: Improving Care at the End of Life.* Cassel CK and Field MJ, eds. Washington, D.C.: National Academy Press.

Institute of Medicine. 1999. *The Unequal Burden of Cancer.* Haynes MA, Smedley BD, eds. Washington, D.C.: National Academy Press.

Johns Hopkins Medicine. Your Guide to Cancer Services. 1999. http://hopkins.med.jhu.edu/PatientInfo/cancer.guide.html.

Kane B, Sands DZ. Guidelines for the clinical use of electronic mail with patients. *Journal of the American Medical Informatics Association* 1998;5(1):104-111.

Lewis R. The Web: a new world opens up. *AARP Bulletin* 1998; 39(2):1, 14.

Loscalzo M. Co-director of the Cancer Pain Service, Johns Hopkins Oncology Center. Personal communication, July 10, 1999.

McClure J. Coordinator of Information Services, National Association of Breast Cancer Organizations. Personal communication, July 25, 1999.

Melton M. Online diagnoses: finding more than a doc-in-a-box. *US News and World Report*, June 21, 1999. http://www.usnews.com/usnews/issue/990621/nycu/drugs.b.htm.

NCCS (National Coalition of Cancer Survivorship). CanSearch: Online Guide to Cancer Resources, 1999. http://www.cansearch.org/canserch/canserch.htm.

Nye L. Head of Social Work, Johns Hopkins Medical Institutions. Personal communication, June 28, 1999.

Pfeifer MP et al. The discussion of end-of-life medical care by primary care patients and physicians: a multicenter study using structured qualitative interviews. *Journal of General Internal Medicine* 1994;9(2):82-88.

Portenoy RK, et al. The Memorial Symptom Assessment Scale: an instrument for the evaluation of symptom prevalence, characteristics, and distress. *European Journal of Cancer* 1994;30A(9):1326-1336.

RWJF (Robert Wood Johnson Foundation). Last Acts: End-of-Life Grantees in Public Engagement, 1999. http://www.lastacts.org:80/scripts/la_res01.exe.

Ryan B. Chief, VA Community-Based Care, Office of Geriatrics and Extended Care, Veterans Health Administration. Personal communication, July 29, 1999.

Smith TJ, Swisher K. Telling the truth about terminal cancer. *Journal of the American Medical Association* 1998;279(21):1746-1748.

Tattersall MH et al. The take-home message: patients prefer consultation audiotapes to summary letters. *Journal of Clinical Oncology* 1994;12(6):1305-1311.

Thomsen C. Chief, Cancer Information Service, National Cancer Institute. Personal communication, August 3, 1999.

U.S. Congress. 1999a. Conquering Pain Act of 1999. H.R. 2188. http://thomas.loc.gov/cgi-bin/query/C?c106:./temp/~c106c9Hp5D.

U.S. Congress. 1999b. Advanced Planning and Compassionate Care Act of 1999. S. 628. http://thomas.loc.gov/cgi-bin/query/C?c106:./temp/~c106wEvoVE.

Weeks JC et al. (for the SUPPORT Group). Relationship between cancer patients' predictions of prognosis and their treatment preferences. *Journal of the American Medical Association* 1998;279(21):1709-1714.

Yates P, Stetz KM. Families' awareness of and response to dying. *Oncology Nursing Forum* 1999;26(1):113-120.

5

Palliative Care for African Americans and Other Vulnerable Populations: Access and Quality Issues

Richard Payne, M.D.
Memorial Sloan-Kettering Cancer Center

BACKGROUND—CANCER STATISTICS

The incidence rates for cancer among African Americans is 454/100,000 compared to an incidence rate of 394/100,000 for whites. The incidence rate of cancer among African Americans is increasing by 1.2 percent per year compared to a 0.8 percent increase per year for whites. African Americans have a 50 percent higher rate of myeloma and cancers of the esophagus, cervix, larynx, prostate, stomach, liver, and pancreas. The 1994 American Cancer Society (ACS) cancer mortality rate was also higher for African Americans than for Caucasians. Black men and women continue to experience higher incidence of and higher death rates from cancer than whites, according to recently published statistics. (Greenlee et al., 2001). Data generated from the ACS and the National Cancer Institute's Surveillance, Epidemiology and End Results (SEER) databases reveal that the death rate from cancer for blacks is 222 per 100,000 compared to 167 per 100,000 for whites. ACS statistics also show that over an eight-year period (1989-1996) the five-year relative survival rate was 62 percent for Caucasians versus 49 percent for African Americans (Greenlee et al., 2001).

UNDERUTILIZATION OF PALLIATIVE AND HOSPICE SERVICES

In 1997, the death rate from all causes was 139.2 for blacks compared to 86.2 for whites (LaVeist et al., 2000). Despite higher death rates from cancer and presentation at later stages of disease, and similar statistics for chronic obstructive pulmonary disease (COPD), renal diseases and AIDS, minority groups significantly underutilize palliative and hospice services. In 1990, 93 percent of patients utilizing the Medicare hospice nenefit were Caucasian (Christakis et al., 1996). The National Hospice and Palliative Care Organization (NHPCO) has concluded that less than 10 percent of all hospice patients are African American. In addition, less than 10 percent of patients utilizing hospice services in the national for-profit chains are minorities. Medicare data culled over an eight-year period (1992-1996) supports this conclusion: minorities make up only 14 percent of the U.S. population that is taking advantage of the Medicare hospice benefit. Consequently, costs for African Americans who are not taking advantage of the benefit in the last year of life are substantially greater. According to the Medicare Payment Advisory Commission (MedPAC), the average cost for African Americans in the last year of life was approximately $32,000 compared to $25,000 for Caucasians (Medicare Payment Advisory Commission, 2000). The MedPAC data did not show higher costs in the last year of life for other minority groups. In addition, MedPAC statistics also revealed a higher percentage of non-hospice inpatient deaths for minorities compared with Caucasians. These last two points need more careful review to understand the full implications for financing health care for African Americans and other minorities facing terminal disease.

Barriers to Utilization of Palliative and Hospice Care

If care is to be improved for African-American and other underserved groups when there is a diagnosis of a life-threatening disease or chronic debilitating illness that may end in death, knowledge of the reasons for the current underutilization of palliative care and end-of-life services must be clearly understood. Unequal access to care in general or a lack of access to palliative and end-of-life care services may be one reason for underutilization. Few physicians know about palliative care alternatives, so they are unable to advise their patients adequately and sufficiently. Another reason for underutilization of palliative care services in the African-American community may stem from a lack of knowledge of federal, state, and local benefits associated with end-of-life health care needs. A failure to address specific cultural and spiritual needs of patients that may not be articulated well or at all by the patient and family could also contribute to underutilization of these services.

Historical Perspective

Historical and societal factors also may act as barriers to the use of palliative and hospice care today in the African-American community

(Crawley et al., 2000). Abuses suffered during slavery and its aftermath (Jim Crow laws, segregated, second-class medical care systems, etc.) resulted in poorer management of diseases and more reliance on alternative or folk medicine. Medical experimentation, such as that documented in the National Public Health Service Syphilis Study at Tuskegee, has left a legacy of mistrust vis-à-vis clinical trials and other "experimental" forms of medical treatment that other groups may embrace as a last opportunity for cure, but that African Americans may view as denial of good medical care (Freimuth et al., 2001; Shavers et al., 2000). Added to this history are recent reports of unequal treatment or mistreatment and denial of best practices in the health care system (Freeman and Payne, 2000). Documentation such as this indicates that the mistrust reported by African Americans about the U.S. health care system is well founded in many instances.

This distrust may prevent many from being initiators of end-of-life care dialogues with their physicians or acceptors of offers such as palliative or hospice care; the former is not well understood, and the latter is deemed a "death sentence" and "giving up." This distrust may be particularly acute in settings where so few of the health care professionals who enter these discussions with minority patients are themselves minority (Massad, 2000).

Because African Americans tend to have a higher incidence of violent deaths and higher death rates from cancer, AIDS, and other chronic illnesses, it is imperative that these communities be educated about palliative care and end-of-life preparatory issues. At present, denial of death (even terminal illness) may be viewed by the African-American community as a "healthy response," as fighting to live at all costs. Communities must be educated to the choices that are (or should be) available and that a denial of death may not be the healthiest response to the end of life's journey. Indeed, such a response may result in not getting the best care at the end of life. Conversely, it must be explained that palliative care does not mean "giving up" and dialogues about palliative care and end-of-life care are not a subterfuge for further denial of access to good medical care. Cultural and personal values must be respected, and physicians, allied health care professionals, and clergy must be trained to handle these discussions and the decisions patients and their families must face.

MINORITY ISSUES IN PALLIATIVE AND HOSPICE CARE

What role does a lack of access to health care play in shaping attitudes about end-of-life care? Studies report that African Americans are admitted to intensive care units (ICUs) less often than whites (Yergan et al., 1987). African Americans are less likely to opt for discontinuation of life support measures (Caralis et al., 1993). There is a strong perception that they will be treated differently and receive inferior care if advanced directives have been signed (McKinley et al., 1996). Blacks are also more likely to opt for aggressive treatment interventions even in a persistent vegetative state and generally tend to question the "humanitarian motives" of predominately white hospice workers (Neuberger and Hamilton, 1990). Based on results of a survey, it appears that African-American physicians place a higher value on length of life than do Caucasian physicians. This survey also revealed that African-American physicians are more likely to support cardiopulmonary resuscitation (CPR), mechanical ventilation, dialysis, and artificial feeding for themselves if they were in a persistent vegetative state (PVS) (McKinley et al., 1996; Mebane et al., 1999).

PHYSICIAN INFLUENCE ON END-OF-LIFE CARE

Physicians play a critical role in the lives of their terminally ill patients. Yet the majority of physicians were not trained in medical school or in continuing education courses about caring for patients at the end of life, communicating effectively and compassionately with them and their families, understanding the impact of cultural differences in addressing medical treatment at the end of life, or the importance of utilizing the full spectrum of medical support professionals in caring for these patients. There appear to be significant differences in attitudes between African-American and white physicians about care at the end of their patients' lives and their own (Mebane et al., 1999). For example, white physicians more often view tube feedings as "heroic" measures in terminally ill patients than do African-American physicians (58 percent vs. 25 percent). In this same study, 36 percent of white physicians accept physician-assisted suicide (PAS) as a treatment alternative, while only 26.5 percent of African-American physicians do. When asked about care for themselves at the end of life, this study also observed startling differences between white and black physicians. For example, if in PVS, African-American physicians were six times more likely than whites to request aggressive treatment. In a scenario in which the doctors might be brain damaged but not terminally ill, the majority of both groups did not want aggressive treatment, but African-American physicians were five times more likely than whites to request specific aggressive treatment (23 percent vs 5 percent) and white physicians were two times more likely to request PAS than African Americans (22.5 percent vs. 9 percent).

Although African Americans constitute 13.8 percent of the U.S. population only 2.9 percent of the physician work force are African Americans; 30 percent of African Americans are cared for by African-American physicians (Byrd et al., 1994).

IMPROVING ACCESS TO AND QUALITY OF PALLIATIVE CARE FOR AFRICAN AMERICANS—HOW DO WE MOVE FORWARD?

Next Steps: Immediate Implementation

Several activities are needed to improve access to and the quality of palliative and end-of-life care for African Americans and other underserved minority populations. Three activities that can be initiated relatively quickly should be put in place simultaneously across different community settings (urban, inner city, rural, etc.).

1. Palliative care units should be established in hospitals. In inner-city locations, end-of-life care for the poor could be initiated until hospice care becomes a more realistic and accepted option.
2. Teams of health care professionals across different settings need to be trained to understand palliative and end-of-life care and be funded to develop programs to provide this care.
3. Focus groups should be conducted in communities to gain a better understanding of the needs of patients and families.

A model program that incorporates these elements has been started in Harlem, at North General Hospital (NGH), in collaboration with Memorial Sloan-Kettering Cancer Center (MSKCC) (see Box 5-1). NGH was chosen as the site for this model program for three reasons:

1. There are already existing collaborations between NGH and MSKCC, and in fact, a $5 million gift from the Ralph Lauren Foundation was recently announced to support a collaborative cancer center.
2. North General Hospital, a 200-bed institution, is of "manageable" size to initiate and evaluate a program of this type. The educational programs and the pre- and post-intervention surveys are more feasible than they would be in the other two, much larger, Harlem hospitals.
3. NGH is a private hospital (not a part of the New York Health and Hospitals Corporation), and therefore, it will be easier to implement administrative changes and measure their effects in a less bureaucracy-laden system. However, once the effectiveness of these interventions has been documented, the model (or major components of it) could be replicated in public hospitals.

Long-Term Steps

• Research is needed to better understand the needs and preferences for end-of-life care of minorities, medically underserved and other vulner-

---

BOX 5-1
Memorial Sloan-Kettering Cancer Center and North General Hospital: Partners in Pain Management and End-of-Life Care in a Minority Community

North General Hospital (NGH) is embarking on an ambitious and definitive series of activities in the area of pain and palliative care. Under the direction of Dr. Harold Freeman, president and Chief Executive Officer of NGH, and Dr. Richard Payne, chief of the Pain and Palliative Care Program at Memorial Sloan-Kettering Cancer Center (MSKCC), NGH has established a new Pain and Palliative Care Program. This program has been an outgrowth of North General's plan to establish a comprehensive cancer center; that center was recently awarded a $5 million grant from the Ralph Lauren Foundation.

Below is a brief description of the current pain and palliative care initiatives at NGH and the collaborating partners. Evaluation of the outcomes of these developing models of care and service delivery will add significantly to our body of knowledge in these areas.

1. The **Pain and Palliative Care Service** is a comprehensive, multidisciplinary endeavor that opened in June 2000. The center has received support from the Ellen P. Hermanson Foundation, NGH, and MSKCC resources for initial staffing. As part of its mission and operation, the Pain and Palliative Care Service at NGH is training its physician, nursing, and support staff, has revised hospital policy and procedures; and has implemented an inpatient pain management consultative service and a weekly ambulatory clinic. The consultative service on pain management and ambulatory services will be available to North General Hospital patients 24 hours a day. This clinical program serves as a community resource providing expertise in palliative medicine for the greater Harlem area. For example, a series of formal and informal educational programs delivered by staff of the Pain and Palliative Care Service has targeted Harlem physicians and other health care providers.

2. The United Hospital Fund's Community Oriented Palliative Care Initiative has funded a two-year collaborative program at NGH with MSKCC and the Visiting

---

able populations. We need to address health policy and financing barriers that prevent the utilization of end-of-life care support that is available. We need to know if demographics (age, social class, and education level) affect the attitudes and practices of these groups at the end of life.

• The National Cancer Institute (NCI) should increase efforts to address disparities in access to cancer care, including end-of-life care (including many of the recommendations in the recent Institute of Medicine report *The Unequal Burden of Cancer* [IOM, 1999]).

• NCI-designated cancer centers should provide plans to address equal access to cancer care services (including end-of-life care) in vulnerable populations. Demonstration projects should be funded to develop models of care delivery and evaluated to assess the effectiveness of care.

Nurse Service of New York (VNSNY)—the **Harlem Palliative Care Network** (HPCN). HPCN will work to (1) increase access to palliative care services for patients facing life-threatening illnesses and their families who reside in Central and East Harlem; (2) overcome cultural and environmental barriers among minority populations concerning timely intervention for life-threatening illnesses; (3) enhance the continuity and coordination of care through greater integration of community-based and institutional services; (4) improve the quality of life for Harlem patients through better pain and symptom management; and (5) provide support services to meet the emotional and spiritual needs of patients and their families. HPCN will achieve these goals by identifying Network Partners—consisting of faith-based organizations, social and community development agencies, and community health care providers—who will agree to assist in identifying patients and to provide services in the community for those patients.

3. HPCN will target patients with a diagnosis of progressive cancer, congestive heart failure, chronic obstructive pulmonary disease, end-stage renal disease, and AIDS in Central and East Harlem. This geographic area is the primary service area of NGH, and it will be the hub for inpatient, outpatient, and community-based palliative care services.

4. The **"Initiative to Improve Palliative and End-of-life Care in the African-American Community"** is supported by funding from the Open Society Institute's Project on Death in America (PDIA). The *Initiative* brought together a group of professionals to begin to delineate and document historical, social, cultural, ethical, economic, legal, policy, and other factors that affect the attitudes toward, acceptance of, access to, and utilization of palliative and hospice services by African Americans. During a planning meeting in February 2000, four key barriers were identified: (1) mistrust of the health care system, (2) lack of effective end-of-life planning, (3) inattention to the spiritual aspects of healing and dying, and (4) viewing pain as a natural or expected part of dying. Plans have also begun toward a national conference, planned for late 2001, to consolidate and disseminate information concerning barriers to improving end-of-life care for African Americans and to suggest specific strategies for change.

REFERENCES

Byrd WM, Clayton LA, Kinchen K, et al. African-American physicians' views on health reform: results of a survey. *J Natl Med Assoc* 1994;86:191-199.

Caralis PV, Davis B, Wright K, Marcial E. The influence of ethnicity and race on attitudes toward advanced directives, life-prolonging treatments and euthanasia. *J Clin Ethics* 1993;4:155-156.

Christakis NK, Escarce J. Survival of Medicare pateints after enrollment in hospice program. *New Engl J Med* 1996;335:172-178.

Crawley L, Payne R, Bolden J, Payne T, Washington P, Williams S. Palliative and end-of-life care in the African American community. *JAMA* 2000;284:2518-2521.

Freeman H, Payne R. Racial injustice in health care. *New Engl J Med* 2000;342:1045-1047.

Freimuth VS, Quinn SC, Thomas SB, Cole G, Zook E, Duncan T. African American's views on research and the Tuskegee Syphilis Study. *Soc Sci Med* 2001;52:797-808.

Greenlee RT, Hill-Gharmon, MB, Murray T, Thun, M. Cancer Statistics, 2001. *CA Cancer J Clin* 2001;51:15-36.

Institute of Medicine (IOM). 1999. *The Unequal Burden of Cancer*. Haynes MA, Smedley BD, eds. Washington, D.C.: National Academy Press.

LaVeist TA, Bowie JV, Cooley-Qyuille M. Minority health status in adulthood: the middle years. *Minority Health Today* 2000;2:46-53.

Massad LS. Missed connections. *JAMA* 2000;284:409-410.

McKinley E. Garrett J, Evans A, Danis M. Differences in end-of-life decision making among black and white ambulatory cancer patients. *J Gen Intern Med* 1996;651-656.

Mebane E, Oman R, Kroonen L, Goldstein M. The influence of physician race, age and gender on physician attitudes toward advance care directives and preferences for end-of-life decision-making. *J Am Geriatrics Society* 1999;47:579-591.

Medicare Payment Advisory Commission. Medicare Beneficiaries Costs and Use of Care in the Last Year of Life, Final Report, May 1, 2000.

Neuberger BJ, Hamilton CL. Racial differences in attitudes toward hospice care. *The Hospice J* 1990;6:37-48.

Shavers VL, Lunch CF, Burmeister LF. Knowledge of the Tuskegee study and its impact on willingness to participate in medical research studies. *J Natl Med Assoc* 2000;92(12):563-572.

Yergan J, Flood AB, LoGerfo JP, Diehr P. Relationship between patient race and the intensity of hospital service. *Medical Care* 1987;25:592.

6

End-of-Life Care:
Special Issues in Pediatric Oncology

Joanne M. Hilden, M.D.
The Cleveland Clinic Foundation
Cleveland, OH

Bruce P. Himelstein, M.D.
University of Pennsylvania School of Medicine
The Children's Hospital of Philadelphia

David R. Freyer, D.O.
DeVos Children's Hospital, Grand Rapids, MI

Sarah Friebert, M.D.
Case Western Reserve University
St. Vincent's Mercy Children's Hospital
Hospice of the Western Reserve, Cleveland, Ohio

Javier R. Kane, M.D.
University of Texas Health Science Center
Christus Santa Rosa Children's Hospital
Christus Santa Rosa Hospice

OVERVIEW: CHALLENGES UNIQUE TO THE PRACTICE OF PEDIATRIC PALLIATIVE CARE

Despite remarkable progress in the treatment of pediatric malignancy, 30 percent of children with cancer still die of their disease or its complications (Pizzo and Poplack, 1997). Cancer is the most common cause of nontraumatic death in children; 2,200 children die each year from cancer in this country (out of a total of 30,000 pediatric deaths annually). Although this is far fewer than the half-million adults who die, the premature death of a child is a unique tragedy.

This report examines the end-of-life care problems unique to pediatrics and suggests steps that could alleviate them. The solutions center on improved models of care and reimbursement structures, which represents the way toward "informed, shared decisionmaking" that can be accomplished only through time-consuming, detailed conferences. In the case of pediatrics, this is multilayered, involving the health care team, the parents, and the child patient. Models of care and reimbursement structures should value and recognize this.

Palliative care for children involves all-inclusive and compassionate care aimed at preventing and relieving suffering for those with life-threatening illness. Pediatric palliative care is family-centered care, with the child and family enwrapped in the center of a circle of professionals addressing spiritual, social, psychological, and physical needs. The prevalence of children living with active palliative care needs at a given time is estimated at 50 per 100,000 (Goldman and Christie, 1993).

Available resources designed for the care of adults with life-threatening illness do not fit the needs of dying children. Also, despite recent increases in interest in adult palliative care and hospice philosophy, a parallel increase in pediatrics has not occurred—80 percent of children dying with cancer in this country are still suffering, and their symptoms are not being adequately palliated (Wolfe, 2000).

Why are children with terminal malignancy suffering? First and foremost, death in childhood is rare. As a result, medical, psychological, social, spiritual, and other practitioners for children are not likely to have much experience in palliative and terminal care. Then too, professionals providing quality end-of-life care to adults, including hospice staff, are not likely to have sufficient training to handle the complex physical, emotional, and psychological care of dying children and their families.

Children are not just small adults. The malignancies that afflict children differ substantially from the common adult cancers, and expectations of cure are much higher. These expectations for both families and treating professionals are realistically based on relatively better overall outcomes for children compared to adults with cancer (even for similar cancers). Heightened expectation of success leads to a reluctance of parents and health care providers to make a formal transition to non-cure-directed interventions.

Dying children defy the natural order, and pediatric providers are more likely to suffer a sense of failure when children die. Referral to an end-of-life program may be seen as abandoning hope, which may interfere with good communication and clinical care. Families and health care providers alike vary tremendously in their state of readiness for transition to an exclusively palliative approach in treating children, even when the definition of palliative care is well established and understood (Frager, 1996). Discussion of palliative care tends to be deferred, and an artificial distinction between curative and palliative care—when there should be continuity of care—is often made.

Communication across differing chronological ages, developmental levels, and decisionmaking capacities is a complex skill set to acquire and demanding to maintain. Children "have a right to be treated as developing persons, as persons with a developing capacity for rationality, autonomy, and participation in health-care decision making" (AAP, 1995). At any given age, however, they may possess none, some, or all of the capacities necessary to participate in their own health care.

Children are extremely resilient and may rebound from multiple medical crises that would ordinarily be life-ending in an adult. Further, the ability of clinicians to predict timing of death is notoriously poor in the adult population and even worse when it comes to children, particularly those living with chronic illness for many years prior to death. Families and provider teams may be faced with waxing and waning palliative care needs and recurrent conversations over time about the transition to palliative care; this type of need does not fit neatly into the medical, psychological, spiritual, and economic framework established for adult end-of-life care.

Despite current practices to the contrary, extrapolation of adult-derived pharmacokinetic and pharmacodynamic data is often inappropriate and sometimes dangerous for children. Although recent government regulations may change the licensing requirements for new drugs to require pediatric labeling and indications, the rarity of death in childhood still mandates large and often cumbersome multi-institutional trials of symptom control measures for dying children.

Discussions and decisions surrounding end-of-life care have not consistently included the family and the child. In pediatric palliative care, only the individual child and family can determine what is best for them, based on their particular values and life experiences (Liben, 1996). Children need to participate in such discussions and decisions to the fullest extent possible, in order to achieve mastery and control over their own dying. Children have grief work to do and goodbyes to say, just as adults. Inadequate professional training in the ethical, moral, and legal implications of including children in their own care has the potential to rob children of their autonomy and to violate the concept of truth telling in medicine (Bartholome, 1993).

Finally, the death of a child is one of the most significant psychological stressors a person may ever face. The bereavement literature supports the notion that the risk of prolonged, complicated grief or pathological bereavement is substantial for the parents of a child who has died.

This chapter explores the issues in eight major areas:

1. education of providers,
2. education of children and families about the dying process,
3. special issues in communication: adolescents and assent,
4. delays in the initiation of palliative care for children,
5. fragmentation of palliative care services,

6. inadequate relief of pain and other physical symptoms,
7. research issues, and
8. reimbursement and regulatory issues.

EDUCATION OF PROVIDERS

Defining the Problem

Improving the quality of care and quality of life for dying children depends on improving the quality of education in pediatric palliative care. However, there are some basic impediments to teaching about death in childhood, including prognostic uncertainty, the move of pediatric residents to more outpatient experiences, and most importantly, the relative rarity of death in childhood (resulting in less provider experience and fewer opportunities for mentoring trainees). Some of these barriers, however, may represent educational opportunities (Sahler et al., 2000).

Training programs in the health professions have begun to pay increased attention to end-of-life issues, but the focus is on adults, with little content applicable to pediatrics. Examples include the American Medical Association's Education for Physicians on End-of-Life Care (EPEC) curriculum (Emanuel et al., 1999) and the American Academy of Hospice and Palliative Care Medicine's (AAHPM's) "UNIPAC" self-study program for physicians who care for terminally ill patients and their families (AAHPM, 1998). Philosophically, adult and pediatric end-of-life care have much in common, but practical applications are clearly different for adults and children. There is currently no comprehensive end-of-life curriculum for pediatric palliative care, although a UNIPAC module for pediatrics is in preparation.

The lack of curriculum content specific to pediatric palliative care exists at all levels and across health care professions. No national standards for curriculum content in pediatric end-of-life care exist for schools of medicine, nursing, or social work, although more medical schools are including some aspects in pediatric clerkships. The Residency Review Committee "Program Requirements for Residency Education in Pediatrics" does not contain any specific language referring to palliative care or end-of-life care. The End-of-Life Nursing Education Consortium (ELNEC) Project from the American Association of Colleges of Nursing also lacks specific pediatric language, although nursing management courses including those specific to pediatric practice would fall within its curriculum guidelines (Ferrell et al., 2000). Recent revisions to accreditation standards from the Liaison Committee on Medical Education (LCME) include a standard on end-of-life care, but it is very broad in its scope, stating that "clinical instruction should cover all organ systems, and must include the important aspects of preventive, acute, chronic, continuing, rehabilitative, and end-of-life care" (Accreditation Standards, 2000).

Although several academic centers have begun fellowship training programs in palliative care, there are no programs for pediatric palliative care. Reflecting this deficiency, the content outline for the AAHPM certification examination in hospice and palliative medicine lists children only as a special population under the subject heading "Death and Dying."

Hospice and home nurse agencies care almost exclusively for adults, but in the absence of special services for children, by default, dying children are cared for by them as well. These providers need education to prepare them for children's care or, at a minimum, ready access to consultation with experts in pediatric palliation. However, there are only a few programs that educate hospice providers in the unique aspects of caring for dying children (Brenner, 1993).

Although the regulatory language for hospice practice (from the Joint Commission on Accreditation of Healthcare Organizations (JCAHO) does not specifically exclude children from consideration, there is a dearth of detailed information for programs that serve dying children (Accreditation Standards, 2000). A tool to address this problem is the *Compendium for Pediatric Palliative Care*, developed by the Children's International Project on Palliative Care/Hospice Services (ChIPPS) and currently under review (Marcia Levetown, M.D.; personal communication, 2000). Once complete, it will be published by the National Hospice and Palliative Care Organization. The stated goal of the compendium is to "provide information that would enable a hospice with no pediatric experience to care for a child." The effectiveness of this tool must be studied once it is released.

The American Society of Clinical Oncology surveyed adult and pediatric oncologists in 1999 regarding palliative and end-of-life care issues. Only 10 percent of pediatric oncologists who responded reported that they had formal courses in pediatric terminal care in medical school, and only 2.2 percent reported a rotation in a palliative care or hospice service. The most common method of learning about these topics reported by pediatric oncologists was "trial and error," and many reported anxiety about having to work with dying children. These practitioners not only are treating children, but are the role models for future generations of both generalists and specialists, who often look to oncologists for expertise in end-of-life care.

Pediatricians and pediatric issues are underrepresented in national organizations and committees dealing with medical care and reimbursement. For example, although organizations such as the National Hospice and Palliative Care Organization-National Council of Hospice Professionals have some pediatric representatives on subcommittees, no subcommittee addresses the unique educational, fiscal, clinical, regulatory, philosophical, and ethical needs of a pediatric hospice population. Similarly, although organizations dedicated to pediatric care have work groups devoted to end-of-life care (e.g., the Children's Oncology Group [COG], the American Academy of Pediatrics [AAP], and Children's Hospice International) and continue to advocate for the needs of dying children, unifying, collaborative national efforts to bring provider education to the forefront do not exist.

Finally, there are only a handful of quality textbooks targeted to pediatric palliative care, and the subject is underrepresented in the classic adult textbooks such as *Supportive Care in Oncology* (Weisman, 1998) or the *Oxford Textbook of Palliative Medicine* (Doyle et al., 1998). Examples of essential pediatric texts include *Hospice Care for Children* (Armstrong-Dailey and Goltzer, 1993), *Care of the Dying Child* (Goldman, 1994), and *Cancer Pain Relief and Palliative Care in Children* (WHO, 1998) as well as two explorations of the more spiritual aspects of childhood death, *The Private Lives of Dying Children* (Bluebond-Langer, 1978) and *Armfuls of Time* (Sourkes, 1995).

Next Steps

• **Develop content for pediatric end-of-life care curricula in medical, nursing, chaplaincy, and social work training programs.** The challenges facing creators of curricula include defining educational objectives; outlining the content of training; selecting teaching methods; exploring personal attitudes toward death, dying, and bereavement; promoting interdisciplinary collaboration; evaluating training; and defining the role and function of educators in pediatric palliative care (see Papadatou, 1997, for a discussion of challenges in creating a pediatric palliative care course).

• **Develop curricula with both traditional and alternative teaching methods.** Standard didactic approaches are the tradition in many post-secondary education programs, but these approaches do not optimally address the emotional and psychological needs of students in a complex field such as pediatric palliative care. Alternative methods such as small group discussion, role playing, experiential learning by partnering with mentors, supervised clinical practice, and/or self-directed on-line learning may better suit training at all levels. Small studies have demonstrated the efficacy of nontraditional learning methods, including those derived from the psychology world, in altering attitudes of students regarding end-of-life issues (Razavi et al., 1988, 1991). At the Children's Hospital of Philadelphia, a pilot study is under way to explore the role of an intensive, brief cognitive-behavioral intervention for staff in changing values and beliefs about pediatric palliative care.

- **Evaluate the effectiveness of educational materials and methods in pediatric palliative care.** Curricula such as EPEC would be expected to be effective, but this cannot be assumed without appropriate evaluation. New outcome measures may be required to assess the skills of trainees and practitioners, incorporating assessments not only of knowledge about death and dying, but also of empathy, spiritual balance, educational capacity and effectiveness, or even business acumen.
- **Develop curricula that teach intact medical care teams the tenets of palliative care.** Parents of seriously ill children have indicated that they strongly value the continuity of care achieved when the primary oncology team continues to care for their child through the time of death. While this delivers the desired continuity to parents, it has resulted in inadequate delivery of palliative care. Training of intact teams may improve the delivery of care as well as facilitate involvement of the necessary professionals.
- **Create and fund pediatric palliative care training and fellowship programs.** Effective training in pediatric palliative care will depend upon many factors, including exposure to a wide array of clinical materials relevant to the field of study; good mentorship; well-defined evidence-based curricula; and the availability of a suitable academic environment to support the study of related fields such as bioethics, adult palliative care, epidemiology and biostatistics, or pharmacology. "Centers of Excellence" in pediatric palliative care should be created in which training and fellowship programs can offer education to adult hospice workers who care for the occasional dying child.
- **Add appropriate end-of-life content to general pediatric, pediatric subspecialty, and hospice and palliative medicine certifying examinations.** Content on end-of-life care should be added not only to general pediatric board examinations, but also to subspecialty certifications such as intensive care, cardiology, neurology, and neonatology, which along with oncology have the most pediatric deaths. Hospice and palliative care practitioners must have a minimum fund of knowledge in order to provide comprehensive and compassionate care to dying children.
- **Add language to home health and hospice regulations specifically mandating competencies in pediatric end-of-life care.** Providers should have a minimum fund of knowledge regarding medical, physiological, emotional, and developmental issues of the dying child. The pediatric UNIPAC curriculum (when available) could be made mandatory for providers who will care for children, and successful completion of the curriculum could be a criterion for individual and institutional licensure.
- **Develop national collaborative efforts to advocate for education in pediatric end-of-life care.** To meet the educational needs of professionals caring for dying children, pediatric palliative care training sessions should

be offered in conjunction with national meetings of organizations that care for children with life-threatening illness (e.g., COG, AAP, and the American Society of Pediatric Hematology/Oncology). For adult hospice providers, pediatric end-of-life curricula should be offered at national meetings of the relevant professions. Collaboration between programs and interested individuals dedicated to pediatric palliative care (e.g., members of the American Association of Hospice and Palliative Medicine, the National Hospice and Palliative Care Organization, and Children's Hospice International), as well as funding for these collaborations, must be a national priority.

EDUCATION OF CHILDREN AND FAMILIES ABOUT THE DYING PROCESS

Defining the Problem

Many families who are navigating the health care system during the treatment of their child's cancer often joke that they should receive honorary medical or nursing licenses. This comment, although somewhat tongue-in-cheek, underscores the complexity of the tasks of children and families facing life-threatening illness. From the time of diagnosis to the time of cure or death, families must assimilate an overwhelming amount of information, function as advocates for their child and themselves, make informed decisions (often without adequate information), and negotiate ever-changing systems for delivery of care (including insurance plans). All this must be accomplished while continuing to work or care for other family members at home. These tasks become increasingly burdensome and difficult when a child's prognosis is not good, and families must balance quality-of-life issues with their drive and need to "leave no stone unturned" in pursuing treatment options. In this scenario, provision of accurate, up-to-date, and comprehensive information in an understandable manner is even more crucial.

It is at the stage of diagnosis of a life-limiting prognosis that families are faced with seemingly dichotomous treatment options. The availability of Phase I and II clinical trials for pediatric oncology patients offers continued "aggressive" therapy with a small chance of physical or life-prolonging benefit to the patient, and possibly with altruistic benefits. At the same time, palliative care options need to be discussed so that optimal symptom management can preserve patient comfort and dignity. It is this *simultaneous* provision of potentially curative and palliative medicine that currently escapes us.

If resources for providers of pediatric end-of-life care are lacking, the availability of educational materials for affected children and their families is even further behind. Some examples of information required by families to make good decisions include understanding the diagnosis and prognosis; the likely effects of the disease on the patient; other relevant physical or emotional problems likely to impact the course of illness; other symptoms likely to occur; what death will look and be like with and without artificial interventions; uses and interactions of medications; the availability of pharmacologic and nonpharmacologic interventions to ease suffering; the availability of professional and nonprofessional resources to aid the family; physical modifications and facilities to make home or transportation more accessible; and what changes in functional status are likely to occur. In short, families need a complete appreciation of the effects of a life-threatening illness on the physical, psychological, spiritual, and practical dimensions of care.

An additional educational need regards advance directives. With adults, there is at least a chance that end-of-life wishes will have been considered before being faced with a life-threatening illness, but this almost never occurs in the pediatric setting. Most pediatricians and even pediatric subspecialists are not skilled in discussing advance directives. Research clearly demonstrates that patients and families prefer to be guided in these discussions by practitioners they trust (Frager, 1996; Whittam, 1993). Resources to make decisions concerning withdrawal of life-sustaining treatment (including nutrition and hydration), and covering principles of palliative care and issues of medical futility, are not currently available to pediatric patients and their families. Although there are books available to parents describing leukemia and other cancers, there is not much available to families to help prepare them for the medical and psychosocial details of the death of their child.

Next Steps

• **Develop protocols for use by interdisciplinary teams to explain disease and prognosis in terms that families and patients can understand.** Content of discussions should be spelled out and be accompanied by delivery of the material in written form for later review.

• **Develop materials for child patients at every developmental level and their families with disease-specific information, prognosis, palliative care terminology and options, and clinical trial terminology and options.**

• **Develop resources that detail expected physical changes toward the end of life.**

• **Involve parents and older adolescents (when appropriate) in national organizations developing policy for pediatric hospice and palliative care standards and reimbursement.**

ADOLESCENTS AND ASSENT

Defining the Problem

Caring for Adolescents

Adolescents facing death have palliative care needs substantially different from those of younger children or adults. The unique psychosocial issues for dying adolescents—which relate to the normal developmental tasks of this time of life—include greater focus on physical appearance, reversal of developing independence, lack of control, loss of self-confidence, social isolation, disruption of future plans, and desire to be listened to by their care providers (Carr-Gregg et al., 1997). At initiation and during provision of palliative care, communication with adolescents requires particular sensitivity to the concerns characteristic of this age group.

Adolescents with cancer do not have proportionate access to clinical trials sponsored by national pediatric oncology cooperative groups, a possible factor in the relatively lower survival rates observed in this age group (Bleyer et al., 1997). It is not clear whether similar differences exist for adolescents in their access to pediatric palliative care services or in their qualitative experience while receiving services.

Issues of Assent and Consent

Children who are developmentally capable of participating in their own health care decisionmaking are often prevented from doing so. Historically, children have been declared legally and ethically incompetent to participate in decisions about their own health care. Except for circumstances involving mature or emancipated minors, decisions regarding health care for children under age 18 generally are made by surrogate decisionmakers, usually parents. However, some health care providers (and most ethicists and palliative care professionals) believe that children who have reached the age of assent and are capable of expressing a preference should be given choices and have their wishes respected. This is especially true in the area of end-of-life care, when quality, not quantity, of life is the main focus. After all, who better can decide what constitutes quality of life for an individual than that person? Leikin (1993) writes:

> ...if a minor has experienced an illness for some time, understands it and the benefits and burdens of its treatment, has the ability to reason about it, has previously been involved in decision making about it, and has a comprehension of death that recognizes its personal significance and finality, then that person, irrespective of age, is competent to consent to forgoing life-sustaining treatment.

In pediatrics, consent actually amounts to authorization by the parents for treatments and procedures, reflecting the assumption that parents are the most authentic spokespeople for their children. However, most children are capable of consent after age 14, by which time, with normal development, they possess full decisional capacity and flexible thinking (Brock, 1989). "Assent" refers to a child's agreement with the proposed treatment. Although it is not a term defined in law, assent respects children as individuals with developing capacities for participation in health care decisionmaking. Conversely, "coercion" describes an essentially paternalistic act of forcing participation in treatment or research, which should be avoided.

Assent in pediatric practice consists of four basic elements:

1. demonstrating respect for the child as a patient and as a developing person by assisting the child to develop an appropriate awareness of illness;

2. disclosing the nature of the proposed intervention and what the child is likely to experience (truth telling);

3. assessing the child's understanding of information and the factors influencing his or her evaluation; and

4. demonstrating respect for emerging autonomy and the development of decisionmaking capacity by soliciting expressions of willingness on the part of the child to accept the intervention (Bartholome, 1993).

The American Academy of Pediatrics Committee on Bioethics recommends that assent for treatment should be obtained from the pediatric patient when developmentally appropriate and should be binding when used in the research setting (AAP, 1995). However, guidelines from the National Institutes of Health (NIH) Office for Protection from Research Risks (OPRR) state that assent or dissent is conditional on parental permission if participation in research is potentially beneficial to the child, in which case parental permission overrides the child's dissent (OPRR, 1991).

Legal and ethical debates about the appropriate age of consent for medical treatment or research participation are interesting and important but oversimplify the issues when it comes to caring for adolescent patients. In the first place, decisionmaking capacity itself is not a static phenomenon; it can be intermittent or fluctuating, and it may vary over time with changes in clinical condition. Secondly, people are not static either: like adults, adolescent patients vary significantly in their ability to comprehend what is happening to them. Care providers, therefore, need to be attentive to changing competence in adolescent patients (Friebert and Kodish, 1999).

Next Steps

• **Develop and promote a structure for communication between clinical staff and family, specifically including the child patient, who should be part of the decisionmaking process whenever possible.** The goal is to set up the expectation that a child will be as fully informed as possible, so that when tough decisions come along, the child can participate. An example of this is the "Final Stage Conference" (Nitschke et al., 1997), used at the Children's Hospital of Oklahoma since the 1970s, in which a consistent approach is employed at the time of a child's cancer relapse to communicate essential information regarding disease status, prognosis, and care options. The child is routinely included in the discussion (with the parents' permission), which is tailored to his or her developmental understanding. Available investigational and palliative therapies and expectations for the terminal course are described. In the experience of the authors, the Final Stage Conference has been effective at conveying essential information, enhancing participation of the child and family in reaching a sound decision, facilitating dialogue within the family unit, and maintaining the family's trust.

Several disease- and treatment-related characteristics of children with cancer are relevant when considering discontinuing active therapy (Freyer, 1992). These include

- the medical experience of the child,
- the nature of pediatric cancer therapy,
- the unpredictability of treatment responses,
- parental and/or physician biases, and
- the necessity of palliative care.

For children and adolescents capable of expressing their values and preferences, the use of "modified substituted judgment" (substituted judgment is a legal concept for surrogates' making decisions for previously competent adults) is recommended for enacting decisions consistent with their wishes (Freyer, 1992). This means that parents can apply their child's stated values when decisions are required. When combined with traditional guidelines for end-of-life decisions (such as benefit-burden analysis), the consistent application of these guidelines for children appears to enhance provider-patient or family communication. Clinical studies are required to confirm this.

• **Develop standards for decisionmaking capacity (including advance directives) in the pediatric population based on developmental level or** "illness competency." Pediatric patients should be assessed individually on their desire and ability to participate in decisionmaking, regardless of chronological age, according to a set of standards that have been validated with input from pediatricians, ethicists, legal counsel, and developmental psychologists.

DELAYS IN THE INITIATION OF PALLIATIVE CARE FOR CHILDREN

Defining the Problem

During the care of a child whose cancer becomes refractory to therapy, there comes a point when it is appropriate to initiate palliative care. This transition point is somewhat arbitrary and lacks a universally accepted definition, but it can be considered as the time at which the goals of palliative care become more important than other treatment end points. Defining the exact time is difficult, however, because the transition from anticancer to palliative therapy is gradual for most children, and palliative care may be appropriate very early, in conjunction with potentially curative treatment.

Delaying the initiation of palliative care results in (1) losing the opportunity to promote palliative care principles to the patient and family; (2) being less able to tailor palliative care to the evolving needs of the patient; (3) crisis-oriented management, which exacerbates the sense of vulnerability and helplessness; (4) absence of a framework for preventive, proactive interventions or decisionmaking; and (5) difficulty in supporting the family's strengths and capacity to cope and in the maximizing quality of the remaining time (Frager, 1996; Goldman, 1996; Vickers and Carlisle, 2000). This is consistent with a recent study in which terminally ill children with cancer were more likely to be described by their parents as peaceful and calm during their last month of life if their hospice care decision occurred earlier in the course of their illness (Wolfe et al., 2000).

Several barriers can prevent timely initiation of palliative care. First, the transition from anticancer therapy to palliation is usually gradual, making the decision point ambiguous for starting palliative care. With each relapse, the prognosis for cure decreases. Although the use of second-line (retrieval) and investigational therapy is often available and reasonable, the need for control of physical and psychological symptoms increases with time as the patient's condition deteriorates.

Second, the traditional framework for making the transition to palliative care deals poorly with this reality, such that health care decisions involve exclusive, all-or-none use of either anticancer therapy or palliative care, separated by a clean break from one to the next at some discrete point in time (Frager, 1996). If families and providers are forced to choose between investigational therapy and palliative care, the result is often delayed implementation of the latter. The study by Wolfe and colleagues (2000) referred to earlier did not assess whether palliative care had been delayed for the 103 children included but did report anticancer treatment very late in the course of disease: Phase I and II investigational drug trials had been received by 24 percent and 38 percent of the patients, respectively, and half of the children had anticancer treatment during the last month of life, which consisted of a bone marrow transplant for 22 percent.

A third barrier to initiating palliative care for some patients is that appropriate services are not available, particularly home-based palliative care. This type of care can be delivered in the inpatient setting (and may be preferred for some patients), but the family's home is the preferred location for most dying children (Collins et al., 1998; Goldman, 1996). Several successful models of home-based palliative care for children have been described (Martinson, 1993a), yet a recent survey by Children's Hospice International (1998) indicates relatively few organized pediatric palliative care services in operation. Adult hospice providers are not experienced with children; parents or providers are understandably reluctant to transition care to such providers. Consequently, it usually falls to the treatment team at the pediatric oncology center to coordinate palliative care. An advantage of this is the continuity through established relationships, but a potential disadvantage is the tendency to delay initiation of palliative care, in part because most pediatric oncologists lack formal training in end-of-life care (Hilden et al., 2001). (See also the the sections on reimbursement and education.)

Fourth, the needs and beliefs of parents may be responsible for delayed implementation of palliative care for children (Children's Hospice International, 1998; Nitschke et al., 2000; Whittam, 1993). Compared with adults, death in children is considered unnatural and especially tragic. It is difficult for most parents not to equate stopping cancer treatment with "giving up" on their child, resulting in continued treatment beyond significant hope of cure or recovery. Nor are physicians invulnerable to the difficulties in refocusing the therapeutic goal from cure to comfort care (Whittam, 1993). Leading obstacles to providing hospice services to children were an association of the hospice concept with death rather than life enhancement, lack of clarity regarding when to refer, and physician reluctance in making the referral (Children's Hospice International, 1998). Additionally, cross-cultural beliefs and practices may influence attitudes toward death and discourage the use of palliative care for some dying children (Die Trill and Kovalcik, 1997; Sagara and Pickett, 1998). In any case, the need for parents to choose aggressive curative therapy for their child is real, not "unrealistic." Our systems of care must accommodate this reality, rather than trying to change parents.

Fifth, the lack of parental awareness and accurate knowledge about palliative care may prevent its early initiation. There is little evidence regarding parental knowledge of optimal care standards for dying children, but in the Children's Hospice International (1998) survey, parents' lack of familiarity with hospice services was rated as an important obstacle to referral. The education and training of pediatric physicians is acknowledged to be deficient in the skillful provision of palliative care (Khaneya and Milrod, 1998; Sahler et al., 2000). It seems reasonable to assume that this deficiency would result in parents' lack of awareness of the option.

Finally, cost may deter early implementation of home-based palliative care. Even though it appears substantially less expensive to care for dying children at home than in a hospital (Martinson, 1993b), the cost of home care may be a barrier for some patients, especially those whose care is publicly funded (Children's Hospice International, 1998; Schweitzer et al., 1993). In addition, "hidden" costs to the family of a child dying at home, in terms of lost wages and out-of-pocket expenses for nonmedical supplies, may be a barrier. Furthermore, some insurance programs do not cover the concurrent provision of anticancer treatments and palliative care (Whittam, 1993).

Next Steps

- **Disseminate to health care professionals clear, widely accepted clinical criteria for determining when palliative care should be initiated for a child with cancer.** The physician and nursing groups from COG, APON (Association of Pediatric Oncology Nurses), and ASPHO (American Society of Pediatric Hematology/Oncology) should collaborate on the development of these criteria.
- **Fund research to determine referral patterns for palliative care services.** If we are to test the hypothesis that earlier referral to palliative care services will improve quality of life for dying children, baseline data are needed, including variation according to geographical area and third-party payer status.
- **Develop a new model for the transition to palliative care, permitting a gradual blending of anticancer and palliative therapies, with the latter becoming more dominant as the child's course proceeds** (Frager,1996).
- **Increase the availability of satisfactory home palliative care services for children, recognizing that multiple models have been used successfully and that there is no single model that is best for all pediatric oncology centers, communities, or regions.** Rural areas are in particular need of improved access to pediatric home palliative care services. In such areas, where the maintenance of a centralized, traditional palliative care program is not feasible, an effective model has utilized trained, community-based

home care providers working in close collaboration with a coordinating palliative care service for children (Martinson, 1993a). Large-scale development of this approach requires mechanisms to ensure appropriate training and funding for the direct care providers, who will be experienced with adult rather than pediatric patients.

• **Develop formal training in palliative care for oncology teams.** This issue is covered in a separate section on provider education. Avoiding delay in referral for palliative care should be included in the educational content of the training programs.

• **Organize efforts to improve coverage of pediatric palliative care services, especially those provided in the home, where cost-effectiveness has been demonstrated** (Martinson, 1993b). This issue is covered in a separate section on reimbursement.

FRAGMENTATION OF PALLIATIVE CARE SERVICES

Defining the Problem

Delivery of palliative care to children routinely involves multiple professionals from various disciplines and spans two months or longer (Children's Hospice International, 1998; Collins et al., 1998; Wolfe et al., 2000). Ideally, the services should be coordinated and seamless, but in practice, lack of coordination leads to fragmentation and poorly timed delivery. The magnitude of this problem is unclear from the literature, but its importance is implied by palliative care guidelines from SIOP (International Society of Paediatric Oncology) (Masera et al., 1999) and the International Work Group on Death, Dying, and Bereavement (1993), which explicitly state the need for a well-coordinated system of care for these patients.

Recent studies indicate that fragmentation of care may contribute to the distress of dying children and their families. In a recent study, parents of children with cancer who had died at home suggested better coordination of care as a way of improving palliative care services (Collins et al., 1998). In the same study, some families reported difficulty in arranging for readmission of children to the hospital for control of symptoms. Conflicting information from caregivers constitutes another form of fragmented care and has been associated with increased pain and non-pain-related suffering in children who died of cancer; the same was true for lack of involvement by the primary oncologist (Wolfe et al., 2000). Similarly, parents of children dying of cancer express a strong need to feel cared for and connected to their treatment team but often experience feelings of abandonment as death nears (James and Johnson, 1997).

Regardless of where care is delivered, *the lack of a designated coordinating entity contributes most to fragmented care*. In its absence, few practicing physicians can fill this gap (Hilden et al., 2001; Khaneya and Milrod, 1998; Sahler et al., 2000). In current medical care structures, providers are tied to particular sites and services (i.e., cardiology or intensive care unit). A family will see different chaplains, social workers, and providers at different sites and on different shifts, and often loses contact with these individuals upon discharge. Even when palliative care or pain teams are involved, their communication over time and sites is discontinuous. Furthermore, in rural regions the wide geographic distribution of dying children makes it untenable for them to be aided by palliative care programs based in metropolitan centers.

Unfortunately, fragmentation also occurs where established palliative care services are available. Although it has not been studied formally, one reason seems to be undefined channels of communication between the family and care providers. In most instances, direct care problems (e.g., development of new symptoms) should be addressed to a home care team. However, families may communicate these problems to personnel more familiar to them at the treatment center. In these situations, fragmentation can result from a failure of one health care team to give prompt notification of the clinical problem to the other. Although less common nowadays, the inability to provide certain interventions in the home setting (e.g., local blood bank policies proscribing transfusions outside a licensed hospital) also can result in fragmentation of care and the need to travel from home to the medical facility. Poor working relationships or communication channels between in-home care providers and the hospital may result in difficulty gaining readmission for management of difficult symptoms during the final stage.

There are some models in place or in the planning stages to remedy these problems. At Boston Children's Hospital the Pediatric Advanced Care Team (PACT) coordinates the essential elements of end-of-life care across the continuum of inpatient, outpatient, and home care settings for children with limited life expectancy. The goals of PACT are to improve family and caregiver communication, lessen pain and suffering, and emphasize meaningfulness during the end-of-life period. Interventions have focused on four main areas: (1) patient care, (2) education, (3) bereavement, and (4) outreach. As of 2000, the program had consulted on 80 patients, and the experience so far suggests that caregivers and families value the service. In a survey of providers following each consult, all physicians and nurses and 93 percent of psychosocial clinicians found the consults helpful (Wolfe, 2000).

The Pediatric Palliative Care Project at Children's Hospital and Regional Medical Center in Seattle, Washington, is another model, begun in 1998 and funded by the Robert Wood Johnson Foundation (http://www.seattlechildrens.org/pedpalcare/). It is evaluating the use of symptom control algorithms, a decisionmaking and charting tool, and a case manager who works with payers. In the first 18 months of the project, 60 children were referred for consideration and 20 enrolled in the program (the others received consultation or referral to appropriate services). The results of these evaluations are not yet available, but one initial impression is that at the time of referral, children are often at a point where symptom control is complex, requiring more sophisticated symptom control algorithms (Beth Forbes, personal communication, 2000).

Children's Hospice International has issued a call for proposals for its "Program of All-Inclusive Care for Children" (PACC), modeled after the adult Program for All-Inclusive Care of the Elderly (PACE), which is being supported by a congressional appropriation. According to the program description (www.chionline.org), "PACC will offer and manage all health care, medical, social services and support services needed by families to care for children diagnosed with life threatening and potentially life-limiting conditions, from the time of diagnosis through end of life care, and support their families, including bereavement care." The first grant cycle is limited to five states but will expand as more funding is available.

The PACC concept, with the addition of a care coordinator (trained to oversee specific communication content), is being tested with adult patients in the National Advanced Illness Coordinated Care (NAICC) program. Pilot results from the NAICC experience are encouraging. In a Department of Veterans Affairs Medical Center in New York State, NAICC patients had an 85 percent completion rate for advance directives, compared to 22.5 percent for a diagnostically matched control sample, and a 90 percent documentation rate for final stage of disease discussions, compared to 40.7 percent for control patients. Also, average inpatient costs were $1,923 less per patient per year for Advanced Illness Coordinated Care Program (AICCP) patients. In addition, providers at sites around the country are highly satisfied with the NAICC training they have received and report meaningful changes in their end-of-life care practices. Several commercial insurers have agreed to reimburse six NAICC visits per patient at selected sites (Daniel Tobin, M.D., personal communication, 2000). A NAICC model for children is under development.

Potential Solutions

• **Develop comprehensive pediatric palliative care services that include a family-oriented, relationship-centered focus.** This should include programs to provide continuity of care over transitions that now result in fragmentation. New roles, such as care coordinators, should be developed and evaluated.

• **Define essential features of a pediatric palliative care service** (Goldman, 1996; Martinson, 1993a):

1. *Continuous (24-hours per day, seven days a week) access to care* providers able to make regular and unscheduled home visits (this will usually be a registered nurse)

2. *Continuous access to pediatric palliative care experts for management suggestions and continuity*

3. *Ability to deliver all reasonable palliative interventions in the home setting without administrative or financial restrictions* (e.g., transfusion of blood products, availability of pharmacy and durable pediatric medical supplies)

4. *Respite care for the family*

5. *Immediate access to hospital or inpatient hospice facility if needed for symptom control*

6. *Bereavement care during and after the death of a child*

• **Develop initiatives to address the special challenges to pediatric hospice and palliative care faced in rural or other underserved areas.** At least one model for pediatric home palliative care has been demonstrated to be effective in this setting (Martinson, 1993b). "Home Care for the Child with Cancer," was a nursing research study initiated in 1976 with funding from the National Cancer Institute to demonstrate the feasibility and benefits of home care for dying children. In that project where approximately 50 percent of the children lived in rural areas, successful use was made of nurses recruited from the patients' communities to provide direct in-home care in collaboration with palliative care experts from the urban center. This model should be implemented on a larger scale (Martinson, 1993b).

• **Develop partnerships between palliative care centers and community-based primary care physicians.** An evolving role has been described for the primary care physician in pediatric palliative care (Howell, 1993; Wessel, 1998), although its cultivation on a large scale will require systematic education initiatives, as well as the active support of established palliative care centers. There is significant potential for these providers to improve continuity of care.

INADEQUATE RELIEF OF PAIN
AND OTHER PHYSICAL SYMPTOMS

Defining the Problem

Despite our best efforts, approximately 30 percent of all children diagnosed with a malignant disease die (Pizzo and Poplack, 1997). Ready access to skilled palliative care is clearly the standard of care for adults dying from malignant disease (Council on Scientific Affairs, 1996), but there is currently no national standard for access to quality palliative care for dying children.

There is considerable evidence that pain is a common symptom in children with terminal cancer (Wolfe et al., 2000). Much effort has gone into developing resources for providing adequate pain relief (Hain, 1997; Schrechter, 1990; WHO, 1998), but they have not been disseminated adequately. For example, of second-year pediatric residents informally surveyed as they started their oncology rotation at the Children's Hospital of Philadelphia, fewer than one-quarter were familiar with the World Health Organization pain ladder (Bruce Himelstein, M.D., unpublished observation, 2000).

Pain therapy in childhood is also limited by the lack of pediatric labeling for drugs that might benefit children; for example, newer long-acting opioid preparations. Investigator-initiated studies are often difficult to carry out in the pediatric palliative care setting, because patients may be geographically separated. There are also inherent difficulties in performing such studies of patients who are largely homebound. The lack of clinical trials for children is not limited to palliative care and has been recognized as a general problem. A partial remedy that is in place is a provision of the Food and Drug Administration (FDA) Modernization Act of 1998, which offers incentives to pharmaceutical companies with drugs under patent to obtain pediatric data in exchange for an additional six-month exclusivity. This leaves the problem of appropriate labeling for off-patent drugs, as well as any patented drugs that industry decides not to test.

Symptoms other than pain are actually more troublesome, according to parents and physicians (Wolfe et al., 2000). Fatigue, dyspnea, poor appetite, constipation, nausea, vomiting, and diarrhea are less successfully managed than pain, as reported by parents (but not by physicians). This finding is bolstered by reports by pediatric oncologists, who do not rate their skills in treating non-pain symptoms highly and who are more anxious treating difficult non-pain symptoms (Hilden et al., 2001). Unfortunately, little information is available about the incidence of these symptoms in children with cancer (Hain et al., 1995).

The evidence base for interventions for symptoms such as delirium, cough, dyspnea, somnolence, anxiety, and anorexia in the terminally ill pediatric population is also very poor. Without essential data from well-designed clinical trials, practitioners of pediatric palliative care are left to extrapolate from adult studies or to practice anecdotal medicine. Quality of care in any other medical subspecialty under these conditions would be considered substandard. The situation is even worse for interventions to improve nonphysical symptoms. Much has been written about the psychological, spiritual, and emotional aspects of dying, including several outstanding studies of dying children and their families (reviewed in Stevens, 1998a, 1998b), but few interventions that might alleviate distress have been tested adequately.

Late referrals to skilled practitioners of end-of-life care may also play a role in the undertreatment of symptoms, but no one has studied the simple epidemiology of time of referral to time of death in pediatrics (although such data are available for adults).

Potential Remedies

• **Develop care models that integrate palliative care specialists, symptom control specialists, and psychosocial services into the mainstream of pediatric oncology care.** Team care has been shown in the adult hospice literature to decrease pain and symptom severity, as well as to improve cost-effectiveness (Hearn and Higginson, 1998; Mercadante, 1999). This will involve the education of physicians simply in terms of the prompt and appropriate use of pain specialists.

• **Research to assess the efficacy of care models.** Pediatric oncology clinical trials units, in particular the recently formed Children's Oncology Group (a merger of the Children's Cancer Group, Pediatric Oncology Group, National Wilms' Tumor Study Group, and Intergroup Rhabdomyosarcoma Study Group), have a central responsibility to improve the quality of life of children with cancer. Trials of novel models of care to improve quality of life for children with terminal malignancy are critical.

• **Research to assess the efficacy of established and innovative symptom control interventions.** The pediatric oncology trials groups (COG, and/or the Pediatric Pharmacology Research Unit funded by the National Institute of Child Health and Human Development) carry out symptom control studies with new agents. Some therapeutic questions may require nationwide trials to enroll enough terminally ill children. Trials should address both physical and nonphysical (e.g., psychological, emotional, spiritual) conditions.

• **Epidemiological research to determine the incidence and prevalence of symptoms in children with life-threatening illness.**

• **State and federal programs to improve access to palliative care services and appropriate use of symptom control measures.** Recent FDA rulings clearly support the desire to obtain pediatric data with new drugs and biologicals. Federal legislation, such as that advocated by Children's Hospice International, recently passed to support the development of demonstration model programs, is needed to provide quality care for children with life-threatening illness.

REIMBURSEMENT ISSUES IN PEDIATRIC PALLIATIVE CARE

Defining the Problem

The biggest problems related to reimbursement are, first, payment for time spent communicating with parents and children and second, payment for palliative and hospice care for dying children.

Reimbursement for Physician-Family and Patient Communication

Excellent communication between physicians and parents, and between physician and the child patient, is essential to excellent cancer care for all children, but even more so for children who die. This communication is even more time-consuming than it is for adult patients, because of the complexity of communicating with children and the need to communicate complicated information to parents who naturally cling to the hope for cure. It is well established that "cognitive services" are generally poorly reimbursed compared to physical medical interventions, and this phenomenon is exaggerated in pediatrics, not only because of the stated complexity, but also because pediatricians are penalized for the fact that their actual patient—the child—is not always present during long discussions with parents. Moreover, billing codes do not distinguish among the subgroups of seriously ill pediatric patients with chronic disease, cognitive impairment, and/or complex life-threatening illnesses, for whom multiple specialty physicians are involved and for whom advance care planning and coordination of care among multiple physicians and services are labor intensive.

Reimbursement rules are discussed here in the context of dying children, but the principles and difficulties are relevant throughout the course of a child's cancer, regardless of diagnosis or prognosis. This discussion is based on reports from practitioners who belong to the Children's Oncology Group Principle Investigators (COG PIs; responders representing 44 out of 125 institutions), polled specifically for this project, in the complete absence of published data on reimbursement rates and amounts either from previous research or from insurers (who view the information as proprietary).

Prolonged Physician Services

Billing codes for "prolonged physician services" would seem to be the appropriate codes for conversations with patients and families pertinent to death and dying. These conversations take considerable time in pediatrics, since they involve working with children at various developmental ages as well as with parents. So for pediatrics, the "talk time" can be at least twice that of working with an adult patient. In the real world of pediatric medical care, these conversations are *separate* from time spent managing the child's complex medical problems.

The prolonged services codes are intended to be used in conjunction with office visit codes or inpatient visit codes (CPT codes 99201-99215, 99241-99245, 99301-99350). These office or inpatient visits are described as appropriately billed for counseling time if the time spent counseling is more than 50 percent of the physician-patient interaction. The total time for these codes goes up to 40 minutes, and this time most often is consumed doing the exam and reviewing charts and test results, so pediatricians should be able to rely on the prolonged service codes to bill additional time for counseling

There are specific codes for *prolonged physician service with direct face-to-face contact* (99354-99357), which are described as follows (Current Procedural Terminology [CPT], 2000):

> Codes 99354-7 are used when a physician provides prolonged service involving direct (face-to-face) patient contact that is beyond the usual in either the inpatient or outpatient setting. This service is reported in addition to other physician service, including evaluation and management service. 99354 or 99456 are used to report a total duration of prolonged service of 30-60 minutes on a given date. 99355 or 99357 are used to report each additional 30 minutes beyond the first hour.

These descriptions suggest that the codes should cover the extended communication necessary in pediatric care. Although the CPT lists these as billable in 30-minute increments with a maximum of 3 hours total, the reality is that they are relatively poorly reimbursed (and often denied outright by payers) relative to surgical procedures or physical exams, even though they represent a large percentage of time spent by physicians in caring for children with advanced illness. The COG PIs reported as follows: 40 percent do not even bill these codes because experience has shown they will not be reimbursed; 60 percent do bill them, and of these, 25 percent are rejected and 75 percent reimbursed (many are not able to collect information about how much is collected), with practices receiving a median of $91.00 for the first hour of service (range $47.00 to $144.00) and a median of $75.00 for an additional half-hour (range $21.00 to $142.00).

The codes for *prolonged physician service without direct (face-to-face) patient contact* are 99358 and 99359. These services are described as appropriate for non-face-to-face time spent by physicians providing "evaluation and management services at any level" and billable for continuous or discontinuous time in 30- minute increments with no stated maximum. However, the Health Care Financing Administration considers these two codes to be bundled into office and hospital visits. Thus most payers do not reimburse them, despite the example given in the CPT 2000 appendix citing the use of these codes to counsel family members without the presence of the patient. Therefore lengthy counseling time is not being reimbursed at all. COG PIs reported as follows: 77 percent do not bill these because they will not be reimbursed; 23 percent do bill them, reporting amounts paid as low as $10.00-30.00.

Lack of reimbursement or poor reimbursement for the prolonged services codes is a serious problem for pediatrics, but the total nonreimbursement of non-face-to-face time codes is an even greater problem for several reasons. First, the parents of seriously ill children often wish to discuss treatment issues—particularly issues regarding the possible death of the child—without their child present. Second, when the child is an infant or toddler, his or her face-to-face presence is irrelevant to the discussions, and children most often are not present for medically complex conversations. Third, interdisciplinary team management is discouraged by this system. Often, when the physician is with the parents, child life or social work staff are counseling the child patient. There are no codes for the latter staff to charge, so their services are bundled into the physician or team services. As a result, the charges that providers code must support the services of the entire team working with the child and family. The American Academy of Hospice and Palliative Medicine training guide for physicians (Storey and Knight, 1996) states that current reimbursement systems "discourage significant patient-physician interaction by selectively reimbursing for brief, procedure-related visits."

Representative examples from the practices of the authors are presented described below.

• A young girl with a brain tumor had a suspicious lesion on magnetic resonance imaging (MRI) at the end of therapy. The child was scheduled for a biopsy, under anesthesia; the oncology pediatric nurse practitioner did the history and physical that morning. The neurosurgeon performed the biopsy and frozen section confirmed the malignancy that day. An hour later, the pediatric oncologist spent 90 minutes with the parents, reviewing the biopsy results, discussing their sadness and fear, and going over with them the treatment options as well as strategizing about how to tell the 10-year-old child. The oncology billing office stated that there was no way for the pediatric oncologist to bill for this time. It was not face-to-face with the patient, and 99238 or 99239 codes are denied in that state. Codes 99354-99357 could not be used as extended time codes, since the oncologist had not done the history and physical and thus, had not had any face-to-face contact with the child, which is required for those codes. Thus, 90 minutes of time, highly valued by the family, was not reimbursed at all.

• A hospital visit of intermediate complexity, which included assessment of liver enlargement in the context of chemotherapy for acute lym-phoblastic leukemia, and 20 minutes of counseling the family, took place on the same day that the pediatric oncologist did a spinal tap on a child (delivering chemotherapy). The hospital visit code was denied as "global to the 96450" (the spinal tap code). Thus, a complex hospital visit, with the total time for the day at 60 minutes, including a procedure as well as extensive counseling, was reimbursed at $161.00. Compare this to local reimbursement rates for upper gastrointestinal endoscopy ($325.00), sig-moidoscopy ($118.30), mammogram ($94.30), and tonsillectomy/adenoid-ectomy ($390.00).

Even when these codes are reimbursed, the rate is not sufficient to support a clinical practice that includes a multidisciplinary team, despite its value to patients and families:

• A clinic visit (99215) with extra counseling time, totaling 80 min-utes, was reimbursed at $64.62 with the prolonged services code denied.
• A hospital visit with management of a complex medical problem was reimbursed at $78.96 (recall that this allows up to 35 minutes before a prolonged services code is allowed to be charged). The prolonged services code 99356 was reimbursed at $96.32, adding up to $143.58 for 90 min-utes of time. Physicians will be hard pressed to run a clinical service at that rate, let alone utilize the multidisciplinary psychosocial team needed by these families.

Hospital Discharge Services

The care of children with advanced illness requires a multidisciplinary team approach, but reimbursement for the contribution of nonphysician providers is extremely poor. Teams depend on staff such as nurse practitio-ners to do a great deal of teaching at the time of discharge. This teaching can prevent readmissions and increases the parents' sense of control and efficacy. Payers routinely deny nurse practitioner charges for discharge services, despite their being licensed and credentialed to provide this ser-vice.

Case Management Services

Case management services (listed in CPT 2000) consist of team confer-ences and telephone calls, which play a huge role in the management of children with advanced illness. They are reimbursed inadequately or not at all.

TEAM CONFERENCES   Billing codes exist for medical conferences by a physician with the interdisciplinary team present (codes are 99361 for 30 minutes and 99362 for 60 minutes). These conferences are described as follows (CPT, 2000): "Medical conference by a physician with interdisciplinary team of health professionals or representatives of community agencies to coordinate activities of patient care (patient not present)." These services are reimbursed very poorly despite their significant contribution to the care of children with advanced illness. COG PIs report that 75 percent no longer bill this code because of nonreimbursement. Of the 25 percent who do bill this, 64 percent get some reimbursement but few could state amounts. The median reported was $75.00 (range $40.00 to $250.00).

TELEPHONE CALLS   The billing codes for phone management by a physician are described as follows: "telephone call by a physician to patient or for consultation or medical management with other health care professionals," from "simple or brief" to "complex or lengthy to coordinate complex services of several different health professionals working on different aspects of the total patient care plan." This excellent description notwithstanding, these codes are reimbursed poorly or not reimbursed at all. The National Association of Children's Hospitals and Related Institutions (NACHRI) pediatric oncology study group recently conducted a study of time spent in telephone care (NACHRI, 1999). In a four week study, oncology practices logged 18 to 84 *hours* of calls. COG PIs report that 98 percent of them do not bill for telephone calls since they are not reimbursed. The few who billed reported receiving no reimbursement.

Care Plan Oversight Services

Physicians are responsible for the medical care (prescriptions, pain management, nutrition and fluid management, infection management, and management of symptoms to the time of death) of children dying at home in the care of hospice teams. It is well established that parents strongly desire the physician who treated their child's illness to oversee care through the dying process (Liben, 1996; Martinson, 1995). These physicians most commonly are not employed by the hospice and so must bill for professional services according to the usual codes. Most supervision of care takes place over the phone, in a mode compatible with that described by care plan oversight codes.

There are various codes for care plan oversight services (99374, 99375, 99377, 99378, 99379, and 99380). As an example, 99377 is described as follows:

> Physician supervision of a hospice patient (patient not present) requiring complex and multidisciplinary care modalities involving regular physician development and/or revision of care plans, review of subsequent reports

of patient status, review of related laboratory studies, communication with other health care professionals involved in a patient's care, integration of new information into the medical treatment plan and/or adjustment of medical therapy, within a calendar month; 15-29 minutes.

Half an hour per month grossly underestimates the time spent in this activity, especially as symptom control needs escalate at the end of life. It is not practical for physicians to make daily home visits, but daily phone calls are common. These codes are very poorly reimbursed despite the heavy responsibility of managing a dying child at home in the care of a home health agency. While the CPT codebook reflects this complexity, the codes are rejected if billed more than once a month, for time spent up to an hour. COG PIs report that 85 percent did not bill for these codes because of total lack of reimbursement. Of the few who did bill and knew the amount paid, the median was $66.00.

Reimbursement of Hospice and Palliative Care Services

Few children with life-threatening conditions get comprehensive palliative care. In the United States, hospice rules and payments are influenced strongly by the federal government, particularly the Medicare hospice benefit, which requires relinquishing reimbursement for potentially life-prolonging treatment in favor of just palliative treatment (Kinzbrunner, 1998; Vermillion, 1996). Every child suffering from chronic, life-threatening and terminal illness needs palliative care interventions, whether or not the family has given up on a cure. Unfortunately, current hospice admission and reimbursement practices are not consistent with optimal palliative care of seriously ill patients (Field and Cassel, 1997a).

Hospice Admission Guidelines

Hospice is a mechanism for delivering care when the goal to achieve comfort overrides the goal to prolong life. It has become synonymous in the United States with palliative care, mainly because of rules established under the Medicare program requiring patients to choose between potentially life-prolonging treatment and palliative care under hospice. Similarly, current guidelines encourage the provision of expert palliative care to children suffering from serious illnesses and their families only if they agree to be enrolled in hospice. It is very difficult, however, to admit pediatric oncology patients to hospice.

The great majority of terminally ill children and their parents are not willing to sign on to hospice service for a variety of reasons. To accept hospice care, both parents and physicians must have a minimal level of "uncertainty" regarding the child's prognosis and must have exhausted all other resources. Accepting hospice means that families have abandoned hope for a cure and have begun to focus on the fact that the child will eventually die. This acceptance of the reality of death is one of a series of steps in a palliative care approach. Unfortunately, acceptance of terminal illness is also a prerequisite for receiving palliative care services through hospice. This is a no-win situation in which acceptance of death is both a prerequisite for eligibility and an expected outcome of palliative care intervention.

The Medicaid hospice benefit provides reimbursement for expert pain and symptom management, grief and bereavement counseling, pastoral care counseling, and home nursing care. Experience in clinical practice, however, shows that children with chronic, life-threatening and terminal illnesses need these services long before they become eligible to receive hospice care (Kane et al., 2000). This includes patients whose disease is likely to be incurable but who continue to be treated with the intent to cure (e.g., with a Phase I agent), even though the chance that treatment may be of benefit is very small and may entail significant toxicity.

Reimbursement Practices in Hospice and Palliative Care

Hospice financing mechanisms are often inimical to quality palliative care. Hospice organizations—which are usually reimbursed at a fixed per diem rate—will not deliver some expensive services for fear of jeopardizing the solvency of their programs (Field and Cassel, 1997b). From a financial perspective, the "ideal" hospice patient is the one who lives the longest with minimal interventions in both personnel time and pharmacotherapy. Thus, hospice is placed in the situation of favoring admission of patients who will not receive medical interventions that may prolong their life. Also, it is more likely to refuse admission to patients with a disease known to be incurable but who continue potentially life-prolonging interventions. This is particularly detrimental for the pediatric cancer patient. Examples where current guidelines may interfere with effective palliative care include the child receiving therapy for a highly malignant disease for whom long-term disease-free survival is known to be unlikely at diagnosis, the child enrolled in a Phase I or II study or its equivalent, and the child with disease refractory to experimental or conventional treatment who most likely will die from his or her disease but whose parents continue to hope for cure.

A clinical case may serve to illustrate this situation. "AJ" was a 20-year-old patient with acute lymphoblastic leukemia who relapsed in the bone marrow for the fourth time. He had received care from his oncology team for eight years. Without a bone marrow transplantation, the prognosis for long-term survival was poor, and this was known by the medical team, patient, and family. However, there was no suitable bone marrow donor available: he had no siblings, and there were no unrelated donors who matched sufficiently well. Nonetheless, the patient and his family continued to choose treatment with curative intent hoping that his leukemia would stay in remission while the search for a marrow donor continued. At the time of his fourth relapse, he was still refusing hospice services—but he was not in denial of reality. He had decided he wanted all medical interventions necessary to keep him alive for as long as possible, but he refused artificial life support, mechanical ventilation, and cardiopulmonary resuscitation. He had signed an out-of-hospital do-not-resuscitate (DNR) form and discussed advance directives, choosing his mother as a surrogate decisionmaker if he was unable to make his own decisions. At one point in this process, he was placed in a difficult dilemma: choose treatment for your leukemia (oral palliative chemotherapy, transfusion of blood products) or hospice services at home. Hospice refused to admit him because of the high cost of care related to palliative interventions necessary to prolong his life, which he believed continued to be of good quality. This young man eventually died in the hospital from a serious infection. He deserved the benefit of palliative interventions but never received hospice care. This seems to be the case for the majority of pediatric oncology patients who die from progressive disease.

Another problem encountered in pediatrics is the choice parents sometimes have to make between hospice care and home nursing services for their ill child. Children who are eligible for services under state Medicaid waiver programs for medically fragile children (potentially any child with a life-limiting illness) are generally not eligible for hospice benefits under Medicaid or private insurers. This reality puts parents in a no-win situation, forcing them to choose between hands-on nursing support hours versus the holistic family-centered care provided by a supportive care or hospice and palliative care program. Most chronically or terminally ill children would benefit from some hours of home nursing support, as defined by the Medicaid criteria. However, most hospice and palliative care programs do not provide continuous nursing support in the home, unless they're paired in a contractual arrangement with a home care company or unless they have chosen to bear the high cost of maintaining a home care license within a hospice.

"Bridge programs" have attempted to circumvent this issue by covering a severely ill child in a home care model until the child is strictly "hospice eligible." Reimbursement for these comprehensive services is sparse at best, and usually means that hospice and palliative care programs are following families as "self- pay" until the very end of the child's life or until the child is placed in a residential facility when home care needs are too great. Under these circumstances, the only part of the multidisciplinary care plan that is potentially reimbursable is physician billing, and the myriad other important services provided by the rest of the hospice or palliative care team go financially unrewarded. This reality creates something of a paradox. Hospice and palliative care organizations often recognize the importance of establishing a separate pediatric team because of the issues unique to pediatric end-of-life care. However, the ability to lose money on a pediatric program, due to poor reimbursement and high numbers of self-pay (usually meaning "no pay") patients, puts undue pressure on smaller programs and necessitates high levels of private, philanthropic support. The responsibility for providing specialized pediatric palliative care services, therefore, generally falls on agencies that are large enough to absorb financial losses on the pediatric side. Such programs generally have as part of their mission statements a commitment to providing quality end-of-life care to children and do so primarily as a community service or as a marketing tool, neither of which is necessarily sustainable.

In addition to putting families and providers in a difficult situation, the current system is also internally inconsistent. It is acceptable for patients with third-party insurance and no financial eligibility for Medicaid to tap into Medicaid waiver programs for nursing support. However, Medicaid patients cannot have both, forcing families to choose between nursing support and hospice or palliative care services. The justification for this policy is to prevent duplication of services by excluding patients receiving waiver support from being eligible for the hospice benefit and other Medicaid programs. The "duplication of service argument" applies only to low-income patients and should be amended.

Even in situations where pediatric patients are enrolled "on the benefit," the contracted rate of reimbursement pays for only a fraction of the services provided. Patients who are on "full benefit" are entitled to all of the core services *modeled after* the Medicare hospice benefit, but this does not include creative arts therapies (e.g., art, dance and movement, music, and drama therapies), nor does it provide bereavement services beyond 13 months, too short for many families who lose children to illness. Longer follow-up is unlikely to be reimbursed by any formal mechanism other than philanthropic support. Similarly, spiritual care, and child life and expressive therapy are particularly important in the pediatric arena as families struggle with a child's terminal illness. The literature abounds with examples of the importance of art, music, and movement therapy for dying children and their families, particularly siblings, in supporting effective coping and grieving. Yet these disciplines are not reimbursed at all in the current benefit system.

Apart from the issues discussed above, pediatric palliative care faces an additional challenge. While no direct reimbursement for palliative care is available for any patient, adult palliative care programs are able to capture some revenue through physician billing under different codes (e.g., for symptom management) than those used by the primary care provider or other specialists involved in the patient's care. In pediatrics, however, this revenue stream is difficult to capture without the services of a pediatric hospice or palliative care physician. Some hospitals and acute care institutions allow internal medicine and family practice physicians to see pediatric patients (especially adolescents), which affords pediatric patients the benefit of hospice or palliative care expertise and allows practitioners to bill for their services. However, these patients are then not receiving specialized pediatric care. The likelihood of finding expertise in pediatric palliative care and hospice is currently low and drops even further when patients are not within a hospital setting.

One additional problem in pediatric hospice care is the shortage of contracted beds for symptom control or hospice admissions within acute care settings. In large hospitals, adult hospice programs have little trouble securing a few beds to be used for their patients. In pediatrics, however, hospitals are reluctant to commit beds to hospice care because they may be empty much of the time but could be used for other admissions if available.

Potential Remedies

• **Set a minimum reimbursement rate for physician communication time with parents *and* with patients.** Legislation may be required to prevent denial of payment for this basic service.

• **Enforce payment for telephone time and care plan oversight time.**

• **Enforce reimbursement of team conferences with patients and families at a rate that reflects participation of the multidisciplinary team.**

• **Develop and test palliative care codes for reimbursement of physicians and other health care providers for pediatric palliative care interventions offered based on the goals of medical care:**

    1. *Palliative care codes*: services offered for patients with incurable disease receiving treatment with the intent to prolong a life of good quality

    2. *Hospice care codes:* palliative care in which the primary focus of treatment is end-of-life comfort care

    3. *Bereavement care codes:* palliative care in the form of grief and bereavement counseling for surviving family members

• **Develop patient evaluation and management codes for reimbursement of palliative care services in different settings. Include funding mechanisms for the *entire multidisciplinary team, including mental health and bereavement workers.***

• **Create contractual arrangements for a small number of beds in pediatric hospitals to be used for children needing respite or symptom control care, with appropriate reimbursement.**

RESEARCH NEEDS IN PEDIATRIC ONCOLOGY
END-OF-LIFE CARE

The research base in pediatric oncology for dying children is deficient in every area, directly affecting the quality of the care that children receive. In addition to the important work of developing and testing new treatments to reduce the number of children who face death from cancer, research must focus on the children who do, in fact, die. Results of research in the following areas could be of direct benefit in the treatment of dying children.

- **Describe current end-of-life care practice patterns.** The descriptive information available for the care of dying children is inadequate (e.g., very little information on the use of hospice, the use of palliative care teams or pain services, incidence of death at home versus the hospital or other inpatient facility, use of advance directives or DNR orders and the duration these are in effect before death, use of psychosocial multidisciplinary teams, and patient and family satisfaction with these services).
- **Create tools to assess the quality of pediatric end-of-life care.** A single instrument (questionnaire) has been validated for pediatrics, consisting of a two-hour interview, which is not practical for broad use (Wolfe, 2000). New instruments (either completely new or adapted from adult models) for widespread use are needed.
- **Evaluate pediatric models for provider-patient-family communication.** Research is needed to define communication models that prevent psychological harm to *parents and children* and that result in a sense of control and efficacy for parents. Research questions include how to communicate bad news effectively, how to discuss withdrawal of therapies, how to teach what to expect as their child dies, how to communicate goals of care that incorporate both curative and palliative therapies without a feeling of "giving up," and how to facilitate communication across treatment sites.
- **Create and evaluate comprehensive parent educational materials,** including, for example, what to expect during withdrawal of support, what will be experienced during an expected death at home, and how to advocate for symptom control.
- Evaluate models of decisionmaking that are family centered, and emphasize the involvement of the child.
- Evaluate models of care that address the needs of siblings.
- Investigate the barriers to optimal symptom control in pediatric oncology practice.
- Develop and validate symptom (and suffering) assessment tools for the pediatric population to be used for both research and treatment.

• Initiate clinical trials in symptom control within the Children's Oncology Group.

• Incorporate symptom control algorithms into COG clinical trials.

• Develop models of care incorporating the principles of palliative care throughout the mainstream of medical therapy of seriously ill pediatric oncology patients, from the time of diagnosis to the time of death.

• Investigate the impact on care delivery of barriers to optimal care.

• Develop and evaluate a "mobile medical record" for palliative care content that will follow the patient across various treatment sites.

• Assess the needs of medical providers caring for dying children.

• Develop palliative care codes for reimbursement of physicians and other health care providers for pediatric palliative care interventions offered across settings based on the goals of medical care.

• Investigate the financial implications of care models developed as discussed above.

• Develop education strategies for providers.

PEDIATRIC ONCOLOGY END-OF-LIFE CARE: FUTURE DIRECTIONS

• The education of providers must be adapted to meet the unique needs of those caring for dying children, and must include both traditional and nontraditional teaching methods. The recommendations below include mechanisms for accountability.

• Develop educational materials for families that facilitate the most complete understanding of the child's condition and prepare them as much as possible for what will occur as the child dies. In this manner, patients and families will be empowered to participate in treatment decisions.

• Facilitate the involvement of children in their treatment decisions (assent).

• Develop and evaluate models of oncology care that incorporate palliative care principles and facilitate continuity of care by providers educated in pediatric end-of-life care.

• Develop strategies to address the inadequate relief of pain and other symptoms in pediatric oncology patients nearing the end of life.

• Institute regulatory and reimbursement policies that adequately address the complexity and time involved in caring for children with advanced illness.

• Develop research initiatives that will assess current practice patterns, evaluate models of care delivery, evaluate models of communication and decisionmaking, study methods of symptom control, evaluate the feasibility and cost-effectiveness of new reimbursement models, and evaluate innovative educational initiatives.

REFERENCES

AAHPM (American Academy of Hospice and Palliative Medicine). 1998. Hospice/Palliative Care Training for Physicians: UNIPACs. Dubuque, Iowa: Kendall/Hunt Publishing Company.

AAP (American Academy of Pediatrics), Committee on Bioethics. Informed consent, parental permission, and assent in pediatric practice. *Pediatrics* 1995;95:314-317.

Accreditation Standards, 2000. Liaison Committee on Medical Education.

Angell, M., Caring for the dying-congressional mischief (editorial). *N Engl J Med* 1999;341: 1923-1925.

Armstrong-Dailey A, Goltzer SZ (eds). 1993. *Hospice Care for Children*. New York: Oxford University Press.

Bartholome WG. Care of the dying child: the demands of ethics. *Second Opin* 1993;18:25-39.

Bennet DS. Depression among children with chronic medical problems: a meta-analysis. *J Pediatr Psychol* 1994;19:149-169.

Bleyer WA. The U.S. pediatric cancer clinical trials programmes: international implications and the way forward. *Eur J Cancer* 1997;33:1439-1447.

Bleyer WA, Tejeda H, Murphy SB, Robinson LL, Ross JA, Pollock BH, et al. National cancer clinical trials: Children have equal access; adolescents do not. *J Adolesc Health* 1997;21: 366-73

Bluebond-Langner M. 1978. *The Private Lives of Dying Children*. Princeton, NJ: Princeton University Press.

Brenner P. 1993. The volunteer component. In: *Hospice Care for Children*, Armstrong-Dailey A, Goltzer SZ (eds). New York: Oxford University Press, pp.198-218.

Brock DW. 1989. Children's competence for health care decisionmaking. In: *Children and Health Care: Moral and Social Issues*, Kopelman LM, Moskop JC (eds). Boston: Kluwer Academic Publishers, pp. 181-212.

Carr-Gregg MRC, Sawyer SM, Clarke CF, Bowes G. Caring for the terminally ill adolescent. *Med J Aust* 1997;166:255-258.

Castro O, Gordeuk VR, Dawkins F. Letter to the editor. *N Engl J Med* 2000;342:1049-50.

Chevlen E. Letter to the editor. *N Engl J Med* 2000;342:1049-1050.

Children's Hospice International. 1998. 1998 Survey: Hospice Care for Children. Executive Summary Report. Alexandria, VA.

Collins JJ, Grier HE, Kinney HC, Berde CB. Control of severe pain in children with terminal malignancy. *J Pediatr* 1995a;126:653-657.

Collins JJ, Kerner J, Sentivany S, Berde CB. Intravenous amitriptyline in pediatrics. *J Pain Sympt Manage* 1995b;10:471-475.

Collins JJ, Grier HE, Sethna NF, Wilder RT, Berde CB. Regional anesthesia for pain associated with terminal pediatric malignancy. *Pain* 1996a;65:63-69.

Collins JJ, Geake J, Grier HE, Houck CS, Thaler HT, Weinstein HJ, Twum-Danso NY, Berde CB. Patient-controlled analgesia for mucositis pain in children: a three-period crossover study comparing morphine and hydromorphone. *J Pediatr* 1996b;129:722-728.

Collins JJ, Stevens MM, Cousens P. Home care for the dying child. A parent's perception. *Australian Family Physician* 1998;27:610-614.

Collins JJ, Dunkel IJ, Gupta SK, Inturrisi CE, Lapin J, Palmer LN, Weinstein SM, Portenoy RK. Transdermal fentanyl in children with cancer pain: feasibility, tolerability, and pharmacokinetic correlates. *J Pediatr* 1999;134:319-323.

Collins JJ, Byrnes ME, Dunkel IJ, Lapin J, Nadel T, Thaler HT, Polyak T, Rapkin B, Portenoy RK. The measurement of symptoms in children with cancer. *J Pain Sympt Manage* (in press).

Cooper MG, Keneally JP, Kinchington D. Continuous brachial plexus neural blockade in a child with intractable cancer pain. *J Pain Sympt Manage* 1994;9:277-281.

Council on Scientific Affairs, American Medical Association. Good care of the dying patient. *JAMA* 1996;275:474-478.

Department of Health and Human Services, Food and Drug Administration. 1998. Regulations requiring manufacturers to assess the safety and effectiveness of new drugs and biological products in pediatric patients. *Federal Register* p. 66632.

Die Trill M, Kovalcik R. The child with cancer: influence of culture on truth-telling and patient care. *Ann NY Acad Sci* 1997;809:197-210.

Doyle D, Hanks GWC, MacDonald N (eds). 1998. *Oxford Textbook of Palliative Medicine*. Oxford: Oxford University Press, pp.1013-1117.

Emanuel EJ, Weinberg DS, Gonin R, Hummel LR, Emanuel LL. How well is the Patient Self-Determination Act working? An early assessment. *Am J Med* 1993;95:619-628.

Emanuel L, von Gunten C, Ferris F. 1999. The education for physicians on end-of-life care (EPEC) curriculum. Princeton, NJ: Robert Wood Johnson Foundation: Princeton.

Faulkner KW. Talking about death with a dying child. *AJN* 1997;97:64-69.

Fehder WP, Sachs J, Uvaydova M, Douglas SD. Substance P as an immune modulator of anxiety. *Neuroimmunomodulation* 1997;4:42-48.

Ferrell B, Grant M, Coyne P, Egan K, Paice J, Panke J. 2000. End-of-life nursing education consortium (ELNEC) project. American Association of Colleges of Nursing.

Field MJ, Cassel CK (eds). 1997. *Approaching Death. Improving Care at the End of Life*. Washington, DC: National Academy Press.

Frager G. Pediatric palliative care: building the model, bridging the gaps. *J Palliat Care* 1996;12:9-12.

Fredrikson M, Furst CJ, Lekander M, Rotstein S, Blomgren H. Trait anxiety and anticipatory immune reactions in women receiving adjuvant chemotherapy for breast cancer. *Brain Behav Immun* 1993;7:79-90.

Freyer DR. Children with cancer: special considerations in the discontinuation of life-sustaining treatment. *Med Pediatr Oncol* 1992;20:136-142.

Friebert SE, Kodish ED. Kids and cancer: ethical issues in treating the pediatric oncology patient. *Cancer Treat Res* 2000;102:99-135.

Goldman A, Christie D. Children with cancer talk about their own death with their families. Pediatr Hematol Oncol 1993;10:223-31.

Goldman A. Home care of the dying child. *J Palliative Care* 1996;12:16-19.

Goldman A (ed). 1994. *Care of the Dying Child*. Oxford: Oxford University Press.

Hain RDW, Patel N, Crabtree S, Pinkerton R. Respiratory symptoms in children dying from malignant disease. *Palliat Med* 1995;9:201-206.

Hain RDW. Pain scales in children: a review. *Palliat Med* 1997;11:341-350.

Hearn J, Higginson I. Do specialist palliative care teams improve outcomes for cancer patients? A systematic literature review. *Palliat Med* 1998;12:317-332.

Hilden JM, Emanuel EJ, Fairclough DL, Link MP, Foley KM, Clarridge BC, Schnipper LE, Mayer RJ. Attitudes and practices among pediatric oncologists regarding end-of-life care: results of the 1998 American Society of Clinical Oncology survey. *JCO* 2001;19:205-212.

National Hospice Organization. 1997. Hospice Fact Sheet.

Howell DA. 1993. Role of the primary physician. In: *Hospice Care for Children*, Armstrong-Dailey A, Golzer SZ (eds). New York: Oxford University Press, pp. 172-183.

Hunt A, Joel S, Dick G, Goldman A. Population pharmacokinetics of oral morphine and its glucuronides in children receiving morphine as immediate-release liquid or sustained-release tablets for cancer pain. *J Pediatr* 1999;135:47-55.

International Work Group on Death, Dying, and Bereavement. Palliative care for children. *Death Studies* 1993;17:277-280.

James L, Johnson B. The needs of parents of pediatric oncology patients during the palliative care phase. *J Pediatr Oncol Nurs* 1997;14:83-95.

Kane J, Barber RB, Jordan M, Tichenor KT, Camp K. Supportive/palliative care of children suffering from life-threatening and terminal illness. *Am J Hosp & Palliat Care* 2000; 17:165-172.

Kart T, Christrup LL, Rasmussen M. Recommended use of morphine in neonates, infants and children based on a literature review. Part 2-Clinical use. *Paediatr Anaesthes* 1997;7:93-101.

Kazak AE, Blackall G, Himelstein B, Brophy P, Daller R. Producing systemic change in pediatric practice: An intervention protocol for reducing distress during painful procedures. *Fam Syst Med* 1995;13:173-185.

Kazak AE, Penati B, Brophy P, Himelstein B. Pharmacologic and psychologic interventions for procedural pain. *Pediatr* 1998;102:59-66.

Khaneya S, Milrod B. Educational needs among pediatricians regarding caring for terminally ill children. *Arch Pediatr Adolesc Med* 1998;152:909-914.

Kinzbrunner BM. Hospice: 15 years and beyond in the care of the dying. *J Palliat Med* 1998;1:127-137.

Kosary Cl, Ries LAG, Miller B et al. (eds). 1995. Cancer in children. In: *SEER Cancer Statistics Review, 1973-1992*. U.S. Dept of health and Human Services, 1995. NIH publication number 96-2789. Bethesda, MD: National Cancer Institute, pp. 455-465.

Landis SH, Murray T, Bolden S, Wingo PA. Cancer statistics, 1999. *CA Cancer J Clin* 1999;49:8-31.

Leikin S. The role of adolescents in decisions concerning their cancer therapy. *Cancer* 1993; 71(suppl):3342-3346.

Levy MH. Doctor-patient communication: the lifeline to comprehensive cancer care. *ASCO Educational Book.* 1998;195-202.

Liben S. Pediatric palliative medicine: obstacles to overcome. *J Palliat Care* 1996;12:24-28.

Manne SL, Jacobsen PB, Redd WH. Assessment of acute pediatric pain: do child self-report, parent ratings, and nurse ratings measure the same phenomenon? *Pain* 1992;48:45-52.

Martinson IM. Hospice care for children: past, present, and future. *J Pediatr Oncol Nurs* 1993;10:93-98.

Martinson I. 1993. A home care program. In: *Hospice Care for Children*, Armstrong-Dailey A, Golzer SZ (eds). New York: Oxford University Press, pp. 231-47.

Martinson IM. Improving care of dying children. *West J Med* 1995;163:258-262.

Masera G, Spinetta JJ, Jankovic M, Ablin AR, D'Angio GJ, Van Dongen-Melman J, et al. Guidelines for assistance to terminally ill children with cancer: a report of the SIOP working committee on psychosocial issues in pediatric oncology. *Med Pediatr Oncol* 1999;32:44-48.

McCarthy AM, Cool VA, Petersen M, Bruene DA. Cognitive behavioral pain and anxiety interventions in pediatric oncology centers and bone marrow transplant units. *J Pediatr Oncol Nurs* 1996;13:3-12.

Mercadante S. Pain treatment and outcomes for patients with advanced cancer who receive follow-up care at home. *Cancer* 1999;85:1849-1858.

NACHRI (National Association of Chilren's Hospitals and Related Institutions).1999. Patient Hematology and Oncology FOCUS Groups.

Nitschke R, Wunder S, Sexauer CL, Humphrey GB. The final-stage conference: the patient's decision on research drugs in pediatric oncology. *J Pediatr Psychol* 1997;2:58-64.

Nitschke R, Meyer WH, Sexauer CL, Parkhurst JB, Foster P, Huszti H. Care of terminally ill children with cancer. *Med Ped Oncol* 2000;34:268-270.

Office of Protection from Research Risks (OPRR). 1991. Protection of human subjects. Department of Health and Human Services. National Institute of Health. Title 45, *Code of Federal Regulations*, Part 46. Appendix 4, p. 16.

Pain Relief Promotion Act of 1999. H.R. 2260. 106th Congress, 1st session.

Papadatou D. Training health professionals in caring for dying children and grieving families. *Death Studies* 1997;21:575-600.

Pizzo P, Poplack D (eds). 1997. *Principles and Practice of Pediatric Oncology*. Philadelphia: Lippincott-Raven.

Razavi D, Delvaux N, Farvaques C, Robaye E. Immediate effectiveness of brief psychological training for health professionals dealing with terminally ill cancer patients: a controlled study. *Soc Sci Med* 1988; 27:369-375.

Razavi D, Delvaux N, Farvacques C, Robaye E. Brief psychological training for health care professionals dealing with cancer patients: a one-year assessment. *Gen Hosp Psychiat* 1991;13:253-260.

Ross JA, Severson RK, Pollock BH, Robison LL. Childhood cancer in the United States: a geographical analysis of cases from the pediatric cooperative clinical trials groups. *Cancer* 1996;77:201-207.

Ryan ND. Psychoneuroendocrinology of children and adolescents. *Psychiatr Clin North Am* 1998;21:435-441.

Sagara M, Pickett M. Sociocultural influences and care of dying children in Japan and the United States. *Cancer Nurs* 1998;21:274-281.

Sahler OJZ, Frager G, Levetown M, Cohn FG, Lipson MA. Medical education about end-of-life care in the pediatric setting: principles, challenges, and opportunities. *Pediatr* 2000; 105:575-584.

Schechter NL, Altman AJ, Weisman SJ (eds). Report of the consensus committee on pain in childhood cancer. *Pediatr* 1990;86(suppl):813-834.

Schweitzer SO, Mitchell B, Landsverk J, Laparan L. The costs of a pediatric hospice program. *Public Health Reports* 1993;108:37-44.

Shir Y, Shenkman Z, Shavelson V, Davidson EM, Rosen G. Oral methadone for the treatment of severe pain in hospitalized children: a report of five cases. *Clin J Pain* 1998; 14:350-353.

Sirkiä K, Hovi L, Pouttu J, Saarinen-Pihkala UM. Pain medication during terminal care of children with cancer. *J Pain Sympt Manage* 1998;15:220-226.

Sourkes B. 1995. *Armfuls of time: the psychological experience of the child with a life-threatening illness*. Pittsburgh, PA: University of Pittsburgh Press.

Staats PS, Kost-Byerly S. Celiac plexus blockade in a 7-year old child with neuroblastoma. *J Pain Sympt Manage* 1995;10:321-324.

Stevens MM. 1998. Psychological adaptation of the dying child. In: *Oxford Textbook of Palliative Medicine*, Doyle D, Hanks GWC, MacDonald N (eds). Oxford: Oxford University Press, pp. 1045-55.

Stevens MM. 1998. Care of the dying child and adolescent: family adjustment and support. In: *Oxford Textbook of Palliative Medicine*, Doyle D, Hanks GWC, MacDonald N (eds). Oxford: Oxford University Press, pp. 1058-75.

Storey P, Knight C. 1996. UNIPAC six: Ethical and legal decision making when caring for the terminally ill. Gainesville, FL: AAHPM.

Teno JM, Casey VA, Welch L, Edgman-Levitan, S. Patient focused, family centered end-of-life medical care: views of the guidelines and bereaved family members. Draft manuscript for Third Woods Hole conference on measuring quality of life and quality of care at life's end. June 2000.

Vermillion J. 1996. The referral process and reimbursement. In: *Hospice and Palliative Care* Sheehan DC, Forman WB (eds). Sudbury, MA: Jones and Bartlett Publishers, pp 11-20.

Vickers JL, Carlisle C. Choices and control: parental experiences in pediatric terminal home care. *J Ped Onc Nursing* 2000;17:12-21.

Weisman SJ. 1998. Supportive care in children with cancer. In: *Principles and Practice of Supportive Oncology*. Berger A, Portenoy RK, Weissman DE (eds). Philadelphia: Lippincott-Raven, pp. 845-52.

Wessel MA. The role of the primary pediatrician when a child dies [editorial]. *Arch Pediatr Adolesc Med* 1998;152:837-838.

Whittam EH. Terminal care of the dying child: psychosocial implications of care. *Cancer* 1993;71:3450-3462.

WHO (World Health Organization) and International Association for the Study of Pain. 1998. *Cancer Pain Relief and Palliative Care in Children*. Geneva: World Health Organization.

Wolfe J. Personal communication to Joanne Hilden, 2000.

Wolfe J, Grier HE, Klar N, Salem-Schatz S, Emanuel EJ, Weeks JC. Physician-assisted suicide and euthanasia: experiences and attitudes among parents of children who have died of cancer. *Proc ASCO* 1999;18:577a.

Wolfe J, Grier HE, Klar N, Levin S, Ellenbogen J, Salem-Schatz S, Emanuel EJ, Weeks JC. Symptoms and suffering at the end of life in children with cancer. *N Engl J Med* 2000;342:326-333.

Yee JD, Berde CB. Dextroamphetamine or methylphenidate as adjuvants to opioid analgesia for adolescents with cancer. *J Pain Sympt Manage* 1994;9:122-125.

7

Clinical Practice Guidelines for the Management of Psychosocial and Physical Symptoms of Cancer

Jimmie C. Holland, M.D.

Lisa Chertkov, M.D.

Memorial Sloan-Kettering Cancer Center

We are not ourselves when nature, being oppressed, commands the mind to suffer with the body.

King Lear, Act II Sc. IV, Li. 116-119

INTRODUCTION

After years of neglect, care at the end of life is receiving increasing attention and concern. We are beginning to recognize that when death is near, the body is suffering the effects of a progressive and mortal illness and that the person is coping not only with the bodily symptoms, but also with the existential crisis of the end of life and approaching death. As the body suffers, the mind is indeed "commanded . . . to suffer with the body," as Shakespeare so well described. Thus, the suffering encompasses both the mind and the body. The imperative of providing optimal symptom relief and alleviation of suffering is the highest priority in care. However, evidence suggests that we are failing to do this (American Society of Clinical Oncology, 1998; Carver and Foley 2000; Cassel and Foley, 1999; Cassem 1997). Although pain management guidelines have been the most widely disseminated, we know that many patients continue to suffer not only from pain, but from other troubling symptoms in their final days (Ahmedzai, 1998; American Academy of Neurology, 1996; American Board of Internal Medicine, 1996; American Nursing Association, 1991; American Pain Society, 1995; Carr et al, 1994). Despite clear advances in the identification and treatment of psychiatric disorders, we continue to underdiagnose and under-treat the debilitating symptoms of depression, anxiety and delirium in the final stages of life (Breitbart et al., 2000; Carroll et al., 1993; Chochinov and Breitbart, 2000; Hirschfeld et al., 1997; Holland, 1997, 1998, 1999). Also, beyond these physical and psychological symptoms, we fall even shorter of our goals of alleviating the spiritual, psychosocial, and existential suffering of the dying patient and family (Cherny et al., 1994, 1996; Fitchett and Handzo, 1998; Karasu, 2000). Yet the ethical and professional challenge to do so is as important as the obligation to cure (Pellegrino, 2000).

In seeking to provide better care for patients at the end of life, the most effective approach appears to be the use of clinical practice guidelines that establish a benchmark of quality based on the delivery of evidence-based medicine (Chassin, 1998; Field and Lohr, 1990, 1992; Field and Cassel, 1997). This chapter outlines the current status of clinical practice guidelines to guide management of psychiatric, psychosocial, and spiritual distress in the context of managing the physical symptoms at the end of life. The focus is on the management of distress and the interaction of physical symptoms and distress.

Clinical Practice Guidelines in Cancer Care

Public and private agencies in the United States have increasingly focused on the quality of health care being delivered (Emanuel, 1996; Ford et al., 1987; IOM, 1999; Patton and Katterhagen, 1997; Stephenson, 1997). This has been particularly useful in cancer because it has encouraged the scrutiny of care delivered across the disease continuum and the establishment of practice guidelines (Morris, 1996).

Clinical practice guidelines are defined as "systematically developed statements to assist both practitioner and patient decisions about appropriate health care for specific clinical circumstances" (Field and Lohr, 1990, 1992). Guidelines are based on evidence derived from research or clinical trials, or from a consensus of experts when objective evidence is not available. There are two types of guidelines in use. The algorithm or path guideline, the most widely used, directs decisionmaking toward a set standard. The other type is the boundary guideline that defines the appropriate use of a new technology or intervention (often as a cost-saving device). The National Cancer Policy Board (NCPB) noted in *Ensuring Quality Cancer Care* that the use of systematically developed clinical practice guidelines, based on best available evidence, improved the quality of care delivered (IOM, 1999). Smith and Hillner (1998) reviewed the status of clinical practice guidelines, critical pathways, and care maps and found that care improved with the use of explicit guidelines in 55 of 59 published studies and in 9 of 11 studies that assessed defined outcomes.

However, a guideline has no impact on health care unless providers endorse and use it. Directly involving physicians in the development of guidelines, holding them accountable through peer pressure, monitoring their compliance, and providing feedback about performance and potential positive effects on outcome are critical to their being used (Katterhagen, 1996). An important corollary, endorsed by the National Comprehensive Cancer Network (NCCN), which has developed guidelines for all cancer sites and many symptoms, is the importance of regular review to update and revise guidelines to reflect new information that impacts on practice. Since much depends on the human element of physician "buy-in," ways to ensure cooperation, dissemination, implementation at the clinical level, and accountability for applying them will continue as important research questions (Grimshaw and Russell, 1993).

Ensuring full application of practice guidelines poses special challenges when applied to end-of-life care. Comfort care is affected by a range of cultural factors: the customs and ethnicity of the patients and their families; community norms and expectations; religious and philosophical belief systems. Physicians' personal attitudes and beliefs about death also affect their interest and participation in end-of-life care. Development and evaluation of clinical practice guidelines for end-of-life care must take into account the unique aspects of treatment during this period. The task becomes daunting, given the recognized problems with implementation of clinical practice guidelines for pain management and the complexity of developing guidelines that direct both medical and psychological care. The majority of existing clinical practice guidelines in cancer are directed toward the management of specific cancer types and stages of disease. Most have been developed through the American Society of Clinical Oncology (ASCO), NCCN (McGivney, 1998), the American College of Surgeons (ACoS), and the Agency for Health Care Research and Quality (AHRQ, formerly the Agency for Health Care Policy and Research) (Table 7-1; Smith and Hillner, 1998). AHRQ also has developed an Internet-based clearinghouse for all practice guidelines meeting certain criteria.

CLINICAL PRACTICE GUIDELINES FOR END-OF-LIFE CARE

The World Health Organization (WHO, 1996, 1998) defined end-of-life care as "the active, total care of patients whose disease is not responsive to curative treatment." The focus at this point is to attain maximal quality of life through control of physical and psychological, social, and spiritual distress of the patient and family. Hospice philosophy has long supported this integrated approach, as well as giving attention to the caregiver. The wide range of these issues makes the task of developing clinical practice guidelines more formidable but, at the same time, more critical. The 1997

TABLE 7-1 Selected, Publicly Available Oncology Guidelines, by
Sponsoring Group

Group	Guidelines	Comment
National Comprehensive Cancer Network	Path or algorithm guidelines for all common cancers	Evidence based, with consensus; when no consensus possible, options listed Intended for mandatory use for all participating cancer centers No date set for implementation No set benchmarks for care Adopted in the community for use outside of NCCN cancer centers No data yet on compliance or outcomes
American Society of Clinical Oncology	Boundary guidelines for new technologies Hematopoietic growth factors Outcomes important enough to justify treatment Antiemetics Surveillance of breast and colorectal cancer patients Path or algorithm guidelines for specific diseases Management of non-small cell lung cancer Metastatic prostate cancer	Evidence based, with consensus demanded before approval Adopted by the community but no data available on compliance or outcomes Likely that all future guidelines will be boundary guidelines for new technologies, with overlap of ASCO and NCCN methods and topics
Society for Surgical Oncology	Path guidelines for management of common surgical problems	Consensus panels
American Urology Association	Path guidelines for common urology problems	Consensus based on evidence
University of California (UC) Cancer Care Consortium (UC and PONA, Inc.)	Path guidelines for most solid tumors	PONA did systematic reviews, consulted with UC faculty for consensus

SOURCE: Smith and Hillner, 1998.

Institute of Medicine (IOM) report *Approaching Death* stated that ensuring quality of care requires that recommendations be made by experienced professionals; that clear goals of care are established; that patients have access to clinical trials, if desired; that a patient receives the available services in a coordinated manner; that the patient is told and understands the treatment options; that there is available an appropriate range of psychosocial services; that the care be given in a compassionate way; and that the care integrates the physical and psychosocial elements.

The need for guidelines has also been acknowledged by policy analysts, health care professionals, patients, families and third-party payers, and work is progressing toward developing them (see Table 7-2). The ASCO Task Force on Cancer Care at the End of Life set out a basic principle for end-of-life care of "optimizing quality of life . . . with attention to the myriad physical, spiritual and psychosocial needs of the patient and family" (ASCO, 1998). An NCCN panel has begun adapting general guidelines for nausea and vomiting and for pain control for end-of-life care (Dr. Michael Levy, personal communication). Several large institutions, including Memorial Sloan-Kettering Cancer Center, have developed guidelines for end-of-life care. Development of algorithm-based clinical practice guidelines relating to psychiatric, psychosocial, and spiritual domains has the potential to enhance end-of-life care in a major way by defining a gold standard for clinicians in an area not previously subjected to this level of scrutiny.

This chapter outlines the status of clinical practice guidelines that relate to end-of-life care and suggests next steps for policy development.

The areas reviewed in this chapter are:

- communication with patient and family;
- management of distress (psychiatric, psychological, social, existential, spiritual) in the patient and family; and
- management of several physical symptoms that are common at the end of life: pain, fatigue, nausea and vomiting, dyspnea.

A key concept for end-of-life care guidelines is the recognition that the physical and the psychosocial, existential, and spiritual concerns are interrelated and overlapping, so it is critical that the patient experience appropriate attention to both (Twycross and Lichter, 1998; Wanzer et al., 1989).

Communication with Patient and Family

Central to ensuring quality of *all* care at the end of life is communication between the doctor, patient, and family (Girgis and Sanson-Fisher, 1995; Ptacek and Eberhardt, 1996). Identification and management of symptoms—physical and psychological—hinge upon this interaction. Buck-

TABLE 7-2   Clinical Practice Guidelines for End-of-Life Care: Status, Source and Further Development Needed

Symptom	Status	Source	Further Development
Overall end-of-life care	NCCN Practice Guidelines (pending) (NCCN, 2001)	Evidence, consensus, or combination	Pilot testing; modify for end-of-life care
Doctor-patient communication	NCCN Practice Guidelines: breaking bad news (pending) (NCCN, 2001)	Evidence, consensus, or combination	Pilot testing; modify for end-of-life care
Distress	NCCN Practice Guidelines: ambulatory care Definition—Psychosocial, existential or spiritual (NCCN, 1999)		Algorithm for recognition and referral; modify for end-of-life care
Delirium	APA Practice Guidelines: physically healthy (APA, 2000)	Evidence, consensus, or combination	Modify for medically ill and end-of-life care
	NCCN Practice Guidelines: ambulatory care (NCCN, 1999)	Evidence, consensus, or combination	Modify for end-of life care; pilot test
Depressive disorders	APA Practice Guidelines: physically healthy (APA, 2000)	Evidence, consensus, or combination	Modify for end-of-life care
	NCCN Practice Guidelines: ambulatory care (NCCN, 1999)	Evidence, consensus, or combination	Modify for end-of-life care; pilot test
Anxiety disorders	APA Practice Guidelines: panic disorder in healthy patients (APA, 2000)	Evidence, consensus, or combination	Modify for medically ill/end-of-life care
	NCCN Practice Guidelines: ambulatory care (NCCN, 1999)	Evidence, consensus, or combination	Modify for end-of-life care; pilot test
Personality disorders	APA Practice Guidelines (APA, 2000)	Evidence, consensus, or combination	Modify for medically ill and end-of-life care
	NCCN Practice Guidelines: ambulatory care (NCCN, 1999)	Evidence, consensus, or combination	Modify for end-of-life care; pilot test

TABLE 7-2 Continued

Symptom	Status	Source	Further Development
Social problems: practical or psychosocial	NCCN Guidelines for Social Work Services: Ambulatory (NCCN, 1999)	Evidence, consensus, or combination	Modify for end-of-life care; pilot test
Spiritual or religious problems	NCCN Guidelines for Clergy/Pastoral Counselors: ambulatory (NCCN, 1999)	Evidence, consensus, or combination	Modify for end-of-life care; pilot test
Pain	AHCPR Guidelines (AHCPR, 1994)	Evidence, consensus, or combination	Modify for end-of-life care
	APS Guidelines (APS, 1995)	Evidence, consensus, or combination	Dissemination and implementation
	WHO Pain Management (WHO, 1996)	Evidence, consensus, or combination	Compliance and implementation
	NCCN Guidelines (NCCN, 1999)	Evidence, consensus, or combination	Modify for end-of-life care; pilot test; dissemination and compliance
Fatigue	NCCN Practice Guidelines: guidelines for anemia-related fatigue management (NCCN, 1999)	Evidence, consensus, or combination	Modify for end-of-life care; pilot test
Nausea and vomiting	NCCN anti-emesis (for treatment-related nausea and vomiting) (NCCN, 1997)	Evidence, consensus, or combination	Modify for end-of-life care; pilot test
Dyspnea	Descriptive guides to care (Ahmedzai, 1998)	Literature	Develop guidelines; pilot test

NOTE: APA = American Psychiatric Association; APS = American Pain Society; AHCPR = Agency for Health Care Policy and Research; NCCN = National Comprehensive Cancer Network

man (1998), an oncologist who teaches communication skills, noted, "Almost invariably, the act of communication is an important part of therapy: occasionally it is the only constituent. It usually requires greater thought and planning than a drug prescription, and unfortunately it is commonly administered in subtherapeutic doses."

Within the area of communication, teaching how to break bad news has been given the most attention, since it is a common task facing oncologists. An NCCN panel has developed algorithm-based guidelines for delivering bad news, which are being revised for application to end-of-life care (Dr. William Breitbart, personal communication). A review of the literature from 1975 to 1999 (Holland and Almanza, 1999) revealed that of the 166 articles published on this topic, the majority were written in the past five years, reflecting the recent, increased concern about this issue. However, only 14 percent of the studies were based on controlled trials; most papers were based on consensus or clinical experience. Baile and colleagues (1999) proposed guidelines for discussing disease progression and end-of-life care.

Several tenets of importance emerge: finding out what the patient understands; learning how much more or less information does she or he want to know; being sensitive to and empathic with whatever emotions the patient expresses; listening attentively and allowing tears and emotions to be expressed without signs of being rushed; and taking into account the family and its ethnic, cultural and religious roots. All may contribute to decisions about care (Braun et al., 2000; Hastings Center, 1987). These tenets should include attention to the needs of traditionally medically underserved patients: those with little or no English proficiency, for whom care at the end of life is particularly difficult because communication is limited, and patients with chronic mental illness or limited education.

The need for communication guidelines and standards is accentuated because of the awkwardness that many professionals feel in talking with patients about death, as well as the difficulty patients themselves have in expressing their fears and uncertainties about their possible death.

Family members face similar challenges in expressing their feelings and asking questions about prognosis. A series of 19 focus groups held in eight cancer centers comprised either doctors alone, nurses alone, or patients alone. The doctors felt they had more trouble communicating with families than with the patients themselves (Speice et al., 2000). Patients noted that their relatives often felt "left out" and "in the way." These issues are particularly disturbing since impending death has a profound impact on the family who shares the death vigil with the doctor. Family members often recall in exquisite detail the sensitivity (or lack of it) of the doctor and staff as their relative was dying. These memories affect the grieving process, recalling as they do the details of how the family was told by the doctor about what was being done, how it was informed of changes in the medical situation, and especially how attentive the doctor and the staff were in controlling the patient's distress and physical symptoms (Chochinov et al., 1998; Zisook, 2000).

Communication with Patient and Family: Next Steps

1. Training of doctors in communication skills is critical to ensure quality end-of-life care. The best teaching model is one that uses faculty from the physician's own discipline (e.g., oncologists for oncologists) as well as a physician or mental health clinician skilled in teaching communication. Such workshops have proven to have a low priority for voluntary attendance; mandating participation via required risk management lectures is useful. The content of the skills teaching sessions is best acquired when the groups are small in number, when they use videotapes of model patterns of communication, and when they include role playing, which enhances sensitivity to patients' emotional responses and also to the doctor's own responses.

2. Research is needed to determine the best teaching methods. Approaches based on a theoretical model of stress are effective, such as the Transpersonal Model of Stress, which examines physicians' and patients' responses at each phase of the discussion (Ptacek and Eberhardt, 1996).

3. Improving communication with family is recommended, especially in view of the role families now play in physical care at the end of life and the intense psychological impact of this time in their lives and for years to come. We have to explore ways to educate the family in how to manage pain, distress, and other symptoms in the patient and how to communicate with the doctor about their concerns.

Management of Distress in End-of-life Care

A diagnosis of incurable cancer carries with it a necessity for patient and family to look at the meaning they attach to life and death. For many in America, this may be the first unavoidable confrontation with death because, as a society, we prefer to avoid thoughts of death—the last taboo topic. A 1991 Gallup poll found that most people in the United States reported that they never, or almost never, thought about death (Gallup and Newport, 1991). Callahan (1993) observed that much of the public excitement, debate, and furor about physician-assisted suicide and euthanasia is really an attempt to "control death" and thereby avoid facing the actual meaning of death in personal terms.

Given this cultural environment in which the meaning of death is denied and the fact that, in recent decades, oncology research has focused primarily on finding cures as opposed to improving palliative care, it is no surprise that the "human" side of end-of-life care, dealing with the emotional distress of being forced to consider the meaning of death, has received less attention. To meet patients' needs for psychological, social, and existential-religious-spiritual concerns, the primary treatment team should include (or have available to it) a psychosocial team that consists of a social worker, a mental health professional, and a pastoral counselor. Currently, the social worker often performs as the entire psychosocial team, but although long distanced from the treatment team, pastoral counselors must come to be viewed as integral members.

Mental health professionals can play an important role in helping dying patients deal with their distress. However, negative attitudes and stigma related to mental health, especially psychiatry, often limit the availability of these services. Medical staff are reluctant to ask for a psychiatric consultation, even when it is highly appropriate, out of concern that a patient may be offended by the request to see a mental health professional. Sometimes, the family sees it as an affront to the patient at a time of grave illness. These barriers, similar to those in pain management, are compounded by other fears. Patients and families often fear psychotropic medication. They worry that the drugs used will be addictive and "make me a zombie." Their attitudes are expressed by comments such as "I have to be strong" and "what can be done to change things?"

Another barrier is perceived cost. Many institutions regard this human aspect of care as expendable, expensive, and unnecessary. As a consequence, too few social workers, mental health professionals, and pastoral counselors are available to provide the consultation and treatment that would benefit patients and their families when the severity of distress exceeds that readily managed by the primary team. This is especially true of bereavement services, as social workers are reduced as a cost-saving measure.

A major problem in palliative care is the underrecognition, underdiagnosis, and thus undertreatment of patients with significant distress, ranging from existential anguish to anxiety and depression. This situation continues to exist despite the fact that when dying patients themselves were asked their primary concerns about their care, three of their five concerns were psychosocial: (1) no prolongation of dying; (2) maintaining a sense of control; and (3) relieving burdens (conflicts) and strengthening ties (Singer et al., 1999).

Even though patients and families express clearly their wishes for attention to their nonmedical concerns and for the inclusion of this domain as a core element in palliative care, there remains significant evidence that inadequate attention is given to these issues, in spite of lip service and good intentions. The evidence is as follows:

1. There are no standards of care for psychological, social, and existential and spiritual care at the end of life.

2. No training standards exist to formally prepare physicians to identify patients with distress, nor are there standards of competence for those who provide psychosocial and spiritual services at the end of life.

3. Mental health professionals (psychiatrists, psychologists, psychiatric social workers, and nurses) and pastoral counselors are not included in the end-of-life care team.

4. There is, as yet, no accountability for the performance of physicians, staff, and institutions in relation to the psychosocial and spiritual care given at the end of life by any regulatory body.

5. Reimbursement of professional services for psychosocial care is poor to absent (often excluded from medical and behavioral health contracts).

Clinical practice guidelines and standards for the management of distress in end-of-life care must incorporate the psychological, social, existential, spiritual, and religious issues faced by patients—the "human" aspects of care. However, the distress relates to coping with the increasing physical symptoms that, by their own nature, become a major source of distress. Patients and families often say that their greatest fear is having pain that cannot be controlled. Cherny and colleagues (1996) used the word "suffering" to encompass these same issues. They included physical symptoms based on the commonly used term "pain and suffering."

The word "distress" is chosen because it is less stigmatizing and incorporates "normal emotions" such as worry, fear, and sadness. However, distress can increase along a continuum to become a full-blown psychiatric disorder such as a major depression or generalized anxiety. Sadness of separation and anticipatory grief may increase to severe distress in the family. The normal search for meaning may increase to become an existential crisis with spiritual or religious meanings and require the advice of a pastoral counselor (Rousseau, 2000). This concept has been the basis for the NCCN guidelines and standards for the management of distress (Holland, 1999).

The NCCN practice guidelines (Table 7-2; Figure 7-1) give an algorithm for rapid identification of patients with significant distress leading to referral to appropriate services when significant distress is found. They also provide the first practice guidelines for mental health, social work, and pastoral counselors.

Distress is a word that also describes the emotions that reflect an inability to cope with the threat to life and the search for ways to give it tolerable meaning. The model of Folkman (Figure 7-2) is useful because it provides a cognitive model of the universal process by which we cope with an overwhelming situation and the distress that it causes (Folkman, 1997). The

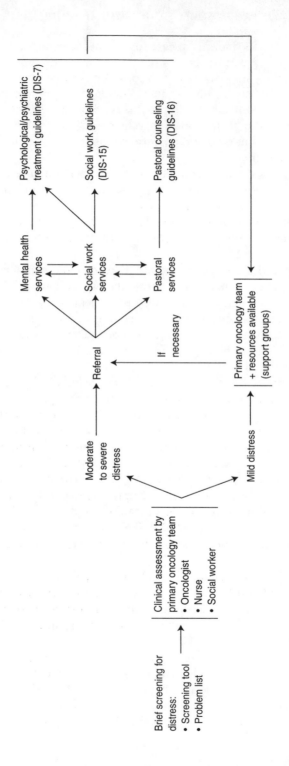

FIGURE 7-1 NCCN Practice Guidelines for Distress: Overview of evaluation and treatment process.
SOURCE: NCCN, 1999.

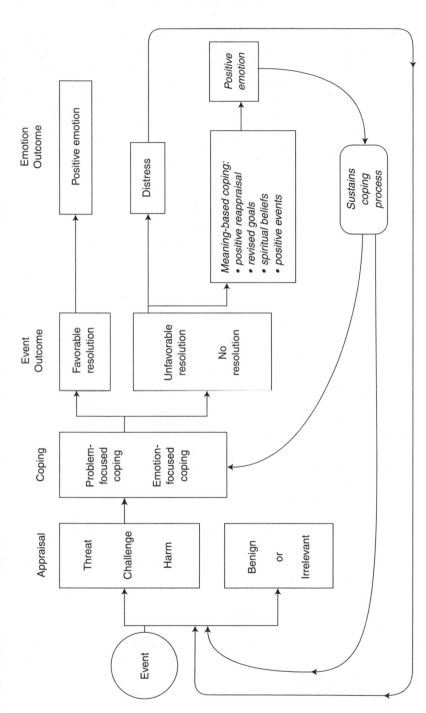

FIGURE 7-2 The process for coping with distress: The Folkman Model.
SOURCE: Folkman, 1997.

model demonstrates how the psychological, social, spiritual, existential and religious are joined in the effort to reduce distress by finding a tolerable meaning in the existential crisis. The effort is to reconcile the meaning of this unresolvable threat to life with the global meaning—the long held values, beliefs, aspirations, and goals that were held prior to the illness. The person seeks a resolution of these two conflicting forces and may cope in several ways: (1) by utilizing positive reappraisal such as viewing death in another way (e.g., "I'll pass on to an afterlife"); (2) by revising or coming to terms with shortened goals (e.g., "I will not see my children marry"); (3) by using spiritual beliefs (e.g., "God—ultimately—will make all things well"); and (4) by finding positive events in the situation (e.g., "I have had some wonderful moments with my children that I never had before"). The particular value of the Folkman model is its demonstration of how the psychosocial and the spiritual or religious domains are integrated in the patient's coping which, when successful, reduces distress.

Development of Standards for Management of Distress

In an effort to improve recognition and treatment of distress, the successful guidelines for pain management have become the model for guidelines to manage distress. The NCCN convened a multidisciplinary panel in 1998 to address the status of psychosocial care in cancer and the need for clinical practice guidelines to guide clinicians. The panel, over two years' time, developed standards of care and an algorithm that triggers referral of a significant level of distress to mental health, social work, or clergy services (Holland, 1999). It also developed clinical practice guidelines for these supportive care disciplines to guide their management of cases. These constitute the first set of clinical practice guidelines for psychosocial and spiritual care developed with full participation of all the supportive care disciplines (psychiatry, psychology, chaplaincy, social work, nursing), as well as oncology and patient advocacy. The principles laid out by this NCCN panel serve as the basis for the end-of-life guidelines outlined below.

• **Standard 1.** The term *distress* is used as a global term to refer to psychosocial or spiritual issues (Holland, 1999). As a nonstigmatizing word, patients can respond without embarrassment. Distress is defined as "an unpleasant experience of an emotional, psychological, social, or spiritual nature that interferes with the ability to cope with cancer treatment. It extends along a continuum, from common normal feelings of vulnerability, sadness, and fear, to problems that are disabling, such as true depression, anxiety, panic, and feeling isolated or in a spiritual crisis."
• **Standard 2.** *The level of distress should be assessed at each visit*, whether this occurs at home, in the clinic or office, or at the hospital or

hospice. A rapid visual analog approach is used by a verbal question, How is your distress today on a scale of 0-10? or by making a hatch mark on the distress thermometer (Figure 7-3). The thermometer is accompanied by a problem list on which the patient marks the nature and source of the distress (physical, social, psychological, or spiritual). The list of physical symptoms assists in targeting patients' major concerns. Patients have found this acceptable, and physicians have found that it serves as a checklist that allows questions to be more directed. Several screening methods are available (Hopwood et al., 1991; Ibbotson et al., 1994; Razavi, 1990).

• **Standard 3.** *When a patient indicates a distress level of 5 or above*, this is the algorithm that triggers referral to one of the specialized supportive services, depending on the problem: mental health, social work, or pastoral counseling. Roth and colleagues (1998) found the level of 5 or above comparable to a significant distress level on the Hospital Anxiety and Depression Scale. Further studies of feasibility and validity are under way with sponsorship from the American Cancer Society.

• **Standard 4.** Standards for professional education and training in end-of-life care must include standards for physicians and nurses, as well as

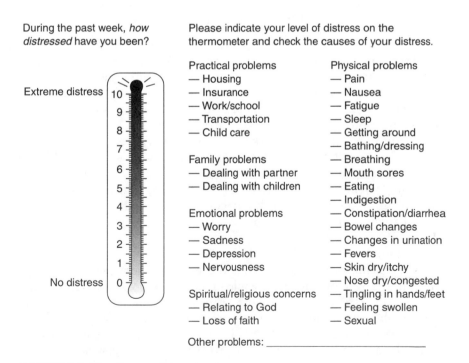

FIGURE 7-3 The distress thermometer.

for social workers, mental health professionals (psychiatry, psychology), and pastoral counselors.

• **Standard 5.** Physicians and nurses must be trained to use rapid screening methods to ensure that patients are asked at each visit about their level of distress and must be able to use the algorithm to refer patients to community resources for psychosocial services. Ready access to community resources is important (e.g., a phone referral list). They must be trained in how to communicate with patients and families in an empathic, compassionate, and supportive manner (Fallowfield et al., 1998; Holland and Almanza, 1999; Maguire, 2000; Maguire and Faulkner, 1988).

• **Standard 6.** Patients and their families, as well as all professionals engaged in end-of-life care, must be educated about the fact that psychosocial and spiritual services are an integral part of total care. Patients should experience no discontinuity between their medical and supportive services.

• **Standard 7.** Appropriate reimbursement for psychosocial services must be considered in all policy planning for end-of-life care.

• **Standard 8.** Evaluation of the quality of end-of-life care must include attention to the management of distress (Kornblith and Holland, 1996).

Clinical Practice Guidelines for Mental Health, Social Work, and Pastoral Services

The multidisciplinary NCCN panel addressed the need for an integration of psychosocial supportive services and the need for practice guidelines for the professionals who provide these services. While the primary care team manages normal levels of distress, higher, more severe levels, presenting as frank psychiatric symptoms or disorders, require management by a mental health professional (e.g., psychiatry, psychology, social work, nursing). Many oncology social workers on the primary treatment team also serve as the mental health professional. A psychiatrist should evaluate a neuropsychiatric disorder or one requiring psychotropic drug management. Significant psychosocial or concrete problems (e.g., transportation, insurance) are referred for social work services (Loscalzo and BrintzenhofeSzoc, 1998). Patients who are experiencing a spiritual or religious crisis are referred to the pastoral counselor or chaplain.

The family and other caregivers are the "secondary patients" since they are experiencing distress along with the patient: worry, sadness, uncertainty, and fatigue of caregiving while maintaining work and home. Managed care has placed an even greater burden on families as hospital length of stay is shortened, more treatments are provided on an outpatient basis, and home care services are reduced. They are a crucial "invisible" piece of the health care continuum. Anticipatory grief is part of their daily distress. Fears of How will he die? and Can I manage? add to the stressors. Studies suggest that while family caregivers persist in their caregiving role, they are subject to increased illness and mortality.

The same guidelines apply to recognition of distress in the family, and the same obligation exists to recognize and treat it, including management of bereavement after the death of the loved one when the staff who knew the patient will have a relationship and can monitor the need for intervention.

Clinical Practice Guidelines for
Management of Common Psychiatric Disorders

Several common psychiatric symptoms or disorders (using the *Diagnostic and Statistical Manual of Mental Disorders*, Fourth Edition [DSM-IV]) are encountered during end-of-life care (Table 7-2). Psychiatrists and psychologists with expertise in problems occurring at this stage can substantially diminish the distress of patients and their relatives. The American Psychiatric Association (APA) Clinical Practice Guidelines are useful for modification for end-of-life care, as are the NCCN guidelines for the management of these disorders specifically in cancer patients (APA, 2000; Holland, 1997; Holland and Almanza, 1999).

Delirium

Delirium is a common psychiatric disorder toward the end of life, estimated to affect as many as 85 percent of patients in their final days (Massie and Holland, 1983). The etiology of delirium in the terminally ill cancer patient is often multifactorial including medication side effects, infection, organ failure, metabolic derangement, and direct central nervous system (CNS) involvement. Older individuals who have mild impairment of cognition are especially susceptible to delirium. In the final stages of life, it is unlikely that the cause of the delirium can be resolved, and attention should focus on comfort. All too often, "quiet delirium" is ignored, but patients may be distressed by delusions that frighten them. Patients' capacity to make health care decisions must be assessed at times and the health care proxy identified. Considerable research has gone into management of delirium by pharmacologic means (see Table 7-2) (Kress et al., 2000).

Delirium is sometimes accompanied by agitation with self-injurious behavior (e.g., pulling out intravenous lines) or less frequently, the risk of injuring others (Johanson, 1993). Sometimes, poor impulse control, confusion, and depression combine to result in poorly planned, impulsive suicide attempts. Loved ones are frightened by a sudden change in behavior, and they need explanation as to the origin—be it related to disease or medication effects or both. Patients also need explanation since they fear, "I'm losing my mind" (Chochinov and Breitbart, 2000).

Thus, appropriate intervention in delirium includes steps to ensure early identification, safety of the patient, interventions (to treat both the delirium and its underlying cause, if possible), and education of patient and family to decrease distress associated with this disturbing symptom (see Table 7-2).

Depression and Depressive Symptoms

Depressive symptoms are common at the end of life, often at the subsyndromal level or as part of an adjustment disorder (Wilson et al., 2000) (Table 7-2). The etiology must first be determined, ruling out metabolic, illness-, or drug-related causes. Irrespective of the etiology, attention is directed to the treatment of the depressive symptoms. A prior history of bipolar disorder or dysthymia suggests a longstanding problem that may be exacerbated during end-of-life care. Evaluation of suicidal ideation and risk is essential, as well as of the capacity to make decisions. The role of depression in requests for physician-assisted suicide makes this a critically important aspect of evaluation and treatment (Burt, 1997). The presence of hopelessness appears to be a separate but related factor, along with depression, in suicidal wishes (Breitbart et al., 2000). The notion that depression is an ordinary aspect of the end of life has been dispelled by careful longitudinal studies by Chochinov and colleagues, who found a high level of fluctuation in suicidal wishes day-to-day, suggesting caution in acting on a patient's stated wish at a particular time (Chochinov and Breitbart, 2000; Passik et al., 1998, 2000; Razavi et al., 1990).

Meeting criteria for true major depression (DSM-IV criteria) is *not* common, but when major depression is present, it should be treated as aggressively as any physical symptom, with psychological support, psychotherapy, and medication. Antidepressants and psychostimulants are of proven value. Existential forms of psychotherapy are under development by the authors and colleagues. Guidelines for treating end-of-life depression are still needed. A start could be made by modifying more general depression treatment guidelines (see Table 7-2). Education for clinical staff about depression, anticipatory grieving, and bereavement is essential for appropriate implementation of guidelines.

Anxiety Disorders

Anxiety is the most common symptom of distress near the end of life. It often stems from fears about shortness of breath, fear of pain, unremitting symptoms, and uncertainty about the future. Reactive anxiety symptoms alone, or mixed with depressive symptoms, constitute the mildest DSM-IV psychiatric disorder, adjustment disorder (APA, 2000). The patient requires careful evaluation for illness or medication-related causes: neuroleptic-induced akathisia, corticosteroids, hypoxia or hypercarbia, glucose imbalance, bronchodilators, drug intoxication or withdrawal, and metabolic changes. All must be considered when failure of vital organs is occurring. Explanation of symptoms and preparation of the patient and family for approaching death are important. Communication about fears plays an essential role in modulating patient and family anxiety and distress. Assessment of patients' safety and supportive psychotherapy, with or without an anxiolytic or antidepressant medication, is indicated.

Generalized anxiety disorder with distressing phobias and panic symptoms, usually antedating the illness, requires titrating medication to control symptoms, along with giving psychological support. Post-traumatic stress disorder (PTSD) may be present at the end of life in patients who have undergone extensive, aggressive treatment with prolonged, poorly controlled pain. Supportive psychotherapy is indicated for these patients along with medication to treat anxiety and sleep problems.

Obsessive-compulsive disorder (OCD) is a type of anxiety disorder that complicates end-of-life care. These patients are often fearful of accepting psychotropic and usually pain medications, have trouble making decisions about treatment and care, and as a result, often suffer more because of inadequate treatment of their symptoms. Family support of decisions and psychotherapy from a mental health professional are of value. End-of-life anxiety guidelines are needed and could be developed by modifying more general anxiety guidelines (see Table 7-2).

Personality Disorders

Patients nearing the end of life may have difficulty in controlling emotions, and underlying personality problems may emerge that require evaluation and intervention. Patients may become angry and hostile, uncooperative and demanding, overly fearful and dependent, indecisive and ambivalent about care, or manipulative and creating conflicts among team members. Such symptoms are best evaluated and recommendations made by a mental health team member. In addition to intervening directly with the patient, a mental health professional can assist staff in managing clinical problems—negotiating behavioral changes, maintaining appropriate boundaries, and addressing conflicts among staff members that arise around caring for such challenging patients. Both the APA Clinical Practice Guidelines for management of personality disorders in physically healthy individuals and the NCCN guidelines for management of distress in ambulatory cancer patients should be revised to provide guidelines for their management in palliative care (see Table 7-2).

Social Work Services Guidelines

The NCCN practice guidelines, developed by social workers and a multidisciplinary panel, determined that the services given by social workers fall into two domains: psychosocial services and concrete services such as transportation. They constitute the first algorithm-based treatment guidelines for delivery of social work services in cancer. These guidelines require only minor revision to apply to end-of-life care. The role of social workers varies enormously across institutions; in some, they provide all of psychosocial services as they address all the psychosocial needs of both patients and families during palliative treatment (see Table 7-2).

Pastoral Services Guidelines

Long an integral part of hospice care, interest is growing in how we can better incorporate the spiritual and religious domains in palliative care in all settings (Post et al., 2000). When life ebbs, beliefs and philosophy take on new meaning so that the clinician should be sensitive to the need to explore these areas with a patient and, if the patient expresses concerns about spiritual or religious matters, to refer him or her to a pastoral counselor (Puchalski and Romer, 2000). The NCCN practice guidelines for management of distress include pastoral counseling as part of psychosocial services to encourage the integration of pastoral services into total support services (Holland, 1999). The common problems referred to pastoral counselors, and for which they counsel, are grief, concerns about death or afterlife, conflicted belief systems, loss of faith, concerns about the meaning or purpose of life, relationship to God, isolation from religious community, guilt, hopelessness, conflicts between religious beliefs and recommended treatment, and ritual needs (Speck, 1998). Clergy who have been trained in pastoral counseling should be available to assist in end-of-life care. Problems such as guilt, hopelessness, and grief may require mental health or social work evaluation, prompting the need for close collaboration among all staff taking care of patients in a palliative setting (see Table 7-2).

IMPROVING MANAGEMENT OF DISTRESS: FUTURE DIRECTIONS

Training of Team   The team giving end-of-life care must be trained in how to recognize, diagnose, and treat distress and in using an algorithm for referrals to mental health, special social work services, or pastoral counseling. A brief curriculum is needed that can be given to staff easily, similar to the curricula in palliative care.

EDUCATION OF PATIENTS AND FAMILIES Patients and their families should be educated to expect attention to and treatment of their distress by their primary care team or by an appropriate resource that is viewed by the patient as an extension of the team. They should experience a seamless flow of medical and mental health services. As nearly as possible, psychosocial and psychiatric services should be given in the same site as medical care to reduce embarrassment and ensure easy access to care for seriously medically ill patients and their families.

PATIENTS' BILL OF RIGHTS This document should explicitly include the patient's right to management of distress as an integral part of comprehensive cancer care.

ACCOUNTABILITY Regulatory bodies (e.g., Joint Commission on Accreditation of Healthcare Organizations, Health Care Financing Administration) must include in their reports for medical centers the quality of doctor-patient communication and their ability to recognize and treat distress and to refer to the appropriate psychosocial resource.

PROFESSIONAL STANDARDS FOR MENTAL HEALTH AND PASTORAL SERVICES It is essential to have standards for training mental health professionals and pastoral counselors in palliative and end-of-life care, as has been done for physicians and nurses. This is particularly true of pastoral services where cost cutting may lead to use of clergy untrained in counseling techniques. The National Association of Professional Chaplains has developed the requisite standards.

MULTIDISCIPLINARY TEAM The team giving end-of-life care must include a mental health professional and a qualified pastoral counselor either on the team, or available to the team for consultation, as well as a psychiatrist for evaluation and management of neuropsychiatric disorders and depression when patients express the desire for hastened death.

REIMBURSEMENT FOR PSYCHOSOCIAL SERVICES Reimbursement for psychosocial services given at the end of life has to be addressed at a public policy level with attention to the inequity in payment for these services compared to medical services.

RESEARCH Clinical practice guidelines and critical care pathways have proven effective in improving quality of care through the use of evidence-based guidelines. There is a great need to apply this approach to managing the problems of distress so that a gold standard will exist for the psychosocial as well as the physical domains.

Studies are needed to provide more evidence-based (as opposed to consensus) guidelines for recognition and management of distress. Empirical studies should explore the best psychotherapeutic approaches; the efficacy of psychopharmacologic interventions through clinical trials (use of neuroleptics, antidepressants, anxiolytics, and psychostimulants in end-of-life care); studies of depression, its predictors, and those associated with requests for physician-assisted suicide; and development of special algorithms for medically underserved populations (e.g., non-English speaking, low income, minorities, chronically mentally ill), with attention to quality-of-life assessment that permits examining patients' quality of life and satisfaction with care. In addition, family members who care for their loved ones during the end of life should be studied to better understand anticipatory grief, distress, the burden of caregiving, and the management of bereavement.

Implementing Needed Changes

1. A multidisciplinary consensus panel (including all disciplines that provide supportive services) should be impaneled to develop an overall taxonomy for the nonphysical domains of patients at the end of life (i.e., the psychological, social, spiritual, existential, religious, and psychiatric dimensions). This area currently suffers from the use of vague, overlapping terms that lack clarity and definition, and is likely to be relegated to a nonsignificant status. The encompassing term "distress" is proposed to incorporate all psychosocial facets to diminish this fragmentation. A consensus panel of experts is needed to promulgate a standard taxonomy (Holland, 1999).

2. The panel should take existing standards of care and clinical practice guidelines developed by NCCN for use with ambulatory cancer patients and modify them for use at end of life. These should be disseminated and tested for feasibility. Given the problems with ensuring implementation of clinical practice guidelines, substantial efforts must be invested in identifying and overcoming barriers to their widespread use.

3. The panel should also examine the NCCN panel's work on guidelines for communication and adapt them to end-of-life care. A current NCCN panel has such work in progress (W. Breitbart, personal communication).

4. The panel should address the major barriers to management of distress as discussed earlier:

- the absence of minimum standards for psychological and social care and for existential, spiritual, and religious needs;
- the absence of oversight by regulatory bodies regarding the perfor-

mance of staff in relation to communication, identification, and management of psychosocial and spiritual problems;

- the negative attitudes of professionals that often demean and discourage integration of these aspects into total care because of the stigmatization of nonphysical "psychological" domains (an equally important barrier is the negative attitudes of patients and families who sometimes feel embarrassed or angered by a consultation by a mental health person, especially a psychiatrist);
- the absence of training of professional staff in the recognition, diagnosis, and management of distress and the absence of an algorithm to trigger referral to supportive services;
- the need for mental health professionals and pastoral counselors to be part of, or be an immediately available resource to, the end-of-life care team to address the psychosocial, spiritual, and religious issues; and
- the absence of reimbursement for these supportive services given to the poor.

5. The panel should outline standards for psychosocial care and obtain endorsement from professional organizations involved in end-of-life care. These should be promulgated in a manner similar to that used with pain management:

- Distress should be assessed at every visit on a 0-10 scale, verbally or with paper and pencil, identifying the level and source of the distress; using the algorithm of scoring 5 or above, patients should be referred to the proper supportive service that can be accessed in a seamless delivery system from the patients' perspective.
- Educational standards must include training of the primary end-of-life care team in the recognition of distress and its management.
- Educational standards must teach mental health professionals how to modify their concepts to include end-of-life care (psychologists, psychiatrists, psychiatric social workers, and nurses) and clergy who are qualified as pastoral counselors).
- Pastoral counseling should be included in psychosocial services, since this should not be fragmented and distanced from other aspects of care during end of life.
- Patients and families must be educated to understand that the psychosocial and spiritual domains are an integral part of their end-of-life care and should not be viewed as disconnected and unrelated.
- Governmental and managed care organizations must be made aware of the inequity in reimbursement for the nonphysical aspects of end-of-life care which impacts negatively on ensuring quality of care to reduce suffering and distress.

6. Professional organizations representing psychology, psychiatry, oncology social work, oncology nursing, and chaplaincy must become familiar with and endorse the clinical practice guidelines modified from existing ones for end-of-life care, to ensure dissemination and education among these disciplines.

7. Any patients' bill of rights must include the right to management of their distress as a symptom of equal concern as a physical symptom that receives prompt and competent care; they must be educated to ask for these services.

8. Accountability: the appropriate regulatory bodies must include performance standards for professionals in relation to their communication and sensitivity to care of the nonphysical symptoms (psychosocial and spiritual) of patients at the end of life.

9. Research should be pursued to test the feasibility and implementation of practice guidelines for management of distress developed for each discipline (mental health, social work, pastoral counseling) giving supportive services. In view of the acknowledged difficulties in implementation of clinical practice guidelines to manage distress and the unique stigma around psychosocial and spiritual services, it is essential that research be undertaken to address these barriers.

10. Delirium, depression, and anxiety are extremely common at the end of life and are frequently underrecognized, underdiagnosed, and undertreated, leading to unnecessary distress for patients and families. Research into recognition and treatment of these symptoms through controlled trials is important to improve care at the end of life.

11. Clinicians are equally responsible for the recognition and treatment of distress in patients' families who bear an increasingly heavy burden of caregiving with its own psychological and physical toll; guidelines for inquiring about distress and educating families must be a part of the research agenda in end-of-life care.

Management of Physical Symptoms

Table 7-2 outlines the status of clinical practice guidelines for management of pain, fatigue, nausea and vomiting, and dyspnea. The focus here is on the emotional distress caused by these symptoms—the physical suffering that we associate with the dying process (Twycross and Lichter, 1998). Patients and families struggle with the concern that these symptoms will not be adequately controlled, with fears about their cause and the potential for their becoming intolerable, and with sadness and anger about diminishing physical function. Thus, the common symptoms of pain, fatigue, nausea, and dyspnea are often the catalyst for severe distress or "suffering of the mind." They lead to severe distress requiring both traditional medical interventions and care targeting the spiritual, existential, psychiatric, and psychosocial distress they precipitate.

Negotiating management of physical symptoms at the end of life is often complex: the first issue is dealing with the meaning of the transition from curative to palliative care. This requires sensitive communication by the physician with opportunity for participation of supportive disciplines that can more fully address the concerns of patients and families.

In addition, medical management for the dying patient is complicated by the interaction of the symptoms of disease and the fact that treatments may produce relief or introduce new problems; for example, analgesics cause troubling constipation. Patient education is an essential component of care to ensure a collaborative approach to symptom management. Clinical practice guidelines usually consider a single symptom in isolation; thus, a guideline addressing a single symptom may apply less well because it fails to take into account many coexisting symptoms. Care of the dying requires creative problem solving, as well as the development of clinical guidelines to address this level of complexity. Palliative treatment should be just as aggressively approached as curative treatment. Many patients' greatest fear is of abandonment, of hearing the echoing words of a physician telling them that there is nothing more that can be done. In fact, treatment of the dying patient continues to the moment of death and beyond, by interventions to assist family members with their grief.

One imperative is improved doctor-patient-family communication about symptoms and more collaborative efforts at symptom management. Uncertainty about the cause of symptoms or what they may signify, fear of future symptoms and worry that symptom control will be inadequate contribute substantially to patients' and families' distress. Many fear unbearable and poorly treated pain and respiratory distress in the final days and hours. Clinicians could be helpful by describing the dying process to patients and families in terms of reassurances about comfort and relief of symptoms. Loved ones usually view Cheyne-Stokes respirations as indicators of substantial discomfort and pain or fear that a gurgling sound indicates the patient is drowning, despite the fact that most patients are no longer conscious in this final stage of dying. Adequate preparation of patient and family about the dying process and anticipated symptoms is essential and must begin with showing a willingness to discuss these matters and address fears and concerns. Treatment of distress caused by fear of potentially uncontrolled physical symptoms will significantly improve quality of life. The public issue that has arisen regarding requests for physician-assisted suicide is prompted considerably by the widespread fear of overwhelming pain and its inadequate control in the care of dying patients (Chochinov and Breitbart, 2000; Sachs et al., 1995).

In addition, psychological, social, and existential or spiritual distress may increase the intensity of physical symptoms. For example, depression and anxiety may increase the experience of pain, and anxiety can increase dyspnea. Conversely, pain and dyspnea increase anxiety and depression.

Prevalence of symptoms at the end of life that cause substantial distress has been identified by the Memorial Symptom Assessment Scale (Portenoy, 2000). Pain, fatigue, nausea and vomiting, and dyspnea are among the most frequently occurring symptoms that reduce quality of life. Others are cachexia, bladder and bowel dysfunction, sleep disturbance, pruritis, constipation, diarrhea, and pressure ulcers (Mercandante, 1994, 1997; Ripamonti, 1994). Anorexia is exceedingly common and emotionally laden, causing patients and families great distress because of the fear that not eating is the cause of cachexia. Patients in the final days of life have diminished hunger and thirst, and oral, parenteral, and enteral force feeding may actually increase suffering (McCann et al., 1994). Development of clinical guidelines for each of these symptoms in end-of-life care is important. Practice guidelines are being developed for anorexia (D. Cella, personal communication).

Symptom management in special populations is a particular problem. In patients with dementia, chronic mental illness, delirium, or deficits in ability to communicate, assessment of the sources of discomfort and the adequacy of palliative interventions is especially problematic. In these cases, clinical experience with comparable situations often must guide palliative care; for example, dosing pain medications based on average needs and then assessing nonverbal cues are recommended. Given the high incidence of terminal delirium and the frequent progressive impairment of cognitive functioning in the final stages of life, palliative care guidelines must address the needs of those patients who cannot speak for themselves to express troubling symptoms.

Pain

Achieving effective pain management has been a priority over the past decade. The American Pain Society (APS), AHRQ, the World Health Organization (WHO), and the NCCN guidelines provide algorithms for decision-making in pain management (AHCPR, 1993; APS, 1995; McGivney,1998; WHO, 1998) (see Table 7-2). Problems remain in implementation; many patients cope with needless suffering. Pain is one of the most prevalent symptoms across terminal illnesses, affecting more than a third of patients. It is also the source of great fear as many patients anticipate final days of agony. Beyond the devastating experience of the symptom itself, pain impairs psychosocial functioning, causes enormous psychological distress (anxiety and depression), and limits patients' capacity for enjoyment and finding meaning in their final days. Studies show pain control remains a challenge for research, with modification of existing guidelines for end-of-life care and accountability to regulatory bodies to ensure compliance.

APS, NCCN, and AHRQ guidelines clearly delineate the principles of effective pain management, providing algorithms for the management of nociceptive and neuropathic pain of varying severity and chronicity (Rischer and Childress, 1996) (see Table 7-2). Identification of the cause and type of pain, use of repeated standardized assessment tools to assess pain severity and response to treatment, evaluation of the effect of pain interventions on mental alertness, and flexibility in revising treatment regimens are the main-stays of effective care. The use of around-the-clock fixed dosing with pa-tient or caregiver "rescues" provides a means of avoiding withdrawal symp-toms and preventing delays in dosing and resulting pain crises (Bottomly and Hanks, 1990). Clinician education about appropriate dosing and medi-cation combinations facilitates better care as well as treatment of depres-sion and anxiety. Use of psychotropic drugs as adjuncts to pain medications and behavioral interventions are effective.

Continuing misconceptions about dependence and addiction, the risks of oversedation, and regulatory problems of opiates have contributed to inadequate implementation of clinical guidelines. In addition, there is a need to educate doctors about the use of opiates and other medications whose use is restricted by Drug Enforcement Agency (DEA) guidelines, in order to resolve the problems of inadequate dosing and reluctance to pre-scribe. Identifying the barriers that have delayed implementation of effec-tive pain management is a continuing research question.

Fatigue

Fatigue is a major end-of-life symptom described as tiredness, heavi-ness, weakness, lack of energy, poor stamina, sleepiness, and poor strength. In the Study to Understand Prognoses and Preferences for Outcomes and Risks of Treatment (SUPPORT), 80 percent of patients complained of fa-tigue in the final three days of life (Phillips et al., 2000). Whether a result of the primary disease process, metabolic abnormalities due to organ failure, treatment side effects, or malnutrition, fatigue limits functional capacity and quality of life. Treatment guidelines have been developed for the man-agement of anemia-related fatigue, but none have addressed fatigue at the end of life. The fatigue related to depression also must be considered in seeking an etiology and choosing an intervention. Despite all efforts, fatigue is often an intractable symptom in the final days of life.

Clinical practice guidelines for this important symptom must build on recent studies documenting the high incidence of fatigue in chronic and terminal illness and its impact on quality of life. Research in the use of stimulants and other new alternatives may offer the potential for future advances (Chochinov and Breitbart, 2000). The complex interplay of psychological and physical complaints is especially significant in the evaluation and treatment of fatigue.

Nausea and Vomiting

Clinical practice guidelines for management of nausea and vomiting have been widely promulgated in the care of cancer patients as advances in antiemetic therapy have vastly reduced the distress associated with chemotherapy. Nausea may be centrally mediated or caused by local factors such as decreased motility, medication effects, or gastrointestinal lesions (Reuben and Mor, 1986). Vomiting may contribute to dehydration, metabolic disarray, and aspiration. Obstruction and gastrointestinal bleeding are particularly difficult to manage and may be the source of great physical and emotional distress. There are practice guidelines for intractable vomiting, including surgery, PEG drainage, restricted oral intake, and symptomatic medications. Patients have described nausea as a particularly demoralizing symptom, affecting self-concept and self-esteem as well as psychosocial functioning. Inability to eat excludes patients from one of the primary sources of social interaction, occurring at meals. Nausea, vomiting, and anorexia are substantial sources of distress for patients and families, often leading to anxiety and depression.

Development of clinical practice guidelines for nausea and vomiting, central in end-of-life care, requires piloting antiemetic regimens that have been successful in the management of chemotherapy-related side effects. Modification to the special needs of patients in the end of life is the next step (see Table 7-2).

Dyspnea

Respiratory distress and shortness of breath are common in the final days of life, affecting more than half of patients. Although the causes of dyspnea are diverse and often multifactorial, there are common approaches to management (Dudgeon and Rosenthal, 1996). The sensation of air hunger causes great anxiety, and the appearance of respiratory distress is traumatic for patient and family (Ahmedzai, 1998). Despite the prevalence of this devastating symptom, there are no formal clinical practice guidelines for its management in end-of-life care.

Palliation of dyspnea, if the underlying cause cannot be addressed, often depends on the use of opiates for cough control and the reduction of air hunger. The use of bronchodilators and oxygen can provide symptom relief depending on the etiology and pathological process. Respiratory secretions can be minimized with scopolamine and atropine if necessary.

Anxiolytics may also make an invaluable contribution in this setting, as may behavioral therapies to assist in relaxation. In the patient who is dying imminently, sedation with intravenous morphine may be most appropriate to treat the distress of severe air hunger. As mentioned earlier, Cheyne-Stokes respiration that often characterizes the final stage before death is especially disturbing to family members who feel that the rapid respiration alternating with apnea must be distressing, although patients are somnolent in this final phase of dying and interventions for comfort are not necessary. However, the suffering of those who care for them must be recognized and psychosocial support and education are essential. Families are often unprepared for the events and symptoms of the final days, and the trauma of this experience is magnified by the uncertainty about the future. Reassurance and education by the medical team are an important component of quality clinical care and can have an enormous impact on the family who otherwise is haunted during its bereavement by images of suffering.

Development and implementation of clinical practice guidelines for dyspnea is especially important, given both the high incidence of this symptom and its emotional impact. Further research on symptom management in the end of life will support evidence-based clinical interventions for terminal dyspnea.

Control of Physical Symptoms: Next Steps

1. Clinical practice guidelines for control of the common symptoms have, at present, been developed largely for the care of ambulatory and hospitalized patients. These must be modified to apply to end-of-life care. Excellent descriptive guides in the literature for symptom management at the end of life must be developed into algorithm-based clinical guidelines. Guidelines should be developed by a multidisciplinary panel to address the spectrum of physical symptoms common at the end of life, modifying and building on existing practice guidelines for symptom management.

2. Education of patients and families, using a practice guideline model, is needed to ensure their understanding of the common symptoms at the end of life and their management. This is essential to minimize distress and to reduce uncertainty and fears about the dying process.

3. Guidelines must be culturally sensitive and address the special concerns around treating underserved medical populations (e.g., non-English speaking, chronically mentally ill, religious, ethnic, and racial minorities).

4. Guidelines must be developed that ensure adequate symptom control to prevent the secondary development of depression and anxiety that further complicate overall management by the presence of greater distress levels.

5. Guidelines must provide for the concept of comprehensive end-of-

life care that integrates the treatment of both physical symptoms and distress in the psychosocial, spiritual, and religious domains, recognizing their interrelationship.

REFERENCES

Agency for Health Care Policy and Research. 1993. Depression Guideline Panel. Depression in Primary Care. Vol. 1, Detection and Diagnosis. Clinical Practice Guideline, No. 5. AHCPR Publication No. 93-0550. Rockville, MD: U.S. Department of Health and Human Services, Agency for Health Care Policy and Research.

Ahmedzai S. 1998. Palliation of respiratory symptoms. In Doyle D, Hanks GWC, MacDonald N (eds.): Oxford Textbook of Palliative Medicine (2nd edition). New York: Oxford University Press; pp. 583-616.

Almanza J, Holland JC. A review of literature on breaking bad news in oncology. Psychosomatics 1999;40:135.

American Academy of Neurology. 1996. Report of the Ethics and Humanities Subcommittee of the American Academy of Neurology: Palliative Care in Neurology. Neurology 1996; 46:870-872.

American Board of Internal Medicine. 1996. Caring for the dying: Identification and promotion of physician competency. Educational Resource Document.

American Nursing Association. 1991. Position Statement on Promotion of Comfort and Relief of Pain in Dying Patients. Kansas City: American Nursing Association.

American Pain Society Quality of Care Committee. Quality improvement guidelines for the treatment of acute pain and cancer pain. JAMA 1995;274:1874-1880.

American Psychiatric Association. 2000. APA Clinical Practice Guidelines for Psychiatric Disorders Compendium 2000. Washington, D.C.: American Psychiatric Association.

American Society of Clinical Oncology. Outcomes of cancer treatment for technology assessment and cancer treatment guidelines. J Clin Oncol 1996;14:671-679.

Baile WF, Glober GA, Lenzi R, Beale EA, Kudelka AP. Discussing disease progression and end of life decisions. Oncology 1999;13:1021-1028.

Bottomly DM, Hanks G. Subcutaneous midazolam infusion in palliative care. J Pain Symptom Manage 1990;5:259-261.

Braun KL, Pietsch JH, Blanchette PL (eds.) 2000. Cultural Issues in End-of-Life Decision Making. Thousand Oaks, CA: Sage Publications.

Breitbart W, Rosenfeld B, Pessin H, Kain M, Funesti-Esch J, Galietta M, Nelson CJ, Brescia R. Depression, hopelessness and desire for hastened death in terminally ill patients with cancer. JAMA 2000;284:2907-2911.

Buckman R. 1998. Communication in palliative care: A practical guide. In Doyle D, Hanks GWC, MacDonald N (eds.): Oxford Textbook of Palliative Medicine (2nd edition). New York: Oxford University Press; pp. 141-156.

Burt RA. The Supreme Court speaks: not assisted suicide but a constitutional right to palliative care. N Engl J Med 1997;337:1234-1236.

Callahan D. 1993. The Troubled Dream of Life: In Search of a Peaceful Death. New York: Simon and Schuster.

Carr JA, Payne R, et al. 1994. Management of Cancer Pain: Adults Quick Reference Guide. No. 9. Rockville, MD: Agency for Health Care Policy and Research, U.S. Department of Health and Human Services.

Carroll BT, Kathol R, Noyes R, et al. Screening for depression and anxiety in cancer patients using the hospital anxiety and depression scale. Gen Hosp Psychiatry 1993;15:69-74.

Carver AC, Foley KM. 2000. Palliative care. In Holland JF, Frei, III E, Bast Jr. RC, Kufe DW, Pollock RE, Weichselbaum R (eds.) *Cancer Medicine (5th edition)*. Hamilton, Ontario, Canada: B.C. Decker; pp. 992-1000.

Cassel CK, Foley KM. 1999. *Principles for Care of Patients at the End of Life: An Emerging Consensus Among the Specialties of Medicine*. New York: Milbank Memorial Fund.

Cassem NH. 1997. The dying patient. In Cassem NH, Stern TA, Rosenbaum JF, Jellinek MS (eds.): *Massachusetts General Hospital Handbook of General Hospital Psychiatry (4th edition)*, St. Louis: Mosby-Year Book; pp. 605-636.

Chassin MR, Gavin RW. The urgent need to improve health care quality: Institute of Medicine Roundtable on Health Care Quality. *JAMA* 1998;280:1000-1005.

Cherny NI, Portenoy RK. Sedation in the treatment of refractory symptoms: guidelines for evaluation and treatment. *J Palliat Care* 1994;10:31-38.

Cherny NI, Coyle N, Foley KM. Guidelines in the care of the dying cancer patient. In Cherny NI, Foley KM. (eds.): Pain and Palliative Care. *Hematology/Oncology Clinics of North America* 1996;10:262.

Chochinov HM, Breitbart W (eds.). 2000. Handbook of Psychiatry in Palliative Medicine. New York: Oxford University Press.

Chochinov HM, Holland JC, Katz LY. 1998. Bereavement: A special issue in oncology. In Holland JC (ed.): *Psycho-oncology*, New York: Oxford University Press; pp. 1016-1032.

Derogatis LR, Morrow GR, Fetting D, et al. The prevalence of psychiatric disorders among cancer patients. *JAMA* 1983;249:751-756.

Dudgeon DJ, Rosenthal S. Management of dyspnea and cough in patients with cancer. In Cherny NI, Foley KM (eds.): Pain and Palliative Care. *Hematology/Oncology Clinics of North America* 1996;10:159.

Emanuel EJ, Emanuel LL. What is accountability in health care? *Ann Intern Med* 1996;124: 229-239.

Fallowfield L, Lipkin M, Hall A. Teaching senior oncologists communication skills: results from phase 1 of a comprehensive longitudinal program in the United Kingdom. *J Clin Oncol* 1998;16:1961-1968.

Field MJ, Lohr K (eds.). 1990. *Clinical Practice Guidelines: Directions for a New Program*. Washington, D.C.: National Academy Press.

Field MJ, Lohr K (eds.). 1992. Guidelines for Clinical Practice: From Development to Use. Washington, DC: National Academy Press.

Fitchett G, Handzo G. 1998. Spiritual assessment, screening, and intervention. In Holland JC (ed.): *Psycho-oncology*, New York: Oxford University Press; pp. 790-808.

Folkman S. Positive psychological states and coping with severe stress. *Soc Sci Med* 1997;45: 1207-1221.

Ford LG, Hunter CP, Diehr P, Frelick RW, Yates J. Effects of patient management guidelines on physician practice patterns: the Community Hospital Oncology Program experience. *J Clin Oncol* 1987;5:504-511.

Gallup G, Newport F. Mirror of America: fear of dying. *Gallup Poll Monthly* 1991;304:51-19.

Girgis A, Sanson-Fisher RW. Breaking bad news: consensus guidelines for medical practitioners. *J Clin Oncol* 1995;13:2449-2456.

Grimshaw JM, Russell TI. Effect of clinical guidelines on medical practice. *Lancet* 1993;342: 1317-1322.

Hastings Center. 1987. *Guidelines on the Termination of Life-Sustaining Treatment and the Care of the Dying: A Report*. Briarcliff Manor, N.Y.: Hastings Center.

Hirschfeld RM, Keller MB, Panico S, et al. The National Depressive and Manic-Depressive Association consensus statement on the undertreatment of depression. *JAMA* 1997;277: 333-340.

Holland JC. Preliminary guidelines for the treatment of distress. *Oncology* 1997;11(11A): 109-114.

Holland JC (ed.). *Psycho-oncology.* New York: Oxford University Press.

Holland JC. NCCN practice guidelines for the management of psychosocial distress. *Oncology* 1999;13(5A):113-147.

Holland JC, Almanza J. Giving bad news: is there a kinder, gentler way? *Cancer* 1999;86:738-740.

Hopwood P, Howell A, Maguire P. Screening for psychiatric morbidity in patients with advanced breast cancer: validation of two self-report questionnaires. *Br J Cancer* 1991; 64:353-356.

Ibbotson T, Maguire P, Selby P, et al. Screening for anxiety and depression in cancer patients: the effects of disease and treatments. *Eur J Cancer* 1994;30A:37-40.

Institute of Medicine. 1997. *Approaching Death: Improving Care at the End of Life.* Washington, D.C.: National Academy Press.

Institute of Medicine. 1999. *Ensuring Quality Cancer Care.* Hewitt M, Simone JV, eds. Washington, D.C.: National Academy Press.

Johanson GA. Midazolam in terminal care. *Am J Hosp Palliat Care* 1993;10:13-14.

Karasu B. Spiritual psychotherapy. *Am J Psychotherapy* 2000;53:143-162.

Katterhagen G. Physician compliance with outcome-based guidelines and clinical pathways in oncology. *Oncology* 1996;10(11 Suppl.):113-121.

Kornblith AB, Holland JC: Model for quality-of-life research from the Cancer and Leukemia Group B: the telephone interview, conceptual approach to measurement, and theoretical framework. *J Natl Cancer Inst Monogr* 1996;20:55-62.

Kress JP, Pohlman AS, O'Connor MF, Hall JB. Daily interruption of sedative infusion in critically ill patients undergoing mechanical ventilation. *N Engl J Med* 2000;342:1471-1477.

Loscalzo M, BrintzenhofeSzoc K. 1998. Brief crisis counseling, In Holland JC (ed.): *Psycho-oncology,* New York: Oxford University Press; pp. 662-675.

Maguire P, Faulkner A. Communicate with cancer patients: 1. Handling bad news and difficult questions. *Br Med J* 19998;297:907-909.

Maguire P. 2000. Communication with terminally ill patients and their relatives. In Chochinov HM, Breitbart W (eds.): *Handbook of Psychiatry in Palliative Medicine.* New York: Oxford University Press, 2000; pp. 291-301.

Massie MJ, Holland JC, Glass E. Delirium in terminally ill cancer patients. *Am J Psychiatry* 1983;140:1048-1050.

McCann RM, Hall WJ, Groth-Juncker A. Comfort care for terminally ill patients: the appropriate use of nutrition and hydration. *JAMA* 1994;272:179-181.

McGivney WT. The National Comprehensive Cancer Network: present and future directions. *Cancer* 1998;82(10 Suppl.):2057-2060.

Mercandante S. The role of octreotide in palliative care. *J Pain Symptom Manage* 1994;9:406-411.

Mercandante S, Kargar J, Nicolosi G. Octreotide may prevent definitive intestinal obstruction. *J Pain Symptom Manage* 1997;13:325-326.

Morris M. Implementation of guidelines and paths in oncology. *Oncology* 1996;10(11 Suppl.): 123-129.

NCCN (National Comprehensive Cancer Network) Second Annual Conference. Antiemesis practice guidelines panel presentation. Ft. Lauderdale, FL, March 2-5, 1997.

NCCN (National Comprehensive Cancer Network) Fourth Annual Conference. Practice guidelines and outcomes data in oncology. Update: NCCN Distress Management Guidelines. Ft. Lauderdale, FL, February 26-March 2, 1999a.

NCCN (National Comprehensive Cancer Network) Fourth Annual Conference. Practice guidelines and outcomes data in oncology. Cancer Pain. Ft. Lauderdale, FL, February 26-March 2, 1999b.

NCCN (National Comprehensive Cancer Network) Fourth Annual Conference. Practice guidelines and outcomes data in oncology. Assessment of fatigue: New Measurement Scales. Ft. Lauderdale, FL, February 26-March 2, 1999c.

NCCN (National Comprehensive Cancer Network) Panel. Doctor-Patient Communication (pending, 2001).

Parle M, Maguire P, Heaven C. The development of a training model to improve health professionals' skills, self-efficacy and outcome expectations when communicating with cancer patients. *Soc Sci Med* 1997;44:231-240.

Passik SD, Donaghy KB, Theobald DE, Lundberg J, Holtsclaw E, Dugan, Jr. WM. Oncology staff recognition of depressive symptoms on videotaped interviews of depressed cancer patients: implications for designing a training program. *J Pain Symptom Manage* 2000; 19:329-338.

Passik SD, Dugan W, McDonald MV et al. Oncologists' recognition of depression in patients with cancer. *J Clin Oncol* 1998;16:1594-1600.

Patton MD, Katterhagen JG. Critical pathways in oncology: Aligning resource expenditures with clinical outcomes. *J Oncol Management* 1997;6:16-61.

Pellegrino ED. 2000. Ethical issues in palliative care. In Chochinov HM, Breitbart W (eds.): *Handbook of Psychiatry in Palliative Medicine*. New York: Oxford University Press; pp. 337-356.

Phillips RS, Hamel MB, Covinsky KE, Lynn J (eds.) Findings from SUPPORT and HELP: Study to Understand Prognoses and Preferences for Outcomes and Risks of Treatment: Hospitalized Elderly Longitudinal Project. *J Amer Geriatrics Soc* 2000;48 (Suppl):S1-S233.

Portenoy RK. 2000. Physical symptom management in the terminally ill. In Chochinov HM, Breitbart W (eds.): *Handbook of Psychiatry in Palliative Medicine*. New York: Oxford University Press; pp. 99-129.

Post SG, Puchalski CM, Larson DB. Physicians and patient spirituality: professional boundaries, competency, and ethics. *Ann Intern Med* 2000;132:578-583.

Ptacek JT, Eberhardt TL. Breaking bad news. A review of the literature. *JAMA* 1996;276:496-502.

Puchalski C, Romer AL. Taking a spiritual history allows clinicians to understand patients more fully. *J Palliative Medicine* 2000;3:129-137.

Razavi D, Delvaux N, Farvacques C, et al. Screening for adjustment disorders and major depressive disorders in cancer patients. *Br J Psychiatry* 1990;156:79-83.

Reuben DB, Mor V. Nausea and vomiting in terminal cancer patients. *Arch Int Med* 1986; 146:2021-2023.

Ripamonti C. Management of bowel obstruction in advanced cancer patients. *J Pain Symptom Manage* 1994;9:193-200.

Rischer JB, Childress SB. Cancer pain management: pilot implementation of the AHCPR guideline in Utah. *J Qual Improvement* 1996;22:683-700.

Roth AJ, Kornblith AB, Batel-Copel L, et al. Rapid screening for psychologic distress in men with prostate carcinoma. *Cancer* 1998;82:1904-1908.

Rousseau P. Spirituality and the dying patient. *J Clin Oncol* 2000;18:2000-2002.

Sachs GA, Ahronheim JC, Rhymes JA, et al. Good care of dying patients: the alternative to physician-assisted suicide and euthanasia. *J Am Geriatr Soc* 1995;43:553-562.

Singer PA, Martin DK, Kelner M. Quality end of life care-patients' perspectives. *JAMA* 1999;281:163-168.

Smith TJ, Hillner BE. 1998. Ensuring quality cancer care: Clinical practice guidelines, critical pathways, and care maps. Unpublished background paper. Washington, D.C.: Institute of Medicine, National Cancer Policy Board.

Speck P. 1998. Spiritual issues in palliative care. In Doyle D, Hanks GWC, MacDonald N (eds.): *Oxford Textbook of Palliative Medicine (2nd edition)*. New York: Oxford University Press; pp. 805-814.

Speice J, Harkness J, Laneri R, et al. Involving family members in cancer care: focus group considerations of patients and oncological providers. *Psycho-oncology: Journal of the Psychological, Social and Behavioral Dimensions of Cancer* 2000;9:101-112.

Stephenson J. Revitalized AHCPR pursues research on quality. *JAMA* 1997;278:1557.

Twycross R, Lichter I. 1998. The terminal phase. In Doyle D, Hanks GWC, MacDonald N (eds.): *Oxford Textbook of Palliative Medicine (2nd edition)*. New York: Oxford University Press; pp. 977-992.

Wanzer SH, Federman DD, Adelstein SJ et al. The physician's responsibility toward hopelessly ill patients-a second look. *N Engl J Med* 1989;120:844-849.

Wilson KG, Chochinov HM, de Faye BJ, Breitbart W. 2000. Diagnosis and management of depression in palliative care. In Chochinov HM, Breitbart W (eds.): *Handbook of Psychiatry in Palliative Medicine*. New York: Oxford University Press; pp. 25-49.

World Health Organization. 1996. Report of the WHO Expert Committee on Cancer Pain Relief and Active Supportive Care: Cancer Pain Relief with a Guide to Opioid Availability. Technical Report Series 804 (2nd edition). Geneva: World Health Organization.

World Health Organization. 1998. Symptom Relief in Terminal Illness. Geneva: World Health Organization.

Zisook S. 2000. Understanding and managing bereavement in palliative care. In Chochinov HM, Breitbart W (eds.): *Handbook of Psychiatry in Palliative Medicine*. New York: Oxford University Press; pp. 331-334.

8

Cross-Cutting Research Issues: A Research Agenda for Reducing Distress of Patients with Cancer

Charles S. Cleeland, Ph.D.
University of Texas M.D. Anderson Cancer Center

INTRODUCTION

This chapter reviews the current status of research on end-of-life issues, advanced cancer, and symptom control and explores linkages with research on the distress experienced by other cancer patients in treatment and by many cancer survivors. Relatively little such research is carried out, despite a rich research agenda. The organizational and other barriers to the development, support, and performance of this type of cancer research, which have led to the current situation, are explored, and steps are proposed that could facilitate basic, behavioral, and clinical research on the symptoms and treatment of patients with advanced cancer.

Background

Despite billions of dollars spent on research in cancer biology and cancer therapeutics, there has been little investment in research that might significantly alleviate the physical and psychological distress of patients at the end of life. The types of distress experienced by these patients are shared, in a temporary or more lasting fashion, with patients being treated for cancer and, at least to some extent, by some who survive the disease. This chapter focuses on symptoms in patients who are dying, but the distinction between these symptoms and those experienced at other points in the disease and treatment continuum is artificial, and much of what is described here will also be applicable to distress experienced by cancer patients more generally.

There is ample evidence that patients who are dying have symptoms that devastate them and consume their families. Many patients experience needless pain that could be controlled by the optimal application of existing therapies. Others experience fatigue, cognitive deficits, depression, physical wasting, and other symptoms that are poorly understood and less easily managed with current treatments. There is a need for a broadly based strategic plan for research in this area that will integrate health services research in the improved delivery of distress management with basic and clinical research that develops new therapeutic strategies. New and existing methods of distress management must be tested clinically for their effectiveness to provide for evidence-based practice recommendations.

Compared with the rest of the cancer research establishment, research directed at cancer-related distress is poorly organized, poorly conceptualized, underfunded, and dependent on an insufficient number of well-trained researchers. Increased organizational and public recognition of the suffering that often dominates the end of life for cancer patients has created an opportunity for a sympathetic response to new proposals in this area. New information in cancer biology and neuroscience could be applied directly to alleviating distress if researchers could be encouraged to recognize and explore potential linkages of information.

OVERVIEW OF RESEARCH RELATED TO END OF LIFE, PALLIATIVE CARE, AND SYMPTOM CONTROL

The types of research that are needed to improve care and reduce distress at the end of life fall into three major categories:

1. descriptive and epidemiologic studies that define the specific needs of patients and caregivers, determine the prevalence and severity of the symptom-generated distress that they experience, and point the way to additional investigation of the causes and potential treatment of this distress;

2. studies of the specific symptoms that patients experience and the treatment of these symptoms, primarily from biomedical and behavioral perspectives; and

3. studies of the delivery of care to these patients and ways to improve this care by the optimal use of existing treatments.

This broad research agenda depends on a wide range of investigators and methods, and its performance will depend on a creative combination of funding from different sources as well as the development of a larger group of researchers interested in and trained to deliver the kinds of research needed.

The notion that the distress of cancer patients at the end of life, and also throughout the spectrum of their disease, is a topic worthy of serious research is relatively new. Public support for this kind of research has grown for several reasons, including increasing knowledge of the widespread nature of the severity of this distress, increasing consumer demand that quality of life is a legitimate issue, and the public debate over end-of-life decisions and assisted suicide. There is also an increasing expectation that the control of pain and other symptoms and at least some aspects of suffering should be included in what medical care has to offer, should be a right of patients under the care of the health system, and should be a competency of their health care providers.

This increasing expectation of and support for better management of the distress of cancer and of dying with cancer has created a condition that is in some ways like the emergence of a new disease. Systems are not prepared to deliver the care required, the biology and behavioral aspects of the disease have to be understood, existing treatments have to be tested to see if they are effective, and new ones must be proposed and tested. When a new disease emerges, there are few if any providers competent in its management, and the funding components of the health care system are not prepared to finance its treatment. The research required to understand its biology, its behavioral ramifications, and the best way to treat it is not in place, and investigators have to be attracted to the area, develop appropriate methods of research, and be funded to carry out the requisite research.

While the new disease analogy may be helpful to explain the demand for new types of research, there are special characteristics of the needed research that makes it hard to conceptualize, to organize, and to fund. Some of these special difficulties include

- the subjective nature of many of the measurement and outcome variables,
- the poor fit of current disease models of research for doing this type of health-related investigation,
- the lack of an organizational structure for responding to this type of research demand,
- the high level of interdisciplinary research that is required to do the work, and
- the absence of a high-priority pathway for putting this type of research in place.

Organization of This Review

This review offers examples from two areas of research that are critical to the delivery of better end-of-life and symptom control care:

1. epidemiology, social-behavioral, and health services research that defines the area and its impact, and

2. symptom research that examines components of the problem from a more traditional biomedical perspective.

The review covers recent research findings in each area, examples of needed research, a description of barriers to organizing and funding research, and suggested policy for changes in priority and structure that may improve and focus research of this type.

Methods

The following methods were used to gather data for this chapter:

- review of recent research (Medline databases),
- review of current National Institutes of Health (NIH) funding using the NIH CRISP retrieval system,
- review of currently active clinical trials using the Clinicaltrials.gov database, and
- survey responses from researchers in the field.

Epidemiology and Descriptive Research: Prevalence, Impact, and Management of Symptoms

Patients with advanced cancer typically experience multiple symptoms related to cancer and cancer treatment. These symptoms can include physical (e.g., nausea, dyspnea), cognitive (e.g., delirium, memory problems, impaired concentration), and affective (e.g., depression, anxiety) experiences associated with the disease and its treatments. Symptom severity is related to the extent of disease and the aggressiveness of therapies such as surgery, chemotherapy, radiotherapy, and biological therapies. Common symptoms of cancer and cancer treatment significantly impair the daily function and quality of life of patients. Pain is a good example. When pain is present, it adversely affects patients' mood, activity, and ability to relate to others (Serlin et al., 1995). Similarly, fatigue, gastrointestinal symptoms, cachexia, anorexia, shortness of breath, and psychological distress add tremendously to the distress that patients experience.

At present, the severe distress, multiple symptoms, and inadequate treatment faced by many patients at the end of life are well documented. Several studies have examined cancer-related symptoms in patients with advanced disease. Coyle and colleagues (1990) found that fatigue, weakness, pain, sleepiness, and cognitive impairment were frequent symptoms of patients with terminal disease enrolled in a supportive care program. Fatigue (58 percent) and pain (54 percent) were the most prevalent symptoms. Donnelly and colleagues (1995) prospectively studied the prevalence and severity of these symptoms in 1,000 patients with advanced cancer. Pain, fatigue, and anorexia were consistently found to be among the 10 most prevalent symptoms at all 17 primary cancer sites studied. When pain, anorexia, weakness, anxiety, lack of energy, severe fatigue, early satiety, constipation, and dyspnea were present, a majority of patients rated them as moderate or severe. Similarly, a prospective study of cancer patients in palliative care centers in Europe, Australia, and the United States found that more than half of the patients reported pain and weakness (Vainio and Auvinen, 1996). Weight loss, anorexia, constipation, nausea, and dyspnea were also common.

As part of the Study to Understand Prognoses and Preferences for Outcomes and Risks of Treatment (SUPPORT), McCarthy and colleagues (2000) evaluated more than 1,000 cancer patients during the three days before death and also at one to three months before death, and three to six months before death. As expected, as they progressed toward death, their estimated six-month prognosis decreased significantly and the severity of their disease worsened. Patients' functional status also declined significantly as they approached death, such that most patients had four or more symptoms within the three days before death. Patients with cancer experienced significantly more pain and confusion as death approached. Severe pain was common; more than one-quarter of patients with cancer experienced significant pain three to six months before death and more than 40 percent were in significant pain during their last three days of life. However, dying patients were only modestly depressed and anxious during their last three days of life.

The distress caused by symptoms for cancer patients at the end of life is shared by patients who are not yet terminal. Very few epidemiological studies have examined the multiple symptoms of cancer patients with less progressed disease. However, the symptoms associated with aggressive treatments such as chemotherapy and radiotherapy have been well documented. For example, multiple studies have found that the majority of patients undergoing chemotherapy or radiotherapy report significant fatigue during the course of treatment (Cleeland et al., 2000; Irvine, et al., 1994; Smets et al., 1996). A few studies have assessed multiple symptoms in samples of cancer patients with different stages of disease. Portenoy and colleagues (1994) administered the Memorial Symptom Assessment Scale to a random sample of inpatients and outpatients with breast, prostate, colon, or ovarian cancer. The most frequently reported symptoms for the sample were lack of energy, worry, feeling sad, and pain. Patients with metastatic disease reported more symptom distress than patients with less advanced disease. In a recent study of more than 500 patients in active treatment, more than 20 percent of patients reported a variety of severe symptoms, including fatigue, worry, distress, poor sleep, lack of appetite, and dry mouth (Cleeland et al., 2000).

It is less well recognized that many cancer survivors continue to experience physical, affective, or cognitive symptoms even when their disease is in remission or treatment has ended. These symptoms may be due to physiological changes associated with prior treatments, delayed side effects of treatment, or long-term consequences of the disease. For example, survivors of bone marrow transplantation may report cognitive impairment, physical symptoms, or emotional distress many years after the transplant (Andrykowski et al., 1995; McQuellon et al., 1996; Prieto et al., 1996).

Evidence for Inadequate Symptom Management

Recent studies have described the prevalence and severity of pain due to cancer and have documented that pain is often undertreated with available analgesics (Cleeland et al., 1994). These studies present a model for the study of other major symptoms, such as depression and fatigue. Approximately 55 percent of outpatients with metastatic cancer have disease-related pain, and 36 percent have pain of sufficient severity to impair their function and quality of life despite current analgesic therapy. Despite national and international guidelines for its management, many patients with pain are not prescribed an analgesic appropriate to the severity of their pain (Cleeland et al., 1994). Evidence suggests that patients in minority groups may have an even greater risk for undertreatment of pain (Anderson et al., 2000; Cleeland et al., 1997).

Two studies of outpatients with metastatic or recurrent cancer receiving treatment at Eastern Cooperative Oncology Group (ECOG) institutions found that more than 40 percent of those with pain were not prescribed analgesics strong enough to match the severity of their pain (Cleeland et al., 1994, 1997). A discrepancy between the physician's and patient's rating of the severity of the pain was a major predictor of undermedication for pain (Cleeland et al., 1994). Pain has to be appreciated before it can be treated. In addition, patients seen at centers that treated predominantly minority patients were three times more likely than those treated elsewhere to have inadequate pain management (Cleeland et al., 1997). Other factors that predicted inadequate pain treatment included age of 70 years or older, female sex, and better performance status. These results support the opinion of oncology physicians that poor assessment of symptoms is a major barrier to adequate symptom management (Cleeland et al., 2000; von Roenn et al., 1993). They also suggest that careful and accurate symptom assessment is particularly important for cancer patients from minority groups, elderly patients, female patients, and patients who appear to be functioning well.

A study by Bemabei and colleagues (1998) took advantage of a large database to examine the treatment of pain in cancer patients cared for in nursing homes. Using the Resident Assessment Instrument and the Minimum Data Set (MDS), part of the Health Care Financing Administration's (HCFA's) Demonstration Project, the investigators found that 38 percent of nursing home residents with cancer from a five-state area complained of, or showed evidence of, daily pain. The study found that 26 percent of these patients with daily pain got no analgesics at all. Patients over 85 years were more likely to receive no analgesia, as were minorities. Only about half of the patients in pain were receiving opioids, and only 13 percent of patients over 85 were receiving these stronger analgesics.

Many cancer specialists recognize that symptom control is often suboptimal. Medical oncologists were surveyed about their treatment of cancer pain in a study conducted by ECOG (von Roenn et al., 1993). Only half of the physicians surveyed indicated that cancer pain control was good or very good in their practice setting. Seventy-five percent of the physicians indicated that the most important barrier to cancer pain management was inadequate pain assessment. More than 60 percent of physicians were reluctant to prescribe analgesics or cited the unwillingness of patients to report pain or take opioids as barriers. Inadequate knowledge about cancer pain management was reported by more than half the physicians who responded. The survey acknowledged that a substandard level of education about cancer pain management and a reluctance to address it in practice existed at all levels of professional health care.

A recent study (Cleeland et al., 2000) repeated the ECOG study format with physician members of the Radiation Therapy Oncology Group. On average, physicians estimated that two-thirds of cancer patients suffered pain for longer than one month. Assessing a case scenario, 23 percent would wait until the patient's prognosis was six months or less before starting maximal analgesia, indicating a very conservative approach to pain management. Adjuvants and prophylactic side-effect management were underutilized in the treatment plan for the case presented. Perceived barriers to good pain management were very similar to the ECOG study, with poor pain assessment being ranked number one. Compounded by inadequate training for physicians in the palliative treatment of cancer, these problems influence decisions made in the management of incurable cancer and profoundly affect end-of-life care.

In spite of recent concerns over symptom management at the end of life, provoked in large part by the debate over euthanasia, there is substantial evidence that symptoms that could, in principle, be well managed are undertreated, especially for patients who are still in active treatment. There is evidence that many symptoms could be controlled more adequately if we systematically applied the knowledge that we now have about symptom management.

Impact of Symptoms on Family Caregivers of Advanced Cancer Patients

Family members most often serve as the primary caregiver for the cancer patient, which may lead to a disruption in family relationships. This burden has been shown to produce emotional and physical disturbances in the caregiver. The appearance of patients' symptoms, such as fatigue, nausea, and pain, underlines the severity of the disease and its potential mortality, adding significantly to the burden of family members who may feel unable to help the patient get relief. Numerous studies have examined the caregiving burden experienced by the family members of patients with cancer (Carey et al., 1991; Cassileth et al., 1985; Miaskowski et al., 1997a, 1997b; Oberst, et al., 1989; Stetz, 1987).

A family caregiver's distress is related to the severity of symptoms experienced by the cancer patient. In a cross-sectional study, Miaskowski and colleagues (1997a, 1997b) found that family members of oncology patients with pain report greater tension, depression, and total mood disturbance than family members of patients without pain. Ferrell and colleagues (1991a, 1991b) conducted a qualitative study of 85 family caregivers of cancer patients to describe their perspective toward cancer pain and their role in its management. When asked about their role in managing cancer pain, caregivers reported making treatment decisions such as deciding what medication to give the patient and when to give it. Caregivers expressed their own and their patients' fears about addiction to pain medication and felt that it was their responsibility to help the patient avoid addiction.

Most of the studies of caregivers have been conducted with white middle-class families. Relatively few studies have focused on the experiences and emotions of minority families of cancer patients, particularly those families with limited financial resources or fragmented health care (Juarez et al., 1998). Limited research indicates that ethnicity and social class do affect how patients, family members, and health care providers perceive illness and, more importantly, how family members and health care providers respond to the multiple needs of the patient (Gonzalez, 1997; Guarnaccia et al., 1992; Sales et al., 1992).

A Good Example of Research on End-of-Life Issues

Specific end-of-life issues have been carefully researched. Decisions about advance directives is an example. The SUPPORT database offers a large amount of information about cancer patients' preferences for cardiopulmonary resuscitation (CPR) and the relationship of this preference to patient characteristics. Haidet and colleagues (1998) analyzed SUPPORT data for 520 patients with colorectal cancer to determine preferences for CPR. Sixty-three percent wanted CPR in the event of cardiopulmonary arrest. Factors independently associated with preference for resuscitation included younger age, better quality of life, absence of lung metastases, and greater patient estimate of two-month prognosis. Of the patients who preferred not to receive CPR, less than half had a do-not-resuscitate (DNR) note or order written. Physicians incorrectly identified patient CPR preferences in 30 percent of cases.

A similar study (Covinsky et al., 2000) examined the characteristics of patients who do request DNR orders. Patients who are older, have cancer, are women, believe their prognoses are poor, and are more dependent in activities of daily living functioning are less likely to want CPR. However, there are considerable variability and geographic variation in these preferences. Physician, nurse, and surrogate understanding of their patients' preferences is only moderately better than chance. Most patients do not discuss their preferences with their physicians, and only about half of patients who do not wish to receive CPR receive DNR orders.

Weeks and colleagues (1998) examined the hypothesis that among terminally ill cancer patients, an accurate understanding of a poor prognosis is associated with a preference for therapy that focuses on comfort over attempts at life extension, using SUPPORT data. Subjects were 917 adults hospitalized with Stage III or IV non-small cell lung cancer or colon cancer metastatic to liver. Patients who thought they were going to live for at least six months were more likely to favor life-extending therapy over comfort care, compared with patients who thought there was at least a 10 percent chance that they would not live six months. (Patients overestimated their chances of surviving six months, while physicians estimated prognosis quite accurately.) Patients who preferred life-extending therapy were more likely to undergo aggressive treatment, but their six-month survival was no better than similar patients who did not seek aggressive treatment.

The effects of the Patient Self Determination Act (PSDA; mandated patient education about advance directives at hospital entry) have also been examined within the context of SUPPORT (Teno et al., 1997). There was no evidence that the PSDA substantially increased documentation of advance directives, and it appears that documentation of advance directives is unlikely to be a substantial element in improving the care of seriously ill patients.

Examples of Studies to Change Practice and Improve End-of-Life Care and Symptom Control

The most ambitious research project to understand and improve care at the end of life was the well-publicized SUPPORT (1990). The descriptive information from SUPPORT (reviewed above) is the best information we have about the dying process. Approximately 20 percent of the sample were patients with cancer. The intervention study, supported by the Robert Wood Johnson Foundation, was designed to improve end-of-life decisionmaking and reduce the frequency of a mechanically supported, painful, and prolonged process of dying. The intervention component of this study included 4,804 patients and their physicians randomized by specialty group to the intervention group (N = 2,652) or control group (N = 2,152). A specially trained nurse had multiple contacts with the patient, family, physician, and hospital staff to discuss outcomes and preferences, attend to pain control, and facilitate advanced care planning and patient-physician communication. Compared to the control group, patients in the intervention group experienced no improvement in patient-physician communication or in the six targeted outcomes (i.e., incidence or timing of written DNR orders, physicians' knowledge of their patients' preferences not to be resuscitated, number of days spent in an intensive care unit [ICU], receiving mechanical ventilation, being comatose before death, level of reported pain). There was no reduction in hospital resources for the intervention. The authors concluded that the type of intervention used to improve communication, education, and advocacy was insufficient to change current practice.

In summary, end-of-life care is inadequate, and much research is needed to improve it. As we have seen, there is also ample evidence of inadequate treatment for the symptoms of cancer. The same reasons for inadequate end-of-life care also apply to the management of pain and other symptoms, including poor assessment, inadequately trained health care providers, low priority for this type of care, lack of patient demand for better care, and negative sanctions against aggressive pain management. As is true of many other medical education efforts, relatively passive continuing medical education programs dealing with these issues have had little effect on practice (Cleeland, 1993; Weissman and Dahl, 1995).

There have been a few studies examining the effectiveness of improving the practice of cancer pain management. A training program that includes the active participation of health care professionals and includes "role models" has demonstrated lasting changes in the cancer pain management knowledge of physicians and nurses (Janjan et al., 1996; Weissman et al., 1993). These studies did not examine patient report of pain as an outcome variable but do suggest that durable change in knowledge is possible.

Beginning with publication of the World Health Organization's (WHO's) *Cancer Pain Management* guidelines in 1986 (WHO, 1986), several guidelines have been issued for cancer pain management, including the Agency for Health Care Policy and Research (AHCPR) *Guideline for Cancer Pain Management* (Jacox et al., 1994), guidelines from the American Pain Society (1999), and more recently, guidelines from the National Comprehensive Cancer Network. There is, however, only one published study that evaluates the effectiveness of physician adherence to a pain management guideline for cancer pain (DuPen et al., 1999). In this study, 81 cancer patients were enrolled in a prospective, longitudinal, randomized study from the outpatient clinics of 26 medical oncologists in western Washington State. A multilevel treatment algorithm, based on the AHCPR Guideline for Cancer Pain Management was compared with "standard practice" (control) therapies for pain and symptom management used by community oncologists. The primary outcome of interest was pain. Patients randomized to the guideline group achieved a statistically significant reduction in usual pain intensity when compared with standard community practice.

A second randomized trial, evaluating the effects of an education program for cancer patients with chronic pain (de Wit et al., 1997), also used pain as an outcome variable. Information about pain and pain management was given to patients in the intervention group by several media: verbal instruction, written material, an audio cassette tape, and the use of a pain diary. The pain education program consisted of three elements: (1) educating patients about the basic principles of pain and pain management, (2) instructing patients how to report their pain in a pain diary, and (3) instructing patients how to communicate about pain and how to contact health care providers. Patients in the intervention group participated in the pain education program in the hospital and three and seven days post-discharge by telephone. Results showed a significant increase in pain knowledge and a significant decrease in pain intensity in patients who received the pain education program.

RESEARCH NEEDS

Studies of the prevalence, severity, and treatment of pain present a model of the descriptive research that has to be done in other areas of symptom management and end-of-life care. First, we need to determine the prevalence and severity of various symptoms in patients throughout the course of their disease: at diagnosis, during treatment, when cancer is in remission, and near the end of life. This includes the behavioral, economic, and social impact of these symptoms. There is an urgent need to learn more about how care for advanced disease is reimbursed. It is important to include longitudinal designs in this research so that we can determine changes in symptom patterns over time. We also need to identify the adequacy of care for these symptoms, including identifying what factors (e.g., patient related, clinician related, system related) are predictive of poor symptom management and poor end-of-life care.

Current projects were identified in areas related to end of life, palliative care, and symptom control by searching CRISP, the NIH engine for indexing currently funded research. Key words for the major areas of such research were combined with "cancer." Individual funding abstracts were inspected to see if they were research projects, defined as "matches." Excluded were training grants, fellowships without a specific research topic, meeting grants, cooperative group renewals, or instances where the key-word match was not a fit for the topic. The matches could be classified as (1) descriptive or health services research, (2) studies of interventions or clinical trials, or (3) basic science investigations. The search results are presented in Table 8-1, illustrating the dearth of research on end-of-life issues and symptoms in patients with advanced cancer.

This section reviews recent research on the following cancer-related symptoms: pain, anorexia and cachexia, cognitive failure (including de-lirium and cognitive impairment such as problems with memory and rea-soning), dyspnea, fatigue, gastrointestinal symptoms, and psychiatric symp-toms (including depression and anxiety). It includes information about the current status of treatment, what is known about the mechanisms respon-sible for the symptom, and what types of clinical and basic research should be carried out to improve the management of the symptom.

Biomedical symptom research is closest to the clinical research model in place at NIH and many other funding agencies and is therefore more likely to be funded than descriptive or health services research. However, a search of currently funded grants for each symptom (basic and clinical) suggests little support for these investigations, even though relatively small incre-ments in our basic and clinical knowledge base are liable to substantially improve care for very ill patients.

One somewhat artificial barrier to progress in this type of research is the balkanization of the research establishment. For example, several NIH institutes are working relatively independently on problems in neuroscience, molecular biology, and the general biology of cancer treatment that might contribute to a better understanding of mechanisms common to the expres-sion of these symptoms. An excellent example is the potential role of in-flammatory processes in pain, wasting, cognitive deficit, depression, and fatigue, where relevant research is being funded by several NIH Institutes.

TABLE 8-1   Results of CRISP Searches for Current Research on End-of-Life, Palliative Care, and Symptom Control (numbers of currently-funded projects as of April 2000)

Search Term + Cancer	Hits (Matches)	Descriptive and Health Services Research	Interventions and Clinical Trials	Basic Science
Palliative	54 (7)	4	2	1
End of life	14 (9)	7	2	0
Bereavement	11 (6)	3	3	0
Symptoms	125 (27)	11	13	3

Pain

Of all the symptoms faced by patients with advanced cancer, pain is perhaps the best understood, and research in this area has a higher level of support than the study of other symptoms (see previous section). Several issues related to the subjective measurement of pain have been successfully addressed, and pain-related patient outcome variables can be specified for clinical, health services research, and epidemiologic studies. It is estimated that a majority of cancer patients could have their pain controlled, at least until the last week or two of life.

Current treatment of cancer pain is beginning to be codified into evidence-based and practice-based guidelines (practice based refers to guidelines that blend expert opinion and research evidence, where the evidence alone is not sufficient), which suggests a maturity of knowledge that does not exist for other symptoms. The common syndromes that account for the majority of cancer pain are well described and dictate specific treatment approaches. In contrast to other areas of research under discussion, there is a group of well-trained investigators who are able to conduct both basic and clinical research in the area. As described above, the biggest problems—which are amenable to health services research—are in getting physicians and patients to use pain medications to their best advantage. However, there are still major basic and clinical research issues to be dealt with, and research in cancer pain is also as affected by compartmentalization and lack of organizational support, funding, and structure as is research in other areas of end-of-life care. One approach to alleviating this problem is to facilitate networking among cancer pain investigators and basic scientists who are working in separate disciplines.

Basic research into the mechanisms of cancer pain has been limited by two major gaps in knowledge: (1) a poor understanding of the specific nature of cancer pain and (2) the lack of appropriate animal models.

Nature of Cancer Pain

Cancer pain potentially involves somatic, visceral, and neuropathic components. There have been marked advancements in understanding the mechanisms of cutaneous somatic pain over the past 20 years. These were largely first driven by the landmark studies of Lewis, and later Hardy and colleagues, that described the phenomena of primary and secondary hyperalgesia. The neurochemical basis of pain is becoming better understood; however, clinical applications of these findings have not yet had an impact on treatment.

Neuropathic pain, produced by nerve destruction and prominent in both cancer and AIDS, is poorly understood and difficult to treat (Woolf and Mannion, 1999). Interactions between inflammatory mediators (such as cytokines and neurotrophins) are thought to sensitize pain receptors (nociceptors) to induce the sprouting of nociceptor terminals in inappropriate regions of the dorsal horn, to potentially alter phenotype of nonnociceptive afferent fibers, and to induce changes in the level of myelination of fibers. The mechanisms whereby these processes interact to produce changes in sensation are just beginning to be understood. Although some older drugs (tricyclics) and newer drugs (anticonvulsants, especially gabapentin) seem to help clinically, well-controlled clinical trial evidence in cancer is sparse. Most agree that advances in treating neuropathic pain will depend on understanding what causes it.

Visceral pain, originating from inflammation or damage to internal body structures, is the least understood of the major classes of pain that contribute to the cancer pain state. At present, the pathways by which noxious inputs from the viscera are transmitted and the forebrain structures involved in the processing of this pain remain little studied and technically difficult.

Animal Models

A recent study by Honore and colleagues (2000) is the first to establish a model of cancer pain. The promise of such models has already been demonstrated by the identification of osteoprotegerin as a potential therapy for bone cancer pain. Osteoprotegerin is a secreted "decoy" receptor that inhibits osteoclast activity (the breakdown of bone) and also blocks behaviors indicative of pain in mice with bone cancer. Osteoprotegerin inhibition of tumor-induced bone destruction inhibits neurochemical changes in the spinal cord thought to be involved in the generation and maintenance of cancer pain. In an unrelated clinical study, osteoprotegerin has already been given to humans, suggesting that a pain-focused clinical trial could come soon.

Behavioral Interventions

Behavioral measures for controlling cancer pain are promising but need further clinical testing. For example, there is some evidence to suggest that educational interventions can be effective for the alleviation of chronic cancer pain (see de Wit et al., 1997), but no research has yet been done to isolate the most useful aspects of these complex interventions. Relaxation has been somewhat more intensively researched, and interventions such as guided imagery and progressive muscle relaxation appear to be effective (Sloman, 1995), but the evidence for the value of other relaxation-based methods is less clear. Hypnosis is the best supported technique for alleviating procedure-related pain (Hawkins et al., 1998; Liossi and Hatira, 1999). However, evidence for the effectiveness of hypnosis in relieving chronic cancer pain is sparse (Syrjala et al., 1992).

Despite the existence of guidelines, the treatment of cancer pain remains largely empirical. There is an urgent need to confirm collected anecdotal information on analgesics, adjuvant analgesics, and neuroablative procedures, in randomized clinical trials.

Basic Research Needs

Major questions for basic research include the following:

1. What are the basic mechanisms of visceral and neuropathic pain, and how can we find better ways to treat these conditions?
2. What are the modifications of the nervous system that sustain chronic pain perception?
3. What newer compounds might have more precise analgesic action with fewer side effects?
4. What are the molecular mechanisms of pain signaling, and receptor modification due to pain, and how can they be modified?
5. What are the forebrain structures that modulate responses to "painful" signals?
6. What is the receptor affinity of different opioids?

Clinical Research Needs

The major issue to be addressed in clinical and health services research is, If we have the means to manage the pain of the majority of cancer patients, why do so many patients still have poorly controlled pain? Studies to improve cancer pain management are needed, as they are for other areas of distress at the end of life. Other issues include the following:

1. How effective are current treatments for neuropathic pain?
2. What are the effects of cancer on tolerance to opioid analgesics, and how can pain be managed in already-tolerant patients? What are the roles of type and route of opioids?
3. What opioids have the "best" side-effect profiles?
4. Trials of intrathecal delivery of novel analgesics need to be conducted.
5. What works to improve the practice of pain management?

Review of Current Funding: CRISP Listings

Searching the CRISP database of current federal funding using the terms cancer and pain produces 147 hits. Inspection of the result finds a total of 42 that relate to basic or clinical research that might have relevance to clinical cancer pain. Of these studies, 9 are descriptive (including correlational and behavioral studies), 19 deal with trials of interventions, and 14 are basic science studies.

CURRENTLY FUNDED CLINICAL TRIALS

1. Combination Chemotherapy in Treating Pain in Patients with Hormone-Refractory Metastatic Prostate Cancer
2. Phase III Randomized Study of Mitoxantrone and Prednisone with or Without Clodronate in Patients with Hormone Refractory Metastatic Prostate Cancer and Pain
3. Flecainide in Treating Patients with Chronic Neuropathic Pain
4. Pain Control in Patients with Recurrent or Metastatic Breast or Prostate Cancer
5. Morphine for the Treatment of Pain in Patients with Breast Cancer
6. Treatment of Prostate Cancer with Docetaxel Alone and in Combination with Thalidomide Treating Patients With Stage IV Prostate Cancer
7. Effect of Androgen Suppression on Bone Loss in Patients With or Without Bone Metastases
8. Combination Chemotherapy in Treating Pain in Patients with Hormone Refractory Metastatic Prostate Cancer

Anorexia and Cachexia

Cancer patients often experience a profound loss of appetite (anorexia), especially in the last weeks of life, as well as a deterioration and wasting of body tissue (cachexia). There is clear evidence that cancer patients have undergone metabolic changes in their physiological responses to food. The metabolic changes with cachexia seem to be mediated by a variety of molecules in the body (including proinflammatory cytokines, neuroendocrine hormones, neurotransmitters, eicosanoids, and tumor-related substances) (produced by the tumor itself and by the body in response to the tumor; Barber et al., 2000). Cachexia is the immediate cause of nearly one-third of cancer deaths (Argiles and Lopez-Soriano, 1999).

Pharmacologic agents commonly used to treat cachexia include corticosteroids and progestational drugs (Gagnon and Bruera, 1998). Eight randomized, double-blind, placebo-controlled studies have confirmed that progestational drugs can increase appetite, food intake, and energy level. Additionally, in many patients, these drugs increase weight, and may also have an effect on nausea and vomiting (Body, 1999). Drugs that lessen the process of skeletal muscle protein catabolism that occurs in cachexia patients (e.g., eicosapentaenoic acid and ibuprofen) are more effective than parenteral nutrition in stabilizing weight loss (Tisdale, 1998).

Parenteral nutrition may be used to improve patients' nutritional status and enable them to receive complete doses of chemotherapy or radiation therapy. However, in prospective randomized clinical trials, parenteral nutrition has not had a significant effect either on a patient's survival or on symptoms and toxicities (Body, 1999).

New treatments for cachexia include thalidomide, dronabinol (THC, tetrahydrocannabinol) and cannabis, and melatonin. THC stimulates appetite and increases body weight in patients with HIV and cancer. However, it is unclear whether THC or cannabis is more effective. Gorter (1999) argues that cannabis may be better tolerated than THC alone because cannabis stimulates the appetite like pure THC but includes other cannabinoids that decrease the psychotropic side effects of THC. Neuropeptide agonists and antagonists currently used to treat obesity may also have an effect on cancer anorexia-cachexia, especially when combined with other agents that affect the breakdown of muscle and protein (Inui, 1999). Clinical trials are needed to test the effectiveness of all the treatments discussed above.

Patients with cachexia often have greater concentrations of proinflammatory cytokines (i.e., tumor necrosis factor alpha, interleukin-1, interleukin-6 [IL-6], serotonin, interferon gamma) (Mantovani et al., 1998; Yeh and Schuster, 1999). When the concentrations of these cytokines are reduced, patients often gain weight. According to Tisdale (Tisdale, 1998), IL-6 is the only cytokine that is correlated with the development of cancer cachexia. Although it seems safe to say that cytokines are involved in cancer cachexia, the specific roles of these cytokines in the production of cachexia are still unclear.

Animal models of anorexia and cachexia have been developed. Emery (1999) placed a transplantable Leydig cell tumor in Fischer rats. Rats with this tumor showed a 20-40 percent decrease in food intake and an increase in energy expenditure compared with controls. Potential explanations for these effects include postprandial metabolism of carbohydrate caused by a greater rate of hepatic glycogen synthesis via the indirect pathway and maintenance of this increased rate of hepatic glycogen synthesis for a longer time after a meal. Another animal model of cachexia involves ciliary neurotrophic factor (a type of IL-6), which decreased muscle mass in experimental animals but did not have a direct effect on muscle in vitro (Tisdale, 1998).

A better understanding of the link between cancer cachexia and cytokines should lead to the development and testing of new pharmacologic agents. For example, megestrol acetate downregulates the synthesis and release of cytokines and increases appetite, body weight, and quality of life in patients with cachexia, and medroxyprogesterone acetate reduces the in vitro production of cytokines and serotonin by peripheral blood mononuclear cells of cancer patients; both of these agents reduce the cisplatin-induced serotonin release in vitro from peripheral blood mononuclear cells of cancer patients (Mantovani et al., 1998).

Another promising area in basic research on cachexia is related to the recent identification of peptides involved in food regulatory systems, including the hormone leptin and leptin receptors, uncoupling proteins, agouti protein, melanocortin receptor isoforms, melanin-concentrating hormone, and the proteins responsible for "tub" and "fat" (mouse models of obesity) (Bessesen and Faggioni, 1998).

Basic Research Needs

Major questions for basic research include the following:

1. What are the specific roles of various cytokines in the cachectic process?
2. What are the roles of the food regulatory peptides in the cachectic process?

Clinical Research Needs

Clinical trials should focus on the following types of drugs:

1. proinflammatory mediators;
2. appetite stimulants;
3. anticatabolic agents (e.g., neuropeptide agonists and antagonists, beta 2- adrenoceptor agonists);
4. polyunsaturated fatty acids, n- [omega-] 3 fatty acids, fish oil;
5. anabolic agents (especially hormonal); and
6. anticytokines (e.g., megestrol acetate, medroxyprogesterone acetate, thalidomide, melatonin).

Review of Current Funding: CRISP Listings

Searching the CRISP database of current federal funding using the terms cancer and cachexia produced 28 hits. Inspection of the result found a total of 10 that relate to basic or clinical research possibly relevant to clinical cancer cachexia. Of these studies, none are descriptive (including correlational and behavioral studies), two deal with trials of interventions, and eight are basic science studies.

CURRENTLY FUNDED CLINICAL TRIALS

1. Omega-3 Fatty Acids in Treating Patients with Advanced Cancer Who Have Significant Weight Loss

2. Megestrol and Exercise in Treating Patients with Cancer-Related Weight Loss

3. High-Dose Megestrol in Treating Patients with Metastatic Breast Cancer, Endometrial Cancer, or Mesothelioma

Cognitive Failure
(Delirium, Temporary and Permanent Cognitive Impairment)

Cognitive decline, including poor memory, attention, and problem solving or even frank dementia and delirium, has long been recognized in patients with end-stage disease. As many as one-third of patients admitted to palliative care units show significant cognitive impairment (Power et al., 1993), and the percentage is much higher for patients in the last week or two of life. From 25 to 85 percent of patients with advanced cancer show confusion (Breitbart, 1995) and delirium is the second most common psychiatric diagnosis among hospitalized elderly cancer patients (Stiefel and Holland, 1991). Confusion, which affects decisionmaking and may interfere with a patient's recognition and reporting of other symptoms, is underreported, undertreated, and rarely studied in palliative care (Breitbart, 1995; Pereira et al., 1997). It can also affect patients' families and is often a deterrent to home terminal care (Minagawa et al., 1996).

A number of treatments are in use for patients with cancer-related cognitive impairment, despite a relative lack of reliable evidence regarding their effects. Neuroleptics and benzodiazepines are used to manage delirium (Bruera and Neumann, 1998). Haloperidol may be given in combination with lorazepam for patients with delirium who are experiencing agitation. Diazepam is frequently prescribed, but may cause cognitive impairment or worsen dementia. Opioid rotation (switching drugs when side effects occur or pain is not relieved) and mild hydration may reduce delirium in some patients with advanced disease (Bruera et al., 1995). Stimulant therapy may reverse some of the cognitive impairment (problems with memory, attention, and reasoning) shown by cancer patients. In a study of patients with malignant glioma who developed cognitive deficits, Meyers et al. (1998) found that methylphenidate (10mg twice daily) significantly improved gait, stamina, and cognitive function in half of the subjects despite progressive neurologic injury as documented by magnetic resonance imaging (MRI).

Patients with cognitive impairment often exhibit a generalized slowing on electroencephalograph readings and impaired function of the brain stem and forebrain in sleep testing procedures (Trzepacz, 1994). In as many as 75 percent of cases, the specific cause of cognitive impairment is unknown (Maddocks et al., 1996). Possible mechanisms of cognitive impairment include brain metastases, meningeal carcinomatosis, hypoxia, sepsis, metabolic abnormalities, hepatic and renal dysfunction, and increased drug levels in the brain or bloodstream (due to disruptions in the blood brain barrier and decreased drug metabolism). Research on cognitive impairment in patients with small cell lung cancer suggests that neuropsychological impairment may be caused by the disease process itself (Meyers et al., 1995; van Oosterhout et al., 1995). It has been hypothesized that long acting morphine metabolites are responsible for delirium (Maddocks et al., 1996; Bruera et al., 1995).

Cognitive impairment may also be caused or exacerbated by various anticancer treatments, including high-dose interferon alpha (INF-α) therapy, cranial irradiation, and high-dose chemotherapy. For example, patients treated with INF-α often exhibit a syndrome of mental slowing and memory impairment, accompanied by mood disturbances. These patients' patterns of test responses suggest mild subcortical dementia (Valentine et al., 1998). Patients receiving recombinant IL-2 have also been noted to develop a severe dementia resembling dementia of the Alzheimer's type (Walker et al., 1996). Therapy-induced cognitive impairment may be either acute or chronic. As discussed above, survivors of bone marrow transplantation may report cognitive impairment, physical symptoms, or emotional distress many years after the transplant (Andrykowski et al., 1995; McQuellon et al., 1996; Prieto et al., 1996).

Basic Research Needs

Major questions for basic research include the following:

1. What are the underlying mechanisms of delirium and cognitive impairment?
2. What is the role of the cancer disease process in producing cognitive impairment?
3. What is the process through which biological therapies (e.g., IFN-α, IL-2) produce cognitive impairment?
4. Are there biological markers for those patients most at risk for delirium and cognitive impairment?

Clinical Research Needs

Research in this area should focus on the understanding, prevention, and treatment of delirium, specifically

1. development of and agreement on standardized assessment for delirium;

2. prevalence, nature, and current treatment for delirium and cognitive impairment;

3. clinical trials of drugs now used empirically for delirium (haloperidol) and cognitive impairment (methylphenidate);

4. clinical trials of stimulants to treat cognitive impairment; and

5. clinical trials of anticancer treatments that include neuropsychological assessments as a required measure of treatment toxicity to determine which treatments may cause cognitive impairment.

Review of Current Funding: CRISP Listings

Searching the CRISP database of current federal funding using the terms cancer and delirium or cognitive impairment produced seven hits. Two relate to basic or clinical research that might have relevance to clinical cancer-related delirium or cognitive impairment. Of these studies, one is descriptive, and one is a basic science study. There are no intervention trials.

CURRENTLY FUNDED CLINICAL TRIALS   There are no current trials for delirium or cognitive impairment.

Dyspnea

Between one-fifth and three-quarters of patients with advanced disease experience dyspnea, which is moderate to severe in 10 to 60 percent of these patients (Ripamonti, 1999). Not surprisingly, a greater proportion of newly diagnosed lung cancer patients—70 percent—experience dyspnea (Muers et al., 1993). Dyspnea often occurs in the presence of other symptoms: patients with dyspnea were 39 percent more likely to complain of other symptoms and 55 percent more likely to report other symptoms as being severe (Farncombe, 1997). The frequency and severity of dyspnea increase with the progression of the disease and when death is approaching.

Dyspnea may be related to anticancer treatments, including chemotherapy, radiotherapy, and surgery (Komurcu et al., 2000). Treatment of the underlying cancer or treatment of the underlying pulmonary or cardiac disease may relieve dyspnea. Additionally, radiotherapy and chemotherapy may relieve dyspnea even when there is no tumor response. The most common treatments administered to dyspneic patients in the emergency department at the University of Texas M.D. Anderson Cancer Center in the early 1990s were oxygen (31 percent), beta 2-agonists (14 percent), antibiotics (12 percent), and opioids (11 percent) (Escalante et al., 1996).

Dyspnea is understudied. There is a great need for research on the pathophysiology of dyspnea in cancer patients. Potential mechanisms for dyspnea include respiratory muscle weakness due to anorexia and cachexia, chemoreceptor stimulation, and efferent activity from the respiratory center by direct ascending stimulation.

Despite the various treatments that are used, few clinical trials of their effectiveness for relieving dyspnea in cancer patients have been carried out (LeGrand and Walsh, 1999). Opioids are often used for patients with dyspnea, but there have been too few well-controlled clinical trials to determine the ideal drug, route, or regimen. Corticosteroids are also commonly used, but even less is known about the effectiveness of these drugs in relieving dyspnea. Benzodiazepines or nebulized opioids have not proven effective for the treatment of dyspnea in clinical trials. Transfusion therapy has been used to relieve dyspnea in patients with anemia, but the effectiveness of this treatment is unclear. Bronchodilators are used to improve breathing in many patients with lung cancer and chronic obstructive pulmonary disease (COPD), and may also be helpful for patients without COPD who have dyspnea.

Basic Research Needs

Major questions for basic research include the following:

1. standardization of measurement and assessment of dyspnea,
2. possible animal model for dyspnea,
3. relationship of dyspnea to the anemia of chronic illness,
4. role of respiratory muscle metabolism/function in dyspnea, and
5. establishing a link between cachexia, tumor necrosis factor, muscle fatigue or weakness, and dyspnea.

Clinical Research Needs

Clinical trials should focus on the following:

1. descriptive studies of prevalence, severity, and current treatment;
2. trials examining effectiveness of opioids by different routes;
3. trials of other agents (corticosteroids); and
4. trials of methylxanthine drugs, which may have a role in treating dyspnea by stimulating respiratory muscles.

Review of Current Funding: CRISP Listings

Searching the CRISP database of current federal funding using the terms cancer and dyspnea produced four hits. Only one relates to basic or clinical research that might have relevance to clinical cancer dyspnea, and it is an intervention study.

CURRENTLY FUNDED CLINICAL TRIALS There are no current trials for dyspnea.

Fatigue

Fatigue is the most common symptom among cancer patients (Glaus et al., 1996). Overwhelming fatigue often characterizes patients with far advanced cancer. Because of its prevalence, it is often reported as the symptom that is the most distressing and causes the greatest interference with daily life (Richardson, 1995). Fatigue in cancer patients is associated with psychological disturbance, symptom distress, and decreases in functional status (Irvine et al., 1994).

Symptomatic treatment of fatigue is in its infancy. Severe fatigue is associated with low levels of hemoglobin (Cleeland and Wang, 1999). Fatigue caused by anemia improves if the anemia can be treated with transfusions or epoietin alfa (Glaspy et al., 1997; Demetri et al., 1998). Therapies used for fatigue include changes in a patient's drug regimen, correction of metabolic abnormalities, and treatments for depression or insomnia. Many health care professionals suggest mild exercise as a way of dealing with fatigue, and a reduction in muscle mass has been suggested as a mechanism for fatigue. A recent controlled study found that aerobic exercise prevented increases in fatigue and psychological distress in patients undergoing high-dose chemotherapy (Dimeo et al., 1999). Other nonpharmacological treatments include modification of activity and rest patterns, cognitive therapies, behavioral therapies to modify sleep (sleep hygiene), and nutritional support.

Pharmacologic treatments currently used to treat fatigue include psychostimulant drugs and corticosteroids, which are supported by very limited research (Portenoy and Itri, 1999). It has been suggested that the selective serotonin reuptake inhibitor (SSRI) antidepressants may have a role in fatigue management, but there are no reports of clinical trials of these agents for fatigue. Informal surveys that the authors have conducted at meetings indicate that many oncologists are prescribing stimulants, primarily methylphenidate, to help their patients combat debilitating fatigue, although this practice is not supported by evidence from published clinical trials. However, methylphenidate has been shown in trials to improve opioid sedation used to manage cancer pain (Bruera et al., 1992a, 1992b) and, as already mentioned, has been shown to improve cognitive function in patients with central nervous system tumors (Meyers et al., 1998).

Fatigue may be caused by the cancer itself, or like other symptoms, it may be caused by treatment. Other mechanisms that contribute to fatigue include sleep disturbance, environmental conditions, level of activity, nutritional status, and the demands of treatment (Nail and Winningham, 1993). Treatment-related anemia is well known for its impairment of quality of life and function and is often associated with severe fatigue in cancer patients (Glaspy et al., 1997). In a survey of cancer patients at M.D. Anderson Cancer Center using the Brief Fatigue Inventory (BFI), patients with hematologic malignancies reported greater fatigue than patients with solid tumors (47 percent of the hematologic group reported "worst fatigue" of 7 or greater versus 28 percent of the solid-tumor group) (Mendoza et al., 1999). In patients with hematologic malignancies, low levels of both hemoglobin and albumin were predictive of severe fatigue (Cleeland and Wang, 1999).

Hormonal deficiencies occur in large numbers of patients treated with IFN-α, and the possibility that hypothyroidism or other adrenal or gonadal dysfunction may be associated with fatigue in these patients should be investigated (Jones et al., 1998). IFN-α and other agents used in treating cancer also excite or inhibit the production of cytokines that are known to be related to fatigue. For example, IL-6 is a proinflammatory cytokine that has been shown to mediate endocrine and neural activity. In normal subjects, IL-6 induces fatigue and inactivity as well as poor concentration (Spath-Schwalbe et al., 1998). Future research should explore the role of proinflammatory cytokines in the production of fatigue experienced by patients treated with IFN-α (Dalakas et al., 1998).

Basic Research Needs

1. Explore new agents for treating fatigue (anticytokines).
2. Develop animal models for fatigue.
3. Explore "common pathways" for fatigue and other symptoms.

Clinical Research Needs

There are needs for trials of the following:

1. stimulant therapies,
2. current anticytokines,
3. SSRIs,
4. exercise, and
5. behavioral interventions.

Review of Current Funding: CRISP Listings

Searching the CRISP database of current federal funding using the terms cancer and fatigue produced 34 hits. Eleven relate to basic or clinical research that might have relevance to clinical cancer fatigue. Of these studies, three are descriptive (including correlational and behavioral studies), eight deal with trials of interventions, and none are basic science studies.

CURRENTLY FUNDED CLINICAL TRIALS

1. Blood Transfusions With or Without Epoietin Alfa in Treating Patients with Myelodysplastic Syndrome
2. Phase III Study of Epoietin Alfa with or Without Filgrastim (G-CSF) vs Supportive Therapy Alone in Patients With Myelodysplastic Syndromes
3. Exercise Plus Epoietin Alfa in Treating Cancer Patients Who Have Anemia-Related Fatigue
4. Phase III Randomized Study of *Hypericum perforatum* (St. John's Wort) for the Relief of Fatigue in Patients Undergoing Chemotherapy or Hormonal Therapy for Malignant Disease
5. Methylphenidate in Treating Patients with Melanoma

Gastrointestinal Symptoms

Nausea, vomiting and bowel obstruction are frequent symptoms in patients with advanced cancer. More than 60 percent of patients who are treated with antineoplastic agents also experience nausea and vomiting. Both clinicians and patients identify nausea and vomiting as the most distressing side effects of chemotherapy. Nausea and vomiting are also associated with radiotherapy. Current pharmacologic treatments for nausea include prokinetic drugs, either alone or in combination with corticosteroids (Bruera and Neumann, 1998) and pure THC (which stimulates the appetite). Treatments for vomiting include: dopamine antagonists (such as ondansetron, a 5-hydroxytryptamine [HT] 3 receptor antagonist), phenothiazines, metoclopramide, corticosteroids, cannabinoids, benzodiazapines, antihistamines, and anticholinergics. Behavioral interventions can be effective against nausea and vomiting that occurs before and after treatments.

Future research should focus on the development of standard tools for the assessment of nausea and vomiting as separate symptoms. More research is needed on these symptoms in special populations of cancer patients (such as women, children, and patients of minority status). Clinical trials should be done to determine the effectiveness of the current treatments for nausea and vomiting and the effectiveness of corticosteroids for the treatment of intestinal obstruction. Well-designed clinical trials should also focus on the use of behavioral and other nonpharmacological methods for the management of nausea and vomiting, such as aerobic exercise, guided imagery, progressive relaxation, and acupressure.

The pathophysiology of nausea and vomiting may involve chemical, visceral, central nervous system, and vestibular system processes (Fessele, 1996). In vomiting associated with chemotherapy and radiotherapy, both central (chemoreceptor trigger zone) and peripheral (gastrointestinal) processes may be involved (Stewart, 1990). Chemotherapy (antineoplastic agents) induced nausea and vomiting is mediated, at least in part, by the neurotransmitter serotonin (Hogan and Grant, 1997). The roles of other neurotransmitters in nausea and vomiting are unclear.

Basic Research Needs

The following should be studied:

1. Relationship of terminal nausea to other symptoms of advanced disease, and
2. Mechanisms of terminal and treatment-induced nausea.

Clinical Research Needs

The following are needed:

1. trials of agents for nausea of advanced disease,
2. trials of agents for bowel obstruction, and
3. descriptive studies of prevalence, severity, and current treatment of terminal nausea.

Review of Current Funding: CRISP Listings

Searching the CRISP database of current federal funding using the terms cancer and nausea or vomiting produced 13 hits. Three relate to basic or clinical research that might have relevance to clinical cancer nausea and vomiting. Of these studies, none are descriptive (including correlational and behavioral studies), one is an intervention study, and two are basic science studies.

Searching the CRISP database of current federal funding using the terms cancer and bowel obstruction produced only one hit, and this hit is not related to basic or clinical research on bowel obstruction in cancer.

CURRENTLY FUNDED CLINICAL TRIALS

Bowel Obstruction

1. Endoscopic Placement of Metal Stent in Patients with Cancer-Related Bowel Obstruction
2. Phase I/II Pilot Study of Enteral Wall Stents in Patients with Colonic Obstruction Secondary to Malignancy

3. Octreotide as Palliative Therapy for Cancer-Related Bowel Obstruction that Cannot Be Removed by Surgery

Nausea or Vomiting

1. Lerisetron Compared with Granisetron in Preventing Nausea and Vomiting in Men Being Treated with Radiation Therapy for Stage I Seminoma
2. Drugs to Reduce the Side Effects of Chemotherapy
3. Acupressure and Acustimulation Wrist Bands for the Prevention of Nausea and Vomiting Caused by Chemotherapy

Psychiatric and Affective Symptoms (Anxiety, Depression)

Estimates of the prevalence of depression in cancer vary somewhat with the methods used to assess depression, when the assessments are done, and possibly with the type of cancer. In general, studies have found that approximately 25 percent of patients have depressed mood, and that between 10 and 15 percent of patients have a major depression sometime during their treatment (Cleeland, 2000). Although anxiety is common, it is rarely assessed regularly in cancer patients, and few patients are diagnosed or treated for it (Bottomley, 1998). The risk of patients developing psychological symptoms is increased with advanced disease, with certain cancer treatments, with uncontrolled physical symptoms (e.g., pain) or functional limitations, with inadequate social support, or with a past history of psychiatric disorder (Breitbart, 1995).

Both pharmacologic and nonpharmacologic therapies can be used to treat psychological symptoms in patients with cancer. However, some antidepressants may have serious side effects in patients with a concurrent illness such as cancer. For this reason, McCoy (1996) argues that pharmacologic agents that have many toxicities or act at multiple receptor sites (e.g., trycyclic antidepressants, monoamine oxidase inhibitors) should not be used to treat psychological symptoms in these patients. SSRIs (e.g., fluoxetine, or Prozac) and other new antidepressants may be a better choice for patients with cancer because they have fewer anticholinergic, cardiac, or cognitive adverse effects (McCoy, 1996). Psychotherapy for the treatment of depression may actually have an effect on the course of cancer. Psychotherapy may improve patients' quality of life and help them learn to cope with their illness. In three randomized studies, psychotherapy increased survival time in patients with breast cancer, lymphoma, and malignant melanoma (Spiegel, 1996).

A report from a 1993 National Cancer Institute of Canada panel on neuropsychiatric syndromes and psychological symptoms in cancer patients made recommendations for future symptom control research (Bruera, 1995). To improve epidemiological research in this area, a uniform terminology and taxonomy has to be widely used and accepted, validated tools should be used to assess these symptoms, and new tools must be developed that are appropriate for palliative care settings. Clinical trials using both pharmacologic and nonpharmacologic treatments are also needed. Fluoxetine (Prozac) is one of several effective treatments for depression; it is currently the most frequently prescribed antidepressant in the United States. Unfortunately, evidence on the use of fluoxetine in patients with cancer is inadequate (Shuster et al., 1992). Research should also explore other psychological symptoms that have not been studied much in cancer patients, such as anxiety, posttraumatic stress disorders, sleep disorders, fatigue, and suicidal ideation.

The prevalence of depression varies with cancer diagnosis and treatment, and the physiological mechanisms related to these differences need exploration. Kelsen and colleagues (1995) found that 38 percent of 83 patients with newly diagnosed pancreatic cancer scored within the depressed range on the Beck Depression Inventory before treatment began, a higher percentage than is usually found in studies of patients with other primary malignancies. In a study of 122 patients receiving radiotherapy, the prevalence of mood disorders was nearly 50 percent (Leopold et al., 1998).

Psychological symptoms such as depression and anxiety may be related to changes in the physiologic functioning of the pancreas, such as changes in the secretion of hormones, neurotransmitters, digestive enzymes, or bicarbonate (Passik and Breitbart, 1996). Depression, cognitive dysfunction, and psychosis have all been associated with antiphospholipid antibodies (Brey and Escalante, 1998). There is evidence of depression related to impaired phospholipid metabolism and impaired fatty acid-related signal transduction processes in patients with cancer and other diseases (e.g., diabetes, cardiovascular disease, immunological abnormalities, multiple sclerosis, osteoporosis; and more generally, aging) (Horrobin and Bennett, 1999). These metabolic changes merit study as a possible primary cause of depression.

Basic Research Needs

The following are needed:

1. animal models for cancer-related affective disturbances, and
2. knowledge of the mechanisms of depression unique to cancer and its treatment.

Clinical Research Needs

Clinical research should include the following:

1. descriptive studies of current management of psychological symptoms in advanced disease;
2. trials of standard antidepressants, especially SSRIs;
3. trials of stimulant therapies (methylphenidate);
4. discussion of trials of novel agents ("empathogens"); and
5. trials of agents for terminal agitation or restlessness.

Review of Current Funding: CRISP Listings

Searching the CRISP database of current federal funding using the terms cancer and depression produced 71 hits. Fifteen relate to basic or clinical research that might have relevance to clinical depression in cancer. Of these studies, eight are descriptive (including correlational and behavioral studies), five deal with trials of interventions, and two are basic science studies.

Searching the CRISP database of current federal funding using the terms cancer and anxiety produced 48 hits. Twelve relate to basic or clinical research that might have relevance to anxiety in cancer. Of these studies, six are descriptive (including correlational and behavioral studies), six deal with trials of interventions, and none are basic science studies.

CURRENTLY FUNDED CLINICAL TRIALS—DEPRESSION   There are no current trials for depression.

CURRENTLY FUNDED CLINICAL TRIALS—ANXIETY

1. Diet and prostate-specific antigen (PSA) Levels in Patients with Prostate Cancer
2. St. John's Wort in Relieving Fatigue in Patients Undergoing Chemotherapy or Hormone Therapy for Cancer

STATUS OF END-OF-LIFE AND SYMPTOM RESEARCH

As we have seen, important areas of research could greatly benefit care at the end of life as well as reduce the symptom distress that cancer patients experience as their disease gets worse. That such research is feasible has been demonstrated. Research and symptom epidemiology, behavioral research, health services research, and basic as well as clinical symptom research have already produced benefits that have been translated into better care. The magnitude of the distress experienced by cancer patients with advanced disease has been documented, as has the impact of this distress on both patients and their caregivers. Although the amount of improvement has not been well studied, it is very possible that patients now experience less distress related to medical procedures, that pain is somewhat better managed, and that there is wider recognition of and attention to end-of-life issues, such as patient preference for end-of-life decisions. Research has also documented the gaps between current care and optimal care and has identified very specific obstacles that could be addressed to improve care.

Perhaps less obvious has been a maturation of research methods that should facilitate the rapid progress of research in this area. Increasingly, the subjective reports of patients about their quality of life and about the severity and impact of their symptoms are accepted as reasonable outcome measures for both clinical and laboratory research. Developments in this type of methodology have been funded and have yielded tangible results. Quality-of-life outcomes have become more accepted as clinical trial end points, as has the prevention or reduction of specific symptoms. New technologies have been developed, primarily from other areas of investigation, that give us unique opportunities to understand the nature, mechanisms, and expression of symptoms that were not possible a few years ago. For example, new brain-imaging techniques may allow us to understand the cortical expression of symptoms (such as pain, depression, and cortical impairment) as well as the modification of this expression by treatment. New developments in biology have opened windows to a better understanding of distress, including the nature and interaction of receptors and transmitters. Developments in pharmacology have produced an array of exciting agents that could provide better control of most of the symptoms of the dying process. There is a real possibility that individual variation in symptom expression may be better understood through progress in genetic science. We can no longer say, as was said a few years ago, that we do not have the tools to advance this area.

We also have a wide range of targets for investigation. The understanding of pain, although more advanced than that for other symptoms, still has enormous gaps. Our understanding of other symptoms is much more primitive. We have only a limited understanding of the context of the dying process, including economic, social, and ethical factors. Research examining ways of improving the care given to patients with advanced cancer is just beginning. Ways of examining the more complex subjective needs of patients (spiritual, existential) have to be developed, and methods of qualitative research have to be strengthened. Few of the practices that we depend upon for the care of the dying and for the patient with advanced cancer have been subjected to the scrutiny of careful randomized clinical trials, impeding the provision of evidence-based practice recommendations.

FUTURE END-OF-LIFE AND SYMPTOM RESEARCH: PROBLEMS AND POTENTIAL SOLUTIONS

Despite the progress, substantial barriers impede the research needed to advance end-of-life care and symptom control. The main problems and some potential solutions are presented below. The ideas have come from the author, published literature, and clinicians and investigators in the field contacted by the author specifically for this report (see Appendix 8A). The issues are presented in specific categories, but it is clear that the problems and solutions are interlinked. For example, the level of funding depends on a sufficient number of well-trained research investigators and research groups, infrastructure and organizational support, and public advocacy.

Low Level of Research Support

THE PROBLEM   A low level of research support has been identified as the major barrier to end-of-life and symptom research. In fiscal year 1999, the National Cancer Institute (NCI) spent $24.5 million in extramural funding for all research with components related to palliative care or hospice. Of this total, $18.3 million went to specific projects or programs, and $6.1 million represents fractions of institutional grants. In addition to the research grants, $1.7 million was spent in 1999 on training grants related to end-of-life or palliative care. Altogether, the 1999 NCI expenditure on palliative and hospice care was just over $26 million, or about 0.9 percent of the total 1999 budget of $2.9 billion (see Chapter 1 of this report).

The proportion of congressionally mandated cancer research in this area funded by the Department of Defense (DOD) is also minimal, and the requests for proposals (RFPs) for these programs may actually discourage submissions. The American Cancer Society (ACS) reports that it spends less than 1 percent of its budget on the topics covered here, and it is estimated that other foundations spend the same or less on such research. A major exception has been the substantial investment of the Robert Wood Johnson Foundation in end-of-life issues.

In 1997, industry spent 1.6 billion in cancer-related research (McGeary and Burstein, 1999), primarily in the development and testing of cancer-related drugs and vaccines. With the increasing acceptance of symptom prevention and control, as well as general quality-of-life outcomes as end points for approval of new drugs, there has been a proportional increase in industry investment in the development and clinical testing of drugs for symptom control. Symptom and quality-of-life data are being gathered on large numbers of advanced cancer patients, and new agents of interest are under development. There are, however, many obvious limitations to the product of this kind of effort. The wealth of symptom and quality-of-life data generated are rarely published or shared with non-industry investigators; data gathering is biased against recording events that may negatively affect approval; and the drugs under investigation are ones expected to generate high profits.

Those individuals in agencies who might fund grants in these areas acknowledge that more needs to be spent but point to a lack of interest within their agencies and a lack of organizational structure that promotes this type of research. They also point to a lack of competitive applications. They emphasize the lack of vocal public advocacy for these topics. There has been little political support for this type of research from the major cancer disease groups, cancer survivors, or scientific and professional organizations (aside from specific topics related to their interests). Issues of end-of-life care and symptom control are detached from the mainstream of perceived urgent research needs and are viewed as of substantially less importance than research focused on cure or prevention.

POTENTIAL SOLUTIONS   Packaging may be important. As has been pointed out, end-of-life, palliative care, and symptom control issues are components of the whole enterprise of cancer care, and elements of research in these areas are critical to all cancer patients. The biology of the symptoms of dying shares much with the biology of cancer symptoms throughout the disease spectrum. Research on improving the quality of cancer care in general will benefit those with advanced disease. It is possible that labeling efforts as "end of life" and as "palliative" may unnecessarily restrict funding considerations and enthusiasm for support. This issue is clearly controversial and political and needs substantial discussion. Support for this discussion, perhaps from a private foundation, could move it forward.

Even before a full discussion, there is an immediate need for additional funds earmarked for advanced disease and symptom control research grants and contracts. Thus far, there is very little targeted funding, but in a one-time limited program in 1998 that resulted in a request for applications developed jointly by several groups at the NIH, the response from the research community was enthusiastic (more than 120 applications were received, approximately 20 of which were eventually funded).

Public and private funding agencies and disease advocacy groups must be informed about the needs and opportunities for research in this area, especially the unnecessary suffering that patients with advanced cancer endure because of inadequate care. The same need exists for academic institutions and cancer research organizations. A reasonable and modest investment could be made by a foundation to explore how public advocacy of these research efforts might be improved.

Infrastructure and Organizational Deficits

THE PROBLEM   Currently, there is no institutionalized mechanism or coordination of efforts to develop new treatments for the relief of cancer-related symptoms or for the care of dying patients. There is no group or office at the NIH or NCI with symptom management as a primary responsibility, even though hundreds of thousands of patients are impaired by these symptoms. The lack of such an organizing structure is not difficult to understand: the NIH and NCI have a mandate to cure or to prevent disease. Managing the symptoms of disease has not been an expectation of those who fund the NIH, nor has it been thought of as an important mission of the NIH. At the NCI, as well as throughout the NIH, a disease model is in place that makes organized planning for symptom-related research cumbersome. At the NCI, it is difficult to identify a project officer that has, as his or her primary title, the coordination, promotion, and review of symptom-related and end-of-life research. The focus is, as it should be, the prevention and cure of cancer, but it is yet to be acknowledged that the control of symptoms and amelioration of distress are part of good cancer care and therefore worthy of publicly supported research.

POTENTIAL SOLUTIONS   Symptom management will be addressed appropriately only when there is (1) an organizing group within the NIH that has an interest in and dedication to symptom management and care of the dying patient and the resources for action to improve it, and (2) the formation of groups or task forces to plot the types of basic and clinical research that must be done. Such groups have to generate long-range plans that encompass needs for basic, clinical, and health services research efforts. There has been such a task force for basic research in pain sponsored by the NIH, which might be a model for the management of other symptoms. An effort to make "supradisease" linkages among the institutes that address issues of advanced disease and symptom control is needed. For example, there is a need to link cytokine research in AIDS, cancer. and arthritis—all of which might have implications for the management of cachexia, pain, fatigue, cognitive impairment and depression—or the role of opioid receptors common to several symptoms. The research needed for progress in understanding and treating advanced disease and symptom control is multidisciplinary, and program project and multi-institutional funding would be ideal mechanisms to enhance it.

It is reasonable to ask NCI to provide staff officers, organizational structure and resources to deal with advanced disease and symptom control and to give them appropriate titles so that they can be identified by organizations, the public, and the research community.

Lack of Investigators and Research Groups

THE PROBLEM   Agency representatives report the lack of highly competitive applications in the areas of end of life and symptom control. Funders, as well as reviewers, often state that such applications are not competitive with "mainline" applications. Many health care professionals acutely interested in doing research with very ill populations by virtue of their clinical contacts are not well prepared in clinical research methods. Although they often pose clinically important, reasonable, interesting, and potentially researchable questions, the methods they propose are inappropriate or lacking in scientific rigor. Not surprisingly, most of the studies in the palliative care literature reviewed for this chapter were (1) retrospective chart reviews (2) studies of caregiver's estimates of patient distress, and (3) studies of the attitudes and opinions of health care professionals, most of which would have benefited from improved research methods. Another portion of the literature consists of a presentation of care principles with no support from clinical trials. There is a need for a larger body of well-trained researchers who have advanced disease and symptom issues as their focus of interest to conduct their own studies and to collaborate with clinicians interested in carrying out research

POTENTIAL SOLUTIONS   Both short-term and long-term solutions to the small supply of investigators are required. In the long term, larger numbers of researchers focused on end-of-life and symptom control issues must be trained. A plan for developing these researchers, including estimates of the needs within various basic, behavioral, clinical, and health services research disciplines, should be laid out as soon as possible. There are many training mechanisms and career tracks in place at the NIH, at NCI, and also at the ACS that could provide for the training and development of these researchers, but they have yet to be applied to advanced disease and symptom control.

With so few investigators now in the field, there is also an immediate need for better communication among those doing this kind of research, both from one institution to the next and from one discipline to another. Several possibilities exist (e.g., research interchanges at regularly scheduled cancer research and clinical meetings). There may also be a place for new research organizations that focus on research issues related to advanced disease.

Symptom-focused cross-disciplinary meetings could also greatly facilitate communication. As an example, M.D. Anderson recently sponsored such a meeting on fatigue and cancer. Researchers shared data on fatigue measurement and prevalence, potential mechanisms (including anemia, endocrine disturbances, cytokine levels, neurotransmitters), and current and potential treatment. Institutional and organizational support for interdisciplinary communication should produce great benefit.

The current relative isolation of investigators in this area might also be addressed by taking advantage of current technology to create a "virtual" research network. This could be seen as a very interesting experiment in scientific communication. Mainline cancer research is facilitated by frequent interchanges of ideas and new data among research groups at large institutions, and it is reasonable to assume that this facilitates research progress. Such a virtual network, using current Internet technology, could support frequent video research exchanges, postings of preliminary data, and collective hypothesis generation. It could also sponsor exchanges between clinicians (defining the problems, sharing observations) and basic, behavioral, and health research scientists. It could explore the potential utility of patient and family interchanges with researchers and provide data from patients' experiences with existing and new symptom-related therapies.

Lack of Clinical Trials

THE PROBLEM   The clinical trial database that covers end-of-life care, palliative care, and symptom control is very small. Most guidelines for management of symptoms depend heavily on "expert" opinion because of this deficit, and treatment is often empirical for the same reason. Few active clinical trials deal with single or multisymptom interventions or with practice change interventions. In studies examining single symptoms, pain is the best studied in clinical trials, but many of the trials are industry sponsored, with very few trials of off-patent medications such as morphine that are used routinely in the care of seriously ill patients.

Fatigue is an excellent example of an area in need of clinical trials. We know that some cancer-related fatigue is due to anemia and that anemia can be treated in some patients. Yet anemia is just one of the many causes of fatigue, and little if any clinical or basic science research is being done to discover the causes of this fatigue or to advance new treatments. Many oncologists are using methylphenidate (Ritalin) to treat patients with cancer-related fatigue, but there is not one published randomized trial (although one is now recruiting patients) that examines the effectiveness of this drug, the appropriate doses, or the indications for use. Dyspnea, psychological distress, poor appetite, wasting, psychological distress, nausea and vomiting, and cognitive impairment are all on the list of potential candidates for clinical trials that could be under way. As has been seen, there are few active trials in any of these areas.

Several NCI collaborative groups have attempted symptom management clinical trials, but with mixed results, and several potentially informative trials have failed for various reasons. In the fall of 1999, the Eastern Cooperative Oncology Group (ECOG) held a retreat to evaluate the place of symptom management trials in the cooperative groups. There was a general recognition that symptom management trials were seen by the NCI as relatively low priority, Several barriers to doing this kind of work in the collaborative groups were identified, including the following:

- The main research institutions are evaluated on research toward cure or increased lifespan, and not on the basis of symptom control, reducing the incentive for doing these trials.
- There are rarely staff designated as responsible for these trials, especially persons familiar with symptom measurement, treatment, or recruitment for these trials.
- Staff lack knowledge about these trials, and patients are not informed about them.
- Such trials are viewed as "extra work."
- Some centers have no interest in symptom management trials.
- Symptom management studies do not contribute to the academic advancement of oncologists.
- There is the perception that enthusiasm at NCI for these types of studies is modest, demonstrated in modest trial credits, lack of extra funding for these efforts, and a low priority relative to treatment and prevention trials.

POTENTIAL SOLUTIONS   The collaborative groups sponsored by the NCI could provide the mechanism for large studies of current and proposed symptom management treatments and research in the issues of advanced disease. Findings from this work could make cancer treatment much more tolerable, could greatly improve the quality of life of those who survive cancer, and could provide enhanced comfort for those who die of the disease. Large numbers of patients with advanced cancer are available to members of these groups who are not now eligible for treatment or prevention trials. SUPPORT provides ample evidence that large numbers of very ill patients can be enrolled in randomized trials. In addition to clinical trials, these collaborative groups are the ideal setting for studies of the prevalence, impact, and current treatment of distress in patients with advanced cancer, but such descriptive studies within the collaborative groups are currently discouraged by the NCI.

The ECOG retreat developed a number of recommendations for how to increase these trials in the collaborative groups but recognized that this would require structural change and a cognitive shift for both the groups and the NCI and other sponsors. The recommendations included incorporating symptom management into the senior leadership (and funding for this position), special nurse coordinators for these trials at several sites, and the designation of a subset of motivated sites to carry out this work. This subset might represent a special collaborative group within the framework of the existing groups. In the face of a lack of NCI enthusiasm for this area, it was suggested that the collaborative groups turn to the managed care or pharmaceutical industry to obtain funding for these trials. One possible function of a new type of group could be to undertake open-label trials of potential candidate symptom control agents.

REFERENCES

American Pain Society. 1999. *Principles of Analgesic Use in the Treatment of Acute Pain and Cancer Pain.* (4th ed.) Glenview, Illinois: American Pain Society.

Anderson KO, Mendoza TR, Valero V, Richman SP, Russell C, Hurley J, DeLeon C, Washington P, Palos G, Payne, R, Cleeland, CS. Minority cancer patients and their providers: pain management attitudes and practice. *Cancer* 2000;88:1929-1938.

Andrykowski MA, Greiner CB, Altmaier EM, Burish TG, Antin JH, Gingrich R, McGarigle C, Henslee-Downey PJ. Quality of life following bone marrow transplantation: findings from a multicentre study. *Br J Cancer* 1995;71:1322-1329.

Argiles JM Lopez-Soriano FJ. The role of cytokines in cancer cachexia. *Med Res Rev* 1999;19:223-248.

Barber MD, Ross JA, Fearon KC. Disordered metabolic response with cancer and its management. *World J Surg* 2000;24:681-689.

Bernabei R, Gambassi G, Lapane K, Landi F, Gatsonis C, Dunlop R, Lipsitz L, Steel K, Mor V. Management of pain in elderly patients with cancer. SAGE Study Group. Systematic Assessment of Geriatric Drug Use via Epidemiology [see comments] [published erratum appears in *JAMA* 1999;281:136]. *JAMA* 1998;279:1877-1882.

Bessesen DH. Faggioni R (1998). Recently identified peptides involved in the regulation of body weight. *Semin Oncol* 1998;25:28-32.

Body JJ. The syndrome of anorexia-cachexia. *Curr Opin Oncol* 1999;11:255-260.

Bottomley A. Anxiety and the adult cancer patient. *European Journal of Cancer Care (English Language Edition)* 1998;7:217-224.

Breitbart W. Identifying patients at risk for, and treatment of major psychiatric complications of cancer. *Supportive Care in Cancer* 1995;3:45-60.

Brey RL, Escalante A. Neurological manifestations of antiphospholipid antibody syndrome. *Lupus* 1998;7Suppl 2:S67-S74.

Bruera E. A National Cancer Institute of Canada Workshop on Symptom Control and Supportive Care in Patients with Advanced Cancer: methodological and administrative issues. *Journal of Pain and Symptom Management* 1995;10:129-130.

Bruera E, Franco JJ, Maltoni M, Watanabe S, Suarez-Almazor M. Changing pattern of agitated impaired mental status in patients with advanced cancer: association with cognitive monitoring, hydration, and opioid rotation. *J.Pain Symptom Manage* 1995;10:287-291.

Bruera E, Miller MJ, Macmillan K, Kuehn N. Neuropsychological effects of methylphenidate in patients receiving a continuous infusion of narcotics for cancer pain. *Pain* 1992a;48:163-166.

Bruera E, Miller MJ, Macmillan K, Kuehn N. Neuropsychological effects of methylphenidate in patients receiving a continuous infusion of narcotics for cancer pain. *Pain* 1992b;8:163-166.

Bruera E, Neumann CM. Management of specific symptom complexes in patients receiving palliative care. *CMAJ* 1998;158:1717-1726.

Carey PJ, Oberst MT, McCubbin MA, Hughes SH. Appraisal and caregiving burden in family members caring for patients receiving chemotherapy. *Oncol Nurs Forum* 1991;18:1341-1348.

Cassileth BR, Lusk EJ, Strouse TB, Miller DS, Brown LL, Cross PA. A psychological analysis of cancer patients and their next-of-kin. *Cancer* 1985;55:72-76.

Cleeland CS. Strategies for improving cancer pain management. *Journal of Pain and Symptom Management* 1993;8:361-364.

Cleeland C S. Cancer-related symptoms. *Seminars in Radiation Oncology* 2000;10:175-190.

Cleeland CS, Gonin R, Baez L, Loehrer P, Pandya KJ. Pain and treatment of pain in minority patients with cancer. The Eastern Cooperative Oncology Group Minority Outpatient Pain Study. *Annals of Internal Medicine* 1997;127:813-816.

Cleeland CS, Gonin R, Hatfield AK, Edmonson JH, Blum RH, Stewart JA, Pandya KJ. Pain and its treatment in outpatients with metastatic cancer. *New England Journal of Medicine* 1994;330:592-596.

Cleeland CS, Janjan NA, Scott CB, Seiferheld WF, Curran WJ. Cancer pain management by radiotherapists: a survey of radiation therapy oncology group physicians. *Int J Radiat Oncol Biol Phys* 2000;47:203-208.

Cleeland CS, Mendoza TR, Wang XS, Chou C, Harle MT, Morrissey M, Engstrom MC. Assessing symptom distress in cancer: The M.D. Anderson Symptom Inventory. *Cancer* (in press).

Cleeland CS, Wang XS. Measuring and Understanding Fatigue. *Oncology* 1999;13:91-97.

Covinsky KE, Fuller JD, Yaffe K, Johnston CB, Hamel MB, Lynn J, Teno JM, Phillips RS. Communication and decision-making in seriously ill patients: findings of the SUPPORT project. The Study to Understand Prognoses and Preferences for Outcomes and Risks of Treatments. *Journal of the American Geriatrics Society* 2000;48:S187-S193.

Coyle N, Adelhardt J, Foley KM, Portenoy RK. Character of terminal illness in the advanced cancer patient: pain and other symptoms during the last four weeks of life. *J Pain Symptom Manage* 1990;5:83-93.

Dalakas MC, Mock V, Hawkins MJ. Fatigue: definitions, mechanisms, and paradigms for study. *Semin Oncol* 1998;25:48-53.

de Wit R, van Dam F, Zandbelt L, van Buuren A, van der Heijden K, Leenhouts G, Loonstra S. A pain education program for chronic cancer pain patients: follow-up results from a randomized controlled trial. *Pain* 1997;73:55-69.

Demetri GD, Kris M, Wade J, Degos L, Cella D. Quality-of-life benefit in chemotherapy patients treated with epoetin alfa is independent of disease response or tumor type: results from a prospective community oncology study. Procrit Study Group. *J Clin Oncol* 1998;16:3412-3425.

Dimeo FC, Stieglitz RD, Novelli-Fischer U, Fetscher S, Keul J. Effects of physical activity on the fatigue and psychologic status of cancer patients during chemotherapy. *Cancer* 1999;85:2273-2277.

Donnelly S, Walsh D. The symptoms of advanced cancer. *Semin Oncol* 1995;22 67-72.

DuPen S, DuPen A, Polissar N, Hansberry J, Kraybill BM, Stillman M, Panke J, Everly R, Syrjala K. Implementing guidelines for cancer pain management: results of a randomized controlled clinical trial. *J Clin Oncol* 1999;17:361-370.

Emery PW. Cachexia in experimental models. *Nutrition* 1999;15:600-603.

Escalante CP, Martin CG, Elting LS, Cantor SB, Harle TS, Price KJ, Kish SK, Manzullo EF, Rubenstein EB. Dyspnea in cancer patients. Etiology, resource utilization, and survival-implications in a managed care world. *Cancer* 1996;78:1314-1319.

Farncombe M. Dyspnea: assessment and treatment [see comments]. *Support Care Cancer* 1997;5:94-99.

Ferrell BR, Cohen MZ, Rhiner M, Rozek A. Pain as a metaphor for illness. Part II: Family caregivers' management of pain. *Oncology Nursing Forum* 1991;18:1315-1321.

Ferrell BR, Rhiner M, Cohen MZ, Grant M. Pain as a metaphor for illness. Part I: Impact of cancer pain on family caregivers. *Oncol Nurs Forum* 1991;18:1303-1309.

Fessele K S. Managing the multiple causes of nausea and vomiting in the patient with cancer. *Oncol Nurs Forum* 1996;23:1409-1415.

Gagnon B, Bruera E. A review of the drug treatment of cachexia associated with cancer. *Drugs* 1998;55:675-688.

Glaspy J, Bukowski R, Steinberg D, Taylor C Tchekmedyian S, Vadhan-Raj S. Impact of therapy with epoetin alfa on clinical outcomes in patients with nonmyeloid malignancies during cancer chemotherapy in community oncology practice. Procrit Study Group. *J Clin Oncol* 1997;15:1218-1234.

Glaus A, Crow R, Hammond S. A qualitative study to explore the concept of fatigue/tiredness in cancer patients and in healthy individuals. *Support Care Cancer* 1996;4:82-96.

Gonzalez EW. Resourcefulness, appraisals, and coping efforts of family caregivers. *Issues Ment Health Nurs* 1997;18:209-227.

Gorter RW. Cancer cachexia and cannabinoids. *Forsch Komplementarmed* 1999;6 Suppl 3:21-22.

Guarnaccia PJ, Parra P, Deschamps A, Milstein G, Argiles N. Si dios quiere: Hispanic families' experiences of caring for a seriously mentally ill family member. *Cult Med Psychiatry* 1992;16:187-215.

Haidet P, Hamel MB, Davis RB, Wenger N, Reding D, Kussin PS, Connors AF Jr, Lynn J, Weeks JC, Phillips RS. Outcomes, preferences for resuscitation, and physician-patient communication among patients with metastatic colorectal cancer. SUPPORT Investigators. Study to Understand Prognoses and Preferences for Outcomes and Risks of Treatments. *Am J Med* 1998;105:222-229.

Hawkins PJ, Liossi C, Ewart BW, Hatira P, Kosmidis VH. Hypnosis in the alleviation of procedure related pain and distress in paediatric oncology patients. *Contemporary Hypnosis* 1998;15:199-207.

Hogan CM, Grant M. Physiologic mechanisms of nausea and vomiting in patients with cancer. *Oncol Nurs Forum* 1997;24:8-12.

Honore P, Luger NM, Sabino MA, Schwei MJ, Rogers SD, Mach DB, O'Keefe PF, Ramnaraine ML, Clohisy DR, Mantyh PW. Osteoprotegerin blocks bone cancer-induced skeletal destruction, skeletal pain and pain-related neurochemical reorganization of the spinal cord [see comments]. *Nat Med* 2000;6:521-528.

Horrobin DF, Bennett CN. Depression and bipolar disorder: relationships to impaired fatty acid and phospholipid metabolism and to diabetes, cardiovascular disease, immunological abnormalities, cancer, ageing and osteoporosis. Possible candidate genes. *Prostaglandins Leukot Essent Fatty Acids* 1999;60:217-234.

Inui A. Cancer anorexia-cachexia syndrome: are neuropeptides the key? *Cancer Res* 1999; 59:4493-4501.

Irvine D, Vincent L, Graydon JE, Bubela N, Thompson L. The prevalence and correlates of fatigue in patients receiving treatment with chemotherapy and radiotherapy. A comparison with the fatigue experienced by healthy individuals. *Cancer Nursing* 1994;17:367-378.

Jacox A, Carr DB, Payne R, et al. 1994. *Management of Cancer Pain. Clinical Practice Guideline No. 9. AHCPR Publication No. 94-0592.* Rockville, MD: Agency for Health Care Policy and Research, U.S. Department of Health and Human Services, Public Health Service.

Janjan NA, Martin CG, Payne R, Dahl JL, Weissman DE, Hill CS. Teaching cancer pain management: durability of educational effects of a role model program. *Cancer* 1996; 77:996-1001.

Jones TH, Wadler S, Hupart KH. Endocrine-mediated mechanisms of fatigue during treatment with interferon-alpha. *Semin Oncol* 1998;25:54-63.

Juarez G, Ferrell B, Borneman T. Influence of culture on cancer pain management in Hispanic patients. *Cancer Pract* 1998;6:262-269.

Kelsen DP, Portenoy RK, Thaler HT, Niedzwiecki D, Passik SD, Tao Y, Banks W, Brennan MF, Foley KM. Pain and depression in patients with newly diagnosed pancreas cancer. *J Clin Oncol* 1995;13:748-755.

Komurcu S, Nelson KA, Walsh D, Donnelly SM, Homsi J, Abdullah O. Common symptoms in advanced cancer. *Semin Oncol* 2000;27:24-33.

LeGrand SB, Walsh D. Palliative management of dyspnea in advanced cancer. *Curr Opin Oncol* 1999;11:250-254.

Leopold KA, Ahles TA, Walch S, Amdur RJ, Mott LA, Wiegand-Packard L, Oxman TE. Prevalence of mood disorders and utility of the PRIME-MD in patients undergoing radiation therapy. *Int J Radiat Oncol Biol Phys* 1998;42:1105-1112.

Liossi C, Hatira P. Clinical hypnosis versus cognitive behavioral training for pain management with pediatric cancer patients undergoing bone marrow aspirations. *Int J Clin Exp Hypn* 1999;47:104-116.

Maddocks I, Somogyi A, Abbott F, Hayball P, Parker D. Attenuation of morphine-induced delirium in palliative care by substitution with infusion of oxycodone. *J Pain Symptom Manage* 1996;12:182-189.

Mantovani G, Maccio A, Lai P, Massa E, Ghiani M, Santona MC. Cytokine activity in cancer-related anorexia/cachexia: role of megestrol acetate and medroxyprogesterone acetate. *Semin Oncol* 1998;2545-52.

McCarthy EP, Phillips RS, Zhong Z, Drews RE, Lynn J. Dying with cancer: patients' function symptoms, and care preferences as death approaches. *J Am Geriatr Soc* 2000;48:S110-S121.

McCoy DM. Treatment considerations for depression in patients with significant medical comorbidity. *J Fam Pract* 1996;43:S35-S44.

McGeary M, Burstein M. 1999. *Sources of Cancer Research Funding in the United States.* [Online]. Available: http://www.iom.edu/iom/iomhome.nsf/WFiles/Fund/$file/Fund.pdf [accessed May 14, 2001].

McQuellon RP, Craven B, Russell GB, Hoffman S, Cruz JM, Perry JJ, Hurd DD. Quality of life in breast cancer patients before and after autologous bone marrow transplantation. *Bone Marrow Transplant* 1996;18:579-584.

Mendoza TR, Wang XS, Cleeland CS, Morrissey M, Johnson BA, Wendt JK, Huber SL. The rapid assessment of fatigue severity in cancer patients: use of the Brief Fatigue Inventory. *Cancer* 1999;85:1186-1196.

Meyers CA, Byrne KS, Komaki R. Cognitive deficits in patients with small cell lung cancer before and after chemotherapy. *Lung Cancer* 1995;12:231-235.

Meyers CA, Weitzner MA, Valentine AD, Levin VA. Methylphenidate therapy improves cognition, mood, and function of brain tumor patients. *J Clin Oncol* 1998;16:2522-2527.

Miaskowski C, Kragness L, Dibble S, Wallhagen M. Differences in mood states, health status, and caregiver strain between family caregivers of oncology outpatients with and without cancer-related pain. *Journal of Pain and Symptom Management* 1997a;13:138-147.

Miaskowski C, Zimmer EF, Barrett KM, Dibble SL, Wallhagen M. Differences in patients' and family caregivers' perceptions of the pain experience influence patient and caregiver outcomes. *Pain* 1997b;72:217-226.

Minagawa H, Uchitomi Y, Yamawaki S, Ishitani K. Psychiatric morbidity in terminally ill cancer patients. A prospective study [see comments]. *Cancer* 1996;78:1131-1137.

Nail LM, Winningham ML.1993. Fatigue. In S.L.Groenwald, M. Froggr, M. Goodman, C. Yarbro (eds.), *Cancer Nursing: Principles and Practice* (3rd ed., pp. 608-619). Boston: Jones and Bartlett.

Oberst MT, Thomas SE, Gass KA, Ward SE. Caregiving demands and appraisal of stress among family caregivers. *Cancer Nursing* 1989;12:209-215.

Passik SD, Breitbart WS. Depression in patients with pancreatic carcinoma. Diagnostic and treatment issues. *Cancer* 1996;78:615-626.

Pereira J, Hanson J, Bruera E. The frequency and clinical course of cognitive impairment in patients with terminal cancer. *Cancer* 1997;79:835-842.

Portenoy RK, Itri LM. Cancer-related fatigue: guidelines for evaluation and management [see comments]. *Oncologist* 1999;4:1-10.

Portenoy RK, Thaler HT, Kornblith AB, Lepore JM, Friedlander-Klar H, Coyle N, Smart-Curley T, Kemeny N, Norton L, Hoskins W. Symptom prevalence, characteristics and distress in a cancer population. *Qual Life Res* 1994;3:183-189.

Power D, Kelly S, Gilsenan J, Kearney M O'Mahony, D Walsh, JB Coakley D. Suitable screening tests for cognitive impairment and depression in the terminally ill—a prospective prevalence study. *Palliat Med* 1993;7:213-218.

Prieto JM, Saez R, Carreras E, Atala J, Sierra J, Rovira M, Batlle M, Blanch J, Escobar R, Vieta E, Gomez E, Rozman C, Cirera E. Physical and psychosocial functioning of 117 survivors of bone marrow transplantation. *Bone Marrow Transplant* 1996;17:1133-1142.

Richardson A. Fatigue in cancer patients: a review of the literature. *Eur J Cancer Care (Engl.)* 1995;4:20-32.

Ripamonti C. Management of dyspnea in advanced cancer patients [see comments]. *Support Care Cancer* 1999;7:233-243.

Sales E, Schulz R, Beigel D. Predictors of strain in families of cancer patients. *Journal of Psychosocial Oncology* 1992;10:1-26.

Serlin RC, Mendoza TR, Nakamura Y, Edwards KR, Cleeland CS. When is cancer pain mild moderate or severe? Grading pain severity by its interference with function. *Pain* 1995; 61:277-284.

Shuster JL, Stern TA, Greenberg DB. Pros and cons of fluoxetine for the depressed cancer patient. *Oncology (Huntingt)* 1992;6:45-50 55.

Sloman R. Relaxation and the relief of cancer pain. *Nurs Clin North Am* 1995;30:697-709.

Smets EM, Garssen B, Cull A, and de Haes JC. Application of the multidimensional fatigue inventory (MFI-20) in cancer patients receiving radiotherapy. *British Journal of Cancer* 1996;73:241-245.

Spath-Schwalbe E, Hansen K, Schmidt F, Schrezenmeier H, Marshall L, Burger K, Fehm H L, Born J. Acute effects of recombinant human interleukin-6 on endocrine and central nervous sleep functions in healthy men. *J Clin Endocrinol Metab* 1998;83:1573-1579.

Spiegel D. Cancer and depression. *British Journal of Psychiatry* 1996;Suppl 30:109-116.

Stetz KM. Caregiving demands during advanced cancer. The spouse's needs. *Cancer Nurs* 1987;10:260-268.

Stewart DJ. Cancer therapy, vomiting, and antiemetics. *Canadian Journal of Physiology and Pharmacology* 1990;68:304-313.

Stiefel F, Holland J. Delirium in cancer patients. *International Psychogeriatrics* 1991;3:333-336.

SUPPORT: Study to understand prognoses and preferences for outcomes and risks of treatments. Study design. *Journal of Clinical Epidemiology* 1990;43 Suppl:1S-123S.

Syrjala KL, Cummings C, Donaldson GW. Hypnosis or cognitive behavioral training for the reduction of pain and nausea during cancer treatment: a controlled clinical trial [see comments]. *Pain* 1992;48:137-146.

Teno J, Lynn J, Wenger N, Phillips RS, Murphy DP, Connors AF Jr, Desbiens N, Fulkerson W, Bellamy P, Knaus WA. Advance directives for seriously ill hospitalized patients: effectiveness with the patient self-determination act and the SUPPORT intervention. SUPPORT Investigators. Study to Understand Prognoses and Preferences for Outcomes and Risks of Treatment [see comments]. *Journal of the American Geriatrics Society* 1997;45:500-507.

Tisdale M J. New cachexic factors. *Curr Opin Clin Nutr Metab Care* 1998;1:253-256.

Trzepacz PT. The neuropathogenesis of delirium. A need to focus our research [see comments]. *Psychosomatics* 1994;35:374-391.

Vainio A, Auvinen A. Prevalence of symptoms among patients with advanced cancer: an international collaborative study. Symptom Prevalence Group. *J Pain Symptom Manage* 196;12:3-10.

Valentine AD, Meyers CA, Kling M , Richelson E, Hauser P. Mood and cognitive side effects of interferon-alpha therapy. *Semin Oncol* 1998;25:39-47.

van Oosterhout AG, Boon PJ, Houx PJ, ten Velde GP, Twijnstra A. Follow-up of cognitive functioning in patients with small cell lung cancer. *Int J Radiat Oncol Biol Phys* 1995; 31:911-914.

von Roenn JH, Cleeland C , Gonin R, Hatfield AK, Pandya KJ. Physician attitudes and practice in cancer pain management. A survey from the Eastern Cooperative Oncology Group. *Annals of Internal Medicine* 1993;119:121-126.

Walker LG, Wesnes KP, Heys SD, Walker MB, Lolley J, Eremin O. The cognitive effects of recombinant interleukin-2 (rIL-2) therapy: a controlled clinical trial using computerised assessments. *Eur J Cancer* 1996;32A:2275-2283.

Weeks JC, Cook EF, O'Day SJ, Peterson LM, Wenger N, Reding D, Harrell FE, Kussin P, Dawson NV, Connors AF Jr, Lynn J, Phillips RS. Relationship between cancer patients' predictions of prognosis and their treatment preferences [see comments] [published erratum appears in *JAMA* 2000;283:203]. *JAMA* 1998;279:1709-1714.

Weissman DE, Dahl JL. Update on the cancer pain role model education program. *Journal of Pain and Symptom Management* 1995;10:292-297.

Weissman DE, Dahl JL, Beasley JW. The Cancer Pain Role Model Program of the Wisconsin Cancer Pain Initiative. *Journal of Pain and Symptom Management* 1993;8:29-35.

Woolf CJ, Mannion R J. Neuropathic pain: aetiology, symptoms, mechanisms, and management [see comments]. *Lancet* 1999;353:1959-1964.

World Health Organization. 1986. *Cancer Pain Relief*. Geneva: World Health Organization.

Yeh SS, Schuster MW. Geriatric cachexia: the role of cytokines [see comments]. *Am J Clin Nutr* 1999;70:183-197.

APPENDIX 8-A

Acknowledgments

This report greatly benefitted from the creative editorial assistance, organizational abilities and insight of Martha Engstrom, M.S. of the Pain Research Group at University of Texas, M.D. Anderson Cancer Center, Houston.

The following contributed to the suggestions for specific research needs, the current barriers to research, and recommendations to improve research in this area:

Ira Byock, M.D.
Missoula Demonstration Project
Missoula, MT

Patrick Dougherty, Ph.D.
Associate Professor of Anesthesiology
University of Texas M.D. Anderson Cancer Center
Houston, TX

Debra Dudgeon, M.D.
Director, Palliative Care Medicine Program
Queen's University
Kingston, Ontario

Betty Ferrell, R.N., FAAN, Ph.D.
City of Hope
Duarte, CA

Perry Fine, M.D.
Professor of Anesthesiology
University of Utah Medical School
Medical Director, Vistacare
Salt Lake City, UT

Howard Gutstein, M.D.
Associate Professor of Anesthesiology
University of Texas M.D. Anderson Cancer Center
Houston, TX

Christina Meyers, Ph.D., ABPP
Associate Professor of Neuro-oncology (Neuropsychology)
University of Texas M.D. Anderson Cancer Center
Houston, TX

Judith Paice, R.N., FAAN, Ph.D.
Professor of Cancer Research
Northwestern University
Chicago, IL

Steve Passik, Ph.D.
Director, Community Cancer Care
Indianapolis, IN

Carla Ripomonti, M.D.
Istituto Tumori
Milano, Italy

Donna Zhukovsky, M.D.
Associate Professor, Symptom Control and Palliative Care
University of Texas M.D. Anderson Cancer Center
Houston, TX

9

Professional Education in Palliative and End-of-Life Care for Physicians, Nurses, and Social Workers

Hellen Gelband
Institute of Medicine

INTRODUCTION

In 1997, the Institute of Medicine (IOM, 1997) described a system of professional end-of-life care whose major deficiencies included

- a curriculum in which death is conspicuous mainly by its relative absence;

- educational materials that are notable for their inattention to the end stages of most diseases and their neglect of palliative strategies; and

- clinical experiences for students and residents that largely ignore dying patients and those close to them.

However, it also reported "increasing acknowledgement by practitioners and educators of the compelling need to better prepare clinicians to assess and manage symptoms, to communicate with patients and families, and to participate in interdisciplinary caregiving that meets the varied needs of dying patients and those close to them." The increasing interest had already translated into new programs by professional societies, medical schools, and private foundations, and these continue. However, impressive as the initiatives are, they are small in scale compared with national needs. The IOM report cautioned that "persistence in their implementation, evaluation, redesign, and extension will be necessary to keep the promise from fading once initial enthusiasm subsides," and this caution remains appropriate in 2001. This chapter takes as a starting point one of the 1997 report's major recommendations:

Educators and other health professionals should initiate changes in undergraduate, graduate, and continuing education to ensure that practitioners
have relevant attitudes, knowledge, and skills to care well for dying patients.

Within medicine, nursing, and social work, the recognition of deficiencies in education are well known, and each profession has at least initiated
efforts to improve the status quo. However, the recognition that improvements are needed does not bring the knowledge and tools necessary to
accomplish those ends. This is the task that lies ahead and that will require
persistent effort and increased and sustained funding for a wide range of
activities. Thus far, funding for the major initiatives have been led by
private foundations. With successful programs started and ideas for new
approaches proliferating however, the amount of funding that can be put to
productive use is much greater. Sustained progress at this juncture requires
a substantial commitment of support from the public sector as well as
continued support for innovation from the private sector.

PHYSICIAN EDUCATION IN END-OF-LIFE CARE

Most U.S. physicians—oncologists, other specialists, and generalists
alike—are not prepared by education or experience to satisfy the palliative
care needs of dying cancer patients or even to help them get needed services
from other providers. With half a million people dying from cancer each
year in this country, this is a stark, but robust finding. The strongest sources
of supporting evidence are

• studies during the late 1990s documenting end-of-life and palliative
care content in undergraduate and residency coursework, and
• studies during the late 1990s of medical textbook content on end-of-
life and palliative care.

Consistent with these sources are responses given by oncologists to American Society of Clinical Oncology (ASCO) 1998 survey questions about
their training in end-of-life and palliative care and their abilities to provide
appropriate care of this type (Emanuel, 2000). The evidence is consistent
with a lack of funding for end-of-life and palliative care educational initiatives, which has begun to change only recently. Even in 2001, however, the
programs are small and funded largely by private grant-making organizations, with little contribution by the federal government. Perhaps even more
persuasive is the complete lack of documented disagreement about the poor
state of end-of-life medical education.

End-of-Life Care Education
During Medical School and Residency Programs

The subject of "death and dying" first entered the medical school curriculum in the 1960s, as a topic of discussion in preclinical coursework. Movement toward integrating end-of-life and palliative care into the clinical curriculum has begun much more recently. In 1999, the Medical School Objectives Project identified "knowledge...of the major ethical dilemmas in medicine, particularly those that arise at the beginning and end of life..." and "knowledge about relieving pain and ameliorating the suffering of patients" as subjects that should be mastered by all undergraduate medical students (Medical School Objectives Writing Group, 1999).

Students in some programs may get the training and opportunities needed, but according to the most recent and most complete survey of medical school and residency end-of-life and palliative care curricula, most do not. Barzansky and colleagues (1999) used three annual surveys that collectively cover all medical school and residency programs to analyze end-of-life and palliative care content. Results for undergraduate medical education and residency programs are summarized separately.

Undergraduate Medical Education

Two surveys provide information on medical school curricula: the Liaison Committee on Medical Education (LCME) Annual Medical School Questionnaires for years 1997-1998 and 1998-1999, and the 1998 Association of American Medical Colleges (AAMC) Graduation Questionnaire. The LCME survey goes to the deans of all 125 LCME-accredited medical schools each year, and in the two years described here, all deans responded. The AAMC questionnaire went to all 14,040 students graduating from the 125 medical schools, of whom 88 percent responded.

The LCME survey asked different questions about end-of-life and palliative care in each of the two years. In 1997-1998, the question was whether selected topics related to end-of-life care were included in the curriculum as courses that were required, parts of required courses, electives, or a combination of these. In the second year, schools were asked (1) whether certain topics related to the care of terminally ill patients were covered in required lectures or conferences and (2) whether students spent time during required courses or clerkships in clinical units devoted to care of terminally ill patients. The 1998 AAMC survey asked students to rate the level of time devoted to end-of-life issues (among others) as either inadequate, appropriate, or excessive.

LCME SURVEYS   At all schools, students have some exposure to end-of-life coursework, but it is overwhelmingly in broader courses, not in required courses on end-of-life topics (Table 9-1). More than half the schools do not offer even one elective course devoted to end-of-life issues. The survey provides no information on how much time was spent on relevant topics or how they were covered but does suggest that there are substantial gaps. For instance, 30 percent of the schools appear to have no required instruction on at least one of the three topics asked about in 1997-1998. The 1998-1999 survey also asked about direct experience with patients in hospice care (or other settings in which the focus was on end-of-life or palliative care) (Table 9-2). At 20 percent of the schools, such experience was required, and at another 20 percent, it was not available at all. No information was gathered on the percentage of students who took advantage of the elective opportunity offered in the remaining three-fifths of the schools.

AAMC MEDICAL SCHOOL GRADUATION QUESTIONNAIRE The AAMC annual survey asks graduating medical students to rate the adequacy of instruction in various areas. In 1998, they were asked about death and dying, and pain

TABLE 9-1 LCME Annual Medical School Questionnaire—Course Content (125 Schools = 100%)

Type of Course	Required Course No. (%)	Some Material in Required Course No. (%)	Elective Course No. (%)
1997-1998 Survey			
Death and dying	4 (3%)	121 (97%)	34 (27%)
Pain management	1 (1%)	105 (84%)	34 (27%)
Palliative care	1 (1%)	97 (78%)	24 (19%)
At least one of above 3		125(100%)	
None of above			69 (55%)
1 item only		15 (12%)	30 (24%)
2 items only		22 (18%)	17 (14%)
All 3 items		88 (70%)	9 (7%)
1998-1999 Survey			
Symptom control	NR	96 (77%)	NR
Advance directives	NR	108 (86%)	NR
Communication with patients and families	NR	118 (94%)	NR
Ethical issues	NR	122 (98%)	NR
All 4 items	NR	90 (72%)	NR

NOTE: NR = not reported.

SOURCE: Barzansky et al., 1999.

TABLE 9-2   LCME Annual Medical School Questionnaire: Experience in Hospice or Other End-of-Life Care Setting, 1998-1999 Survey (125 Schools = 100%)

Type of Experience	No. (%)
Required course or clerkship	24 (19%)
Elective—some students	74 (59%)
No such experience offered	27 (22%)

SOURCE: Barzansky et al., 1999.

management (Table 9-3). The responses are subjective, but again, they suggest strongly that students are not prepared to care for dying patients as well as they could be during their undergraduate medical education.

Residency Programs

The 1997-1998 American Medical Association (AMA) Annual Survey of Graduate Medical Education was sent to 7,861 residency programs (all of those accredited by the Accreditation Council on Graduate Medical Education), of which 96.5 percent responded. The survey asked whether each program had a structured curriculum in end-of-life care. (No more specific definitions of what might be included in an end-of-life curriculum were provided, so the term may have been interpreted differently by different respondents.)

Overall, 60 percent of programs reported that they did have a structured curriculum, but there was tremendous variability among programs in different specialties. Of the types of physicians most likely to care for dying patients

- 92 percent of programs in family practice and internal medicine and 98 percent in critical care medicine reported positively, and
- between 60 percent and 70 percent of programs in obstetrics-gynecology, pediatrics, psychiatry, and surgery reported positively.

The results of these recent surveys suggest that undergraduate medical and residency training lacks adequate content in end-of-life care, but without much detail. One would like to know what topics are covered in end-of-life education, the format (i.e., lectures, discussions, clinical experience), how much time is devoted to each subject, and how well students are prepared by the extent and types of training they receive. This information has not been assembled in a comprehensive way, but pieces of it are ex-

TABLE 9-3   AAMC Medical School Graduation Questionnaire: Level of Coverage of Death and Dying and Pain Management 1998 Survey (N = 13,861 responses out of 14,040 eligible)

Topic	Excessive No. (%)	Appropriate No. (%)	Inadequate No. (%)
Death and dying	389 (3%)	9,398 (68%)	4,074 (29%)
Pain management	65 (0.5%)	4,696 (34%)	9,124 (66%)

SOURCE: Barzansky et al., 1999.

plored in the recent literature in different ways. A wide-ranging review of published literature and grant proposals for end-of-life care by Billings and Block (1997) has brought together the relevant material.

Billings and Block (1997) searched the published literature for articles on palliative care and related topics for the years 1980 through 1995 and reviewed palliative care education grants funded by the National Cancer Institute or submitted for funding to the Project on Death in America. One hundred eighty articles—culled from more than 9,000 potentially relevant citations—form the basis of their analysis. Their findings, which complement and support the findings of the recent surveys discussed earlier, are summarized here.

CURRICULUM IN END-OF-LIFE CARE   Some of the literature reviewed by Billings and Block (1997) represented reports of the surveys of medical school deans in years earlier than those characterized by Barzansky and colleagues (1999). The following findings were reported from the 1989 survey of medical school deans, which at the time numbered 124, of whom 111 responded (Mermann et al., 1991).

Twelve of the schools had no curriculum at all in death and dying. In 30 schools, one or two lectures on death and dying were included in other courses. In 51 schools, it was taught as a distinct module in a required course, consisting of four to six lectures or a combined lecture and seminar series with small-group discussion. Eighteen schools offered a separate course on death and dying, which was required in the first two years by nearly half of the schools. The format varied from a one-weekend workshop to semester-long lecture and seminar classes, with the lecture format predominating (15 schools). There was very little contact with dying patients in any program.

The class presidents of all U.S. medical schools were polled in 1991 about terminal care education (Holleman et al., 1994). Among the findings highlighted by Billings and Block are

- more than one-quarter reported one hour or less of class time,
- 39 percent recalled some reading on the topic, and
- 37 percent rated the quality of teaching "ineffective" and 3 percent rated it "very effective."

In contrast to the students' evaluations, a national sample of cancer center directors and directors of nursing oncology reported high levels of satisfaction with supportive care instruction (greater than 90 percent) (Belani et al., 1994). However, in the one institution where students were actually studied, the level of satisfaction was 27 percent.

RELATED FINDINGS   When Billings and Block reviewed the literature in the mid-1990s, they found a number of small, more detailed studies, all of which lend support to the need for more attention to end-of-life care. Their findings span research published from 1980 through 1995; thus, some findings may be less relevant in 2001 than when published, but the pace of change has not been so great that this is necessarily so. Following are some provocative observations from individual studies:

- 30 percent of a random sample of generalists in Oregon recalled medical school training in dealing with dying patients, and 87 percent thought that more such instruction should be given in medical school;
- 39 percent of a sample of young physicians felt they had good or excellent preparation for managing the care of patients who want to die;
- 41 percent of students completing third-year clerkships were never present when an attending physician talked with a dying person, 35 percent had never discussed with an attending physician how to deal with terminally ill patients, 73 percent had never been present when a surgeon told a family about bad news after an operation, and one-third could not identify problems that would arise for family members when a dying patient was discharged to go home.

Articles on end-of-life care during residency reviewed by Billings and Block (1997) are consistent with the more recent survey findings. A similar survey of 1,068 accredited residency programs in family medicine, internal medicine, pediatrics, and geriatrics, published in 1995 (Hill, 1995) found that

- 26 percent of all residency programs in the United States offer a standard course in end-of-life care,
- almost 15 percent of programs offer no formal training in care of terminally ill patients, and
- 8 percent require a hospice rotation and 9 percent offer an elective one.

More than 1,400 residents in 55 internal medicine residency programs were surveyed by the American Board of Internal Medicine about the adequacy of their training in end-of-life care (reported in Foley, 1997). The percentage of residents reporting "adequate training" in specific areas was

- 72 percent, managing pain and other symptoms;
- 62 percent, telling patients that they are dying;
- 38 percent, describing what the dying process will be like; and
- 32 percent, talking to patients who request assistance in dying.

Conclusions

Most new physicians leave medical school and residency programs with little training or experience in caring for dying patients. In most cases, a few lectures are folded into other courses (in many cases in psychiatry and behavioral sciences, ethics, or the humanities). A few schools offer full-length courses on end-of-life care, but they are nearly all electives. According to the limited information available, most end-of-life training is provided in lectures only. Contact with dying patients, particularly for undergraduate medical students, if any, is limited.

Formal curriculum in end-of-life care is presented predominantly in preclinical years. In clinical training, which tends to be more informal and less systematic, teachers may have no special interest or expertise in end-of-life care. The importance of role models and mentors who are enthusiastic about caring for dying patients has largely been overlooked.

There is a tremendous opportunity to train the next generation of physicians in the care of dying patients. At the same time, opportunities must be created to improve the competence of physicians who are already practicing, but who have had inadequate preparation in end-of-life care.

End-of-Life Care in Medical Textbooks

Textbooks play an important role both in educating medical students and in informing practicing physicians of the standard of care for each disease covered. The topics included in textbooks and the way information is organized may be strong influences on the practice of medicine. In the past few years, researchers have looked systematically at the information relating to end-of-life issues that is contained in a variety of medical textbooks. Two landmark studies, one of general medical texts and the other of medical specialty texts, which are the most recent and comprehensive, are presented here (a similar analysis of nursing texts is discussed later in this chapter). Both studies included specific cancers in their analyses.

End-of-Life Content in Four General Medical Textbooks

The study of general medical textbooks (Carron et al., 1999) focused on four widely used books: *Harrison's Principles of Internal Medicine* (Isselbacher et al., 1994), the *Merck Manual* (Berkow, 1992), *Scientific American Medicine on CD-ROM* (SAM-CD, 1994), and *Manual of Medical Therapeutics* (Ewald and McKenzie, 1995; also known as the *Washington Manual*). In addition, the authors reviewed (although not in the same quantitative format as the target texts) William Osler's (1899) *Principles and Practice of Medicine*, and the *Mayo Clinic Family Health Book* (Larson, 1996) a medical reference for nonprofessionals.

Information was sought from each book on 12 of the leading causes of death in the United States, and for each disease, nine "content domains" were assessed (Table 9-4). In addition to displaying the content score for each domain by disease, a rough overall score was calculated for each book by assigning a value of 1 for each "+" rating and 2 for each "++" rating and dividing the total by the total possible score (i.e., a rating of ++ in each category).

The following are some general findings (Carron et al., 1999):

• *Harrison's Principles of Internal Medicine*, the *Merck Manual*, and *Scientific American Medicine* characterized medical interventions and prognostic factors but often did not mention decisionmaking or the effect of death and dying on the patient's family.
• *The Washington Manual* "offered almost no helpful information."
• Dementia, AIDS, lung cancer, and breast cancer received the most comprehensive coverage of issues related to dying. However, "the best

TABLE 9-4   End-of-Life Care in General Medical Textbooks

Diseases Studied	Content Domains
AIDS	Epidemiology
Dementia	Prognostic factors
Chronic obstructive pulmonary disease	Disease progression
Congestive heart failure, chronic renal failure	Medical interventions that change
Cancer: breast, lung, pancreas, and colon	disease course
Cirrhosis	Advance care planning
Diabetes	Mode of death
Stroke	Decisionmaking
	Effect of death and dying on patient's family
	Symptom management

SOURCE: Carron et al., 1999.

coverage...was scored as presenting useful information in only five of the nine domains."

Overall scores ranged from 11 percent for *The Washington Manual* to 38 percent for *Harrison's Principles of Internal Medicine.*

In contrast to the lack of coverage in medical textbooks, the *Mayo Clinic Family Health Book* contains a chapter on death and dying with a comprehensive discussion of "pain control in a terminal patient, the emotions of a dying patient, hospice care, funeral arrangements, when and how to tell the patient about a terminal diagnosis, and what the family should expect" (Carron et al., 1999).

Osler's 1899 textbook was found to be more straightforward about the fact of death but generally not about how to help patients cope with dying. One exception is Osler's admonition to use opiates for patients dying of hemorrhage into the lungs, to suppress terror and dyspnea. This information did not appear in any other text.

End-of-Life Content in 50 Medical Specialty Textbooks

The end-of-life content of 50 top-selling textbooks in a variety of specialties (Table 9-5) was the subject of the second major review (Rabow et al., 2000). The methodology followed closely the methods used by Carron and colleagues in their study of general medical textbooks, but the content domains were expanded and the medical conditions studied necessarily varied from book to book and were chosen to represent the common causes of death in each specialty. The authors also reviewed the tables of contents for chapters dealing specifically with end-of-life care and searched the indexes for 18 relevant key words. In scoring, rather than calculating an overall score for each book (as Carron and colleagues did), the results are presented as the percentage of instances of "absent," "minimal," and "helpful" information.

When the overall scores for each specialty were calculated (the average of the individual textbook scores in each specialty), there were some differences among specialties but a generalized pattern of 50-70 percent absent content and lower scores (i.e., poorer ratings) for minimal or helpful content (see Rabow et al., 2000, figure 1). Although the differences were not large, the authors noted that textbooks with the least end-of-life content were in the specialties of infectious diseases and AIDS, oncology and hematology, and surgery.

Information on how each domain was covered was presented for the six internal medicine textbooks. The 14 conditions analyzed in these texts included three cancers (breast, colon, and lung). The best-covered domains were epidemiology and natural history (i.e., consistent ratings of 2), and the

TABLE 9-5 End-of-Life Care Content of 50 Textbooks: Specialties, Content Domains, Scoring

Specialties Included (No. of books)	Content Domains	Scoring
Cardiology (4)	Epidemiology (vital statistics)	0: Absent
Emergency medicine (4)	Natural history (prognosis, time course, mode of death, symptoms)	1: Minimal
Family and primary care medicine (5)	Pain management	2: Helpful
	Nonpain symptom management (dyspnea, nausea and vomiting, delirium, fatigue, etc.)	
Geriatric medicine (5)	Psychological issues (depression, anxiety, fear, loneliness, grief)	
Infectious disease and AIDS (3)	Social and demographic issues (interpersonal relationships with spouses or partners, family, and friends; race; cultural and economic issues)	
Internal medicine (6)	Spiritual issues (abandonment, completion of tasks, acceptance, religious tasks, choices)	
Neurology (3)		
Oncology and hematology (6)	Family issues (communication of patient and family member wishes, grief and bereavement, informal caregiver role and support, education, economic issues)	
Pediatrics (4)		
Psychiatric medicine (3)	Definition of end-of-life care (definition of death and goals of care)	
Pulmonary medicine (4)	Ethics Law Policies (individual vs. organization ethics, patients' self-determination, double effect, withdrawal and withholding of life support)	
Surgery (3)	Physician after-death responsibilities (pronouncement, autopsy, organ donation)	
	Physician roles (communication with patient and family, personal grief and bereavement)	
	Context of care (advance directives, options for end-of-life care, referral to hospice, funeral arrangements)	

SOURCE: Rabow et al., 2000

worst were social, spiritual, and family issues; ethics, and physician responsibilities. In the remaining domains, minimal information (a rating of 1) was most common.

Ten conditions were appropriate to more than one specialty, and these included two cancers: lung cancer and leukemia. Lung cancer was covered in family and primary care medicine, internal medicine, and oncology-hematology; leukemia in family and primary care medicine and pediatrics, in addition to oncology-hematology. For lung cancer, oncology-hematology had the lowest helpful score (11.6 percent), followed by internal medicine (20.5 percent), and family and primary care had the best helpful score

(28.2 percent). For leukemia, pediatrics and oncology-hematology helpful scores were similar (21.2 percent and 20.5 percent, respectively), and the lowest score was in family and primary care medicine (10.3 percent).

The analysis of key end-of-life index words showed an overall paucity of references, consistent with the content domain analyses.

Comment on Textbook Studies

A physician consulting a textbook on the treatment of a potentially fatal condition is most likely to find no specific information that will help care for the patient who does, indeed, die. In a minority of cases, useful information may be found. In both studies (Carron et al., 1999; Rabow et al., 2000), the scoring was generous, erring on the side of giving higher rather than lower scores, so even these scores may overestimate the useful content. The investigators also did not rate how useful or complete the information was. However, Carron and colleagues found that more often than not, when information about prognostic factors and disease progression was present, it was vague and would not be helpful in caring for a patient (e.g., the admonition that "supportive care is all that can be offered at this point").

Knowing that many physicians have little experience with dying and little training to help them, Carron and colleagues commented that "standard reference textbooks should provide at least the essentials of good practice." Yet, in fact, physicians cannot rely on these texts for much-needed information: on advance care planning, decisionmaking, the effect of death and dying on a patient's family, or symptom management. Most texts do not describe the way that people with a disease generally die.

The findings from these textbook reviews are so stark that they cannot, and in fact have not, been ignored. Partly in response to these studies, some textbook publishers have commissioned updates for particular chapters. In addition, the Robert Wood Johnson Foundation has begun a Textbook Revisions Project with the goal of working with publishers and editors to ensure that end-of-life chapters are added to textbooks and that end-of-life information is added to other chapters as appropriate (Gibson, 2000).

The 1998 ASCO Survey

In 1998, American Society of Clinical Oncology conducted the first and only large-scale survey of U.S. oncologists about their experiences in providing care to dying patients. The questionnaire consisted of 118 questions about end-of-life care under eight headings, one of which was education and training (Hilden et al., 2001). All U.S. oncologists who reported that they managed patients at the end of life, and were ASCO members, were eligible for the survey, a total of 6,645 (the small number of ASCO members from England and Canada was also included). About 40 percent (2,645) responded (see table below) (Emanuel, 2000). No information is available to compare the characteristics of those who responded with those who did not.

This survey documented serious shortcomings in the training and current practices of a large proportion of oncologists who responded. Among the key findings are the following:

• Most oncologists have not had adequate formal training in the key skills needed for them to provide excellent palliative and end-of-life care. Less than one-third reported their formal training "very helpful" in communicating with dying patients, coordinating their care, shifting to palliative care, or beginning hospice care. About 40 percent found their training very helpful in managing dying patients' symptoms.

• Slightly more than half (56 percent) reported "trial and error in clinical practice" as one important source of learning about end-of-life care. About 45 percent also ranked role models during fellowships and in practice as important. Traumatic patient experiences ranked higher as a source of learning than did lectures during fellowship, medical school role models, and clinical clerkships.

Recommendations to Improve End-of-Life Medical Education

In 1997, the Robert Wood Johnson Foundation and the Project on Death in America brought together 94 academic leaders (selected through a structured nomination process) in a national consensus conference on medical education for end-of-life care (Barnard et al., 1999). Their task was to develop recommendations to guide teaching in end-of-life care, based on evidence from the literature and expert opinion. The work was carried out by eight working groups in the following areas:

1. Preclinical years
2. Primary care and ambulatory care
3. Acute care hospitals
4. Pediatrics
5. Emergency medicine
6. Intensive care
7. Long-term institutional care
8. Home care and hospice care

Each working group addressed five questions:

1. How do death and dying manifest themselves in your setting?
2. What are the tasks of end-of-life care in your setting?
3. What are the major opportunities and barriers to learning about end-of-life care?
4. What can be done to improve teaching about end-of-life care in your setting?
5. What currently available and new resources are needed to facilitate change?

A set of guiding principles for undergraduate medical education provides a framework for the recommendations of all the working groups (Billings and Block, 1997). The recommendations at the end of this chapter address how these principles might be advanced. This report does not make recommendations about the precise content of educational materials or programs, but the general skills and knowledge required are summarized well in the IOM report, *Approaching Death* (IOM, 1997).

Basic Principles for Enhancing
Undergraduate Medical Education in Palliative Care[1]

1. The care of dying persons and their families is a core professional task of physicians. Medical schools have a responsibility to prepare students to provide skilled, compassionate end-of-life care.

2. The following key content areas related to end-of-life care must be appropriately addressed in undergraduate medical education *(NOTE: this list will differ depending on the setting and to some extent, patient population, e.g., children vs. adults.)*

3. Medical education should encourage students to develop positive feelings about dying patients and their families and about the role of the physician in terminal care.

4. Enhanced teaching about death, dying, and bereavement should occur throughout the span of medical education.

5. Educational content and process should be tailored to students' developmental stage.

6. The best learning grows out of direct experiences with patients and families, particularly when students have an opportunity to follow patients longitudinally and develop a sense of intimacy and manageable personal responsibility for suffering persons.

---

[1]The section is taken verbatim from Billings and Block (1997).

7. Teaching and learning about death, dying, and bereavement should emphasize humanistic attitudes.

8. Teaching should address communication skills.

9. Students need to see physicians offering excellent medical care to dying people and their families, and finding meaning in their work.

10. Medical education should foster respect for patients' personal values and an appreciation of cultural and spiritual diversity in approaching death and dying.

11. The teaching process itself should mirror the values to which physicians aspire in working with patients.

12. A comprehensive, integrated understanding of and approach to death, dying, and bereavement is enhanced when students are exposed to the perspectives of multiple disciplines working together.

13. Faculty should be taught how to teach about end-of-life care, including how to be mentors and to model ideal behaviors and skills.

14. Student competence in managing prototypical clinical settings related to death, dying, and bereavement should be evaluated.

15. Educational programs should be evaluated using state-of-the-art methods.

16. Additional resources will be required to implement these changes.

Programs and Activities Needed to Advance End-of-Life Medical Education[2]

Faculty Development

Few medical faculty, at either the undergraduate or the graduate level, are knowledgeable and enthusiastic about end-of-life care and therefore are not likely to be effective teachers. To compound this, there is little end-of-life care included in the grand rounds, teaching conferences, or journal clubs of traditional continuing medical education (CME) programs.

The end-of-life skills of interns and residents, who often act as role models for medical students in hospitals, may be lacking and should also be enhanced through special programs for house staff (Weissman et al., 1999).

More intense faculty development programs should be offered to improve communication, mentoring, and other teaching skills. Educators need ready access to end-of-life educational resource materials (e.g., handouts, pocket guides).

---

[2]Drawn and adapted largely from Block et al. (1998) except as noted.

Improved Educational Materials

New materials have to be created and existing materials improved for training new and practicing physicians. This includes adding end-of-life content to medical textbooks, producing pocket guides and other references for interns and residents, and developing continuing education materials for practicing physicians.

Coordination of Medical Schools and Teaching Hospitals

Medical education takes place in a number of settings throughout the schooling process. Each medical school should develop a plan for teaching end-of-life care. This could be overseen by a committee with responsibility to review content across the entire curriculum, including preclinical and all phases of clinical education in outpatient, acute care hospital, long-term care, and home and hospice settings.

Coordination should also emphasize the need for interdisciplinary teamwork in caring for dying patients. Students should experience working together with physicians of different specialties, nurses, social workers, psychologists, other mental health workers, and clergy. They should also be instructed in caring for, and have opportunities to interact with, dying patients and their families (Weissman et al., 1999).

Residency Program Guidelines

The residency review committees that establish guidelines for clinical training have generally not mandated the inclusion of end-of-life and palliative care instruction. Perhaps presaging change, however, the internal medicine residency review committee has revised its guidelines to require instruction in palliative care and recommend clinical experience in hospice and home care.

Evaluation of Clinical Competence in End-of-Life and Palliative Care

Competence in these areas should be tested in the same way as for other clinical topics. Structured clinical examinations should be designed to assess the relevant skills in clinical care, decisionmaking, reasoning, and ethical problem solving.

In the hospital setting, communication and clinical decisionmaking skills can be observed by attending physicians or residents and they can give immediate feedback to students. Students' attitudes can be assessed by consulting hospital staff, patients, and family members, and medical charts can be reviewed to evaluate clinical practice (Weissman et al., 1999).

Licensing and Certifying Examinations

Both undergraduate licensing and graduate certification examinations have begun to include more questions on end-of-life care, but the content is still minimal. More questions on these exams will likely promote appropriate additions to the curriculum.

Improving the Research Base for Palliative Care Education

In addition to the many unanswered clinical questions surrounding end-of-life care, there is research to be done that could directly benefit the education process. The "epidemiology of dying" would describe where, how, and under whose care patients die in different settings, including the interactions of physicians, nurses, social workers, clergy, family, and other caregivers. Information about the effect on physicians (and others) of caring for dying patients could also help guide medical education.

The transition period of "prognostic uncertainty," when choices must be made in the face of an uncertain outcome, is relatively unstudied in terms of the choices for patients and physicians.

Activities of Professional Organizations

Medical societies of various kinds, as well as societies of medical educators, can take a leadership role in placing end-of-life care prominently on the educational agenda. They can assess the educational needs of their members, develop clinical practice guidelines, encourage research, highlight end-of-life care at annual and other meetings, and undertake other activities (Weissman et al., 1999).

Standard-setting organizations, such as the Joint Commission on the Accreditation of Healthcare Organizations (JCAHO) can promote more comprehensive end-of-life care requirements for hospitals, nursing homes, and other institutions. They also can help to educate medical administrators about quality end-of-life care (Weissman et al., 1999).

Recent and Ongoing End-of-Life Medical Education Project: Funding and Aims

Work on many of the identified needs has been started, mainly through foundation grants. These projects have succeeded in raising awareness of the need for improvement and stimulating innovative ideas. The major projects and funding sources are characterized in Table 9-6. The National Cancer Institute also funded a group of grants through a one-time initiative but has no ongoing program for soliciting proposals in this area.

TABLE 9-6   Recent and Ongoing End-of-Life Medical Education Projects

Name, Funding Source, Duration	Description and Aims
Project on Death in America Faculty Scholars Program	Five to eight two-year fellowships of up to $70,000 per year are made to institutions on behalf of the Scholars Program. Fellowship funds are used to support the scholar's salary and benefits and to provide up to $5,000 in travel funds for national meetings, research assistance, summer stipends, and other costs related to work on the scholar's project. Each scholar carries out a significant project that addresses a critical issue in the care of the dying in his or her own institution or community.

RWJF Funded or Supported Projects

The EPEC Project—Education for Physicians on End-of-Life Care (EPEC) Funding with AMA 2/1/97-5/31/00 $1,541,943 from RWJF	Designed to teach practicing physicians "the essential clinical competencies required to provide quality end-of-life care" (AMA, 2000). The focus of EPEC is a curriculum to be presented to groups by individuals who have been trained specifically in the course. In 1999, six regional workshops were held, at which 500 physician-educators were trained in running the program. Videotapes and printed material, in addition to didactic and interactive sessions, are used. The format consists of four 30-minute plenary modules and twelve 45-minute workshop modules.
Harvard Medical School Palliative Care Education Center 7/1/98-6/30/03 $997,873 from RWJF	Center for training faculty from around the country in palliative and end-of-life care
Stanford University Medical School Faculty Development Program 10/1/98-9/30/02 $831,931	Train-the-trainer program for medical faculty from across the country
New York State Medical School Curricula Project in Palliative Care 3/15/99-9/14/00 $268,792	Developing a consensus on core curriculum for all medical schools in the state that schools will begin to incorporate into their programs. A "report card" on implementation will be completed for each school at the end of the project.

TABLE 9-6   Continued

Name, Funding Source, Duration	Description and Aims
RWJF Funded or Supported Projects (continued)	
Faculty Development in the Veterans Health Administration 6/1/98-6/30/00 $982,595	Establishes a faculty development program in the Department of Veterans Affairs health system to improve care for dying patients.
Medical College of Wisconsin: Improving Residency Training in EOL Care 4/1/98-3/31/99 $71,448	Pilot project (completed) for end-of-life educational interventions in internal medicine residency training programs.
Promoting End-of-Life Care Content in Medical Textbooks 4/1/98-3/31/03 $216,638	Promote inclusion of EOL content in 50 of the most commonly used medical textbooks, including both general and specialty texts.
Recommendations for EOL Issues in the Medical Licensure Examination 4/1/98-12/31/01	Bringing together the National Board of Medical Examiners with palliative care experts to review the U.S. medical licensing examination for end-of-life content and prepare questions to increase their quality and quantity.
NCI-Funded End-of-Life Education Projects[a]	
Teaching Palliative Care to 4th Year Medical Students Pennsylvania State University, Hershey Medical Center 9/1/96-8/31/99 $86,523	A fourth-year clerkship in which medical students will learn how to manage medical problems in palliative care and how to function as a member of an interdisciplinary hospice team.
Palliative Care Role Model Program Harvard University Medical School 1/1/99-12/31/99 $100,203	An educational partnership among the Division of Primary Care of Harvard Medical School (HMS), the Department of Ambulatory Care and Prevention of HMS and Harvard Pilgrim Health Care, the Brigham and Women's Hospital, the Dana Farber Cancer Institute, and Massachusetts General Hospital to develop and implement a Palliative Care Role Model Program to train clinical leaders in these institutions.

continues on next page

TABLE 9-6 Continued

Name, Funding Source, Duration	Description and Aims

Network Project
Sloan Kettering Institute
  for Cancer Research
4/1/99-3/31/00
  $129,078
	To continue and expand a cancer education and training program in pain management, rehabilitation, and psychosocial issues; an interdisciplinary multicomponent cancer pain education and training program.

Dying, Death, and Grief—
  Internet Project
Northwestern University
5/1/99-4/30/00
  $124,820
	Internet outreach program in palliative medicine education, using material of multidisciplinary faculty of the Robert H. Lurie Cancer Center Program in Palliative Medicine and Education at Northwestern University. Curriculum will address the complex medical, psychological, social, religious, cultural, and ethical dimensions of dying, death, and bereavement. Available to physicians, nurses, allied health providers, and students.

Supportive Oncology—
  Reducing the Burden of
  Cancer
Fox Chase Cancer
  Center
5/1/97-4/30/99
  $70,425
	To improve the knowledge, skills, and attitudes of Fox Chase Cancer Center (FCCC) medical oncology fellows toward the supportive care needs of cancer patients and families. Fellow training will be through a series of didactic lectures and a one-month rotation within the newly formed FCCC Supportive Oncology Program.

Enhancing Cancer Education—
  Medical and Nursing
  Students
University of South Florida
7/1/99-6/30/00
  $144,162
	To improve the care of persons at risk for or diagnosed with cancer by improving the skills of primary care providers through an innovative educational curriculum that allows medical and graduate nursing students to participate in both combined and separate learning experiences. The learning experiences will be provided as part of the required curriculum and as elective coursework and will involve both classroom and clinical experiences.

Hospice Educational Program
  for the School of Medicine
University of Maryland
7/1/98-?
  $67,472 + $110,526
	Renewal of project whose long-term goals are to design, implement, evaluate, and institutionalize a comprehensive program of hospice and palliative care education at the University of Maryland School of Medicine for medical students and physicians (residents and faculty) and to integrate modern hospice and palliative care practices within the University of Maryland medical academic treatment and educational centers.

TABLE 9-6 Continued

Name, Funding Source, Duration	Description and Aims
Comprehensive Educational Program in Palliative Care University of Colorado Health Sciences Center 2/3/98-? $67,472 + $69,496	Renewal of an interdisciplinary educational program in palliative care at the University of Colorado Health Sciences Center.
Equipping Medical Students to Manage Cancer Pain University of Kentucky 1998 $110,063	The Structured Clinical Instruction Module (SCIM) has been piloted as a format for enhancing the teaching of clinical skills pertinent to the diagnosis of cancer pain in the multidisciplinary care of the patient with cancer. The current study is developing and implementing the SCIM for medical students, with the teaching of clinical skills critical to the diagnosis and multidisciplinary management of the cancer pain patient.
Physician Hospice/Palliative Care Training—UNIPACS American Academy/Hospice And Palliative Medicine 9/30/99-9/29/00 $149,413	To promote physician competence in end-of-life care by developing practical, clinically oriented educational materials that can be used in training medical students, residents, and practicing physicians to care for dying patients.
Cancer Pain Role Model Program Medical College of Wisconsin 9/1/99-8/31/00 $125,873	Continuation of an education project of the Wisconsin Cancer Pain Initiative; 180 physicians and nurses involved in medical education will be recruited each year for five years to attend one of three model conferences a year.

NOTE: NCI = National Cancer Institute; RWJF = Robert Wood Johnson Foundation

aFunding information from Begg (2000).

NURSING EDUCATION IN END-OF-LIFE CARE

Nurses are expected to provide physical, emotional, spiritual, and practical care for patients in every phase of life. They spend more time with patients near the end of life than do any other health professionals. Yet, like physicians, most nurses in the United States do not receive the training and practical experience they need to carry out these duties in the best fashion. The nursing curriculum has been less studied than the medical curriculum, but this has been changing, particularly in response to debates about assisted suicide and euthanasia (Ferrell et al., 2000).

The 1997 Institute of Medicine report (IOM, 1997) reviewed studies of the nursing curriculum and found that coursework varied greatly from school to school. Nurses were found to have had little supervised clinical experience with dying patients and had been given minimal guidance on handling their personal reactions and involvement with dying patients. Criticisms were also raised that the end-of-life curriculum is out of date and not based on current models of death education.

End-of-Life Nursing Curriculum and Nurses' Preparedness for End-of-Life Care

Analytical studies of the U.S. nursing curriculum for end-of-life content have not yet been done, but a recent survey of nursing faculty and members of state nursing boards about their perceptions of this content provides a useful starting point (Ferrell et al., 1999). The survey is part of a larger project (funded by the Robert Wood Johnson Foundation) in which the three main nursing education associations are taking part, and the members of these three organizations were surveyed: the National Council of State Boards of Nursing, Inc.; the American Association of Colleges of Nursing; and the National League for Nursing Accreditation Commission.

Of the 725 respondents (the number surveyed was not reported), one-third were deans or chairpersons of schools of nursing, just over half were faculty members, and four percent were consultants or staff of state nursing boards (the rest had various roles). The key finding was that the adequacy of end-of-life content in these schools was rated at 6-7 on a scale of 0 (not adequate) to 10 (very adequate). This held for each of 10 specific content areas (e.g., death and dying, pain management, ethical issues).

The survey respondents also called for resources to help faculty improve end-of-life content in the form of

- Case studies
- Access to clinical sites
- Internet resources
- Audiovisuals
- Access to speakers, experts
- Lecture guides or outlines on end-of-life topics
- Computer-assisted instruction
- Textbooks
- Standardized curriculum

As part of the same overall project, a sample of nurses completed a survey on a number of end-of-life topics, including their assessment of the effectiveness of nursing education in this area. The nurses surveyed included volunteers (300 who mailed in the survey, which was published in two general nursing journals) and 2,033 oncology nurses solicited directly (out of 5,000 who were mailed the survey), so the results should be considered descriptive only. They were asked about nine aspects of nursing education:

1. pain management,
2. overall content,
3. role and needs of family caregivers,
4. other symptom management,
5. grief and bereavement,
6. understanding the goals of palliative care,
7. ethical issues,
8. care of patients at time of death, and
9. communication with patients and families.

Less than 13 percent of those responding rated their education in all nine aspects as adequate. Most frequently rated as not adequate were pain management (71 percent), overall content (62 percent), and roles and needs of family caregivers (61 percent), but more than half reported "not adequate" education in each of the nine areas.

Most other relevant studies have focused on nurses' knowledge in the area of cancer pain management and palliative care, and these have found major deficiencies, most likely resulting from deficiencies in training (see, e.g., Ferrell and McCaffery, 1997; McCaffery and Ferrell, 1995).

End-of-Life Care in Nursing Textbooks

A major review of nursing textbooks for end-of-life content was completed recently (Ferrell et al., 1999b). Fifty current nursing textbooks, both general and specialty, used heavily in nursing programs were selected for analysis (Table 9-7). "Critical content areas" were identified as key items that should appear in complete discussions of each content area (the pharmacology texts were treated somewhat differently, appropriate to their different scope), and included:

- Palliative care defined
- Quality of life
- Pain
- Other symptom assessment and management
- Communication with dying patients and their family members
- Role/needs of caregivers in end-of-life care
- Death
- Issues of policy, ethics, and law
- Bereavement

TABLE 9-7   End-of-Life Care Content in 50 Nursing Textbooks

Categories	No. Texts Reviewed	Chapters Devoted to End-of-Life Content/ Total Chapters	Pages Related to End of Life/ Total Pages
AIDS/HIV	1	0/16	20.0/26
Assessment/diagnosis	3	0/80	15.3/1783
Communication	2	0/35	38.0/767
Community/home health	4	0/116	21.3/3108
Critical care	4	2/181	80.8/4116
Emergency	2	1/69	14.5/1006
Ethics/legal issues	5	4/88	143.0/2018
Fundamentals	3	3/140	114.9/4353
Gerontology	5	2/72	84.8/2515
Medical-surgical	2	2/298	146.3/9969
Oncology	2	7/149	107.5/3264
Patient education	3	0/26	8.0/636
Pediatrics	4	2/70	33.5/2599
Pharmacology	3	0/236	22.0/3476
Psychiatry	3	1/127	35.3/2886
Nursing review	4	0/47	17.0/2661
TOTAL	50	24/1750 (1.4%)	901.9/45,683 (2%)

SOURCE: Ferrell et al., 1999b.

For each critical content area, a list of specific types of information were prespecified as important for inclusion in a text. For examples, under "Pain," the topics identified were:

- definition of pain;
- assessment of pain—physical;
- assessment of meaning of pain—scales;
- pharmacologic management of pain at end of life (classes of analgesics);
- use of invasive techniques;
- principles of addiction, tolerance, and dependence;
- nonpharmacologic management of pain at end of life;
- physical pain versus suffering;
- side effects of opioids;
- barriers to pain management;
- fear of opioids hastening death or opioids near death;
- equianalgesia; and
- recognition of nurses' own burden in pain management.

The authors tallied the presence of end-of-life information in various ways, including examining tables of contents and indexes for mentions, as well as analyzing each text for the critical content areas. Among the key findings are the following:

- 1.4 percent of all chapters (24 out of 1,750) and 2 percent of all content (902 out of 45,683 pages) were devoted to any end-of-life topic;
- 30 percent of the texts had at least one chapter devoted to end-of-life issues (the vast majority were devoted only to pain);
- the strongest coverage was in the two areas of pain and issues of policy or ethics; end-of-life topics with the poorest coverage were quality of life issues and role and needs of family caregivers; and
- overall, 74 percent of the prespecified content was absent, 15 percent was present and 11 percent was present and useful or commendable.

The authors also qualitatively analyzed the information that was found in the texts, drawing a number of conclusions, among them:

- most end-of-life content focused only on cancer and AIDS;
- although pain was frequently discussed, the text referred mainly to acute or chronic pain, and not pain at the end of life; minimal content was found on pain assessment, neuropathic pain, or pain assessment in the cognitively impaired or nonverbal patient;
- outdated drug approaches were frequently recommended, and there was virtually no information on pain management at the end of life;
- minimal information was found on symptoms other than pain at the end of life; and
- the four pharmacology texts all included erroneous information and lacked information on current approaches to pain and symptom management.

The overarching finding was a lack of content on essential topics for end-of-life care.

Ongoing Programs and Initiatives

As is the case for education programs for physicians, much of support for nursing education comes from private foundations (Table 9-8).

SOCIAL WORK EDUCATION IN END-OF-LIFE CARE

Social workers are central to counseling, case management, and advocacy services for the dying and for bereaved families. With their focus on

TABLE 9-8   Major Recent and Ongoing End-of-Life Nursing Education
Projects

Name, Funding Source, Duration	Description and Aims
RWJF Funded or Supported Projects	
Strengthening Nursing Education in Pain Management and End-of-Life Care City of Hope National Medical Center 11/1/97-10/31/00 $793,014	Three-pronged project, including review of 50 most commonly used nursing textbooks for end-of-life content; in collaboration with National Council of State Boards of Nursing, review of end-of-life content of nursing licensure examination; and work with nursing education accrediting bodies to incorporate end-of-life care standards into nursing education.
Strengthening End-of-Life Care in Nursing Practice Oncology Nursing Certification Corporation 1/1/99-6/30/00 $165,125	Three main goals are (1) determine adequacy of content of end-of-life nursing care through specialty nursing certification examinations, (2) improve end-of-life content in nursing continuing education programs; and (3) support specialty nursing certification organizations to promote competence in end-of-life care.
EOL Educational Materials for Nursing School Faculty and Practicing Nurses University of Washington School of Nursing 5/1/99-4/30/03 $1,584,242	To create, develop, and market educational materials for interactive learning of palliative care nursing in two versions—one for nurse educators and a self-study version for practicing nurses.
End-of-Life Nursing Education Consortium (ELNEC) City of Hope National Medical Center and American Association of Colleges of Nursing 2/1/00-7/31/03 $2,224,543	ELNEC is a project for nursing parallel to EPEC for physician education. The goal is to create a comprehensive end-of-life curriculum for nurses, which will be implemented in this project; by 450 undergraduate nursing programs, 225 continuing education providers, and the 100 state boards of nursing.

NOTE: EPEC = Education for Physicians on End-of-Life Care; RWJF = Robert Wood Johnson
Foundation.

the psychosocial aspects of the dying process, they work not only with patients but with those around them in making decisions about treatment options, marshaling resources, helping families cope with terminal illness and death of a relative, and generally encouraging the best quality of life for all concerned. The demands on social workers have changed over time. A major reason is the shift from largely hospital-based care for those who are dying to home, hospice, and other settings, which has required social workers to coordinate a broadening array of services and providers and to navigate a more complex set of rules and regulations.

Just as nursing and medicine have begun to do, the social work profession has been examining its education process for preparing practitioners to care for dying patients and their families. Efforts to improve undergraduate and master's level social work training in this area are just getting under way in the United States, in comparison to the more mature field in Canada and England, and in comparison to medical and nursing education. Quite recently, opportunities have been identified, and some programs initiated, to begin making the needed changes.

End-of-Life Care Training in Social Work Education[3]

Studies in the 1990s began to look at the end-of-life content of social work education and the preparedness of social workers to care for dying patients and their bereaved families. Four small but prominent studies set the stage for the most definitive review of this issue, by Christ and Sormanti (1999).

Briefly, of the four earlier studies, one was a survey of 108 hospice social workers from around the country, which found a uniform lack of preparation at the master's level for end-of-life care (Kovacs and Bronstein, 1998). The second consisted of a focus group of 10 oncology social work supervisors who described serious gaps in the social work curriculum related to end-of-life care (Sormanti, 1995).

A survey of social work programs found that in most, the end-of-life content was folded into courses on "human behavior and the social environment" or into gerontology courses. Less than a quarter of all students enrolled in these courses when they were electives (Dickinson et al., 1992). The last study was based on a questionnaire given to 50 M.S.W. students at the beginning of the second year, who reported feeling "a little" or "somewhat" prepared to deal with dying patients and their families (Kramer, 1998).

Though small and of varied types, these studies suggest that, like medi-

---

[3]This section is largely based on the work of Christ and Sormanti (1999).

cine and nursing, social work students have insufficient training—both didactic and practical—to provide the best care at the end of life. (No studies of social work textbooks for end-of-life care content have yet been carried out.)

Christ and Sormanti (1999) extended the earlier efforts with surveys and focus groups designed to address the following issues (of which the last two are of most interest in this section):

1. barriers to effective social work practice in palliative care and care of the bereaved,

2. the adequacy of M.S.W. practitioners' preparedness for this work, and

3. the extent of social work educators' experiences in teaching and research in bereavement and end-of-life care.

The first survey involved 48 oncology social workers attending the 1998 annual meeting of the Association of Oncology Social Workers. Regarding education, they were asked about their preparation in M.S.W. programs and about postgraduate training and educational opportunities. The practitioners uniformly reported insufficient training in end-of-life issues to prepare them for the work they were doing. None except for the few who had trained in hospice settings had clinical experience with dying patients. The respondents were asked about their preparation in 10 skill categories, with the result that in only two—supportive counseling and advocacy—did less than half rate their preparation as "unsatisfactory." At least 50 percent rated end-of-life training in symptom management, communication, bereavement, education, ethics, case management, decisionmaking, and discharge planning as unsatisfactory.

Only one continuing education program associated with a school of social work was identified among the 48 participants. Overall, most lacked access to continuing education programs that were at all satisfactory. Even where programs exist, finding funds to attend and being able to take time away from work are significant barriers. In addition, most programs highlight medicine and nursing, and few social workers speak in the relevant courses. Five focus groups were held with social workers who provide end-of-life services, and they largely corroborated the findings of the survey.

Finally, 35 faculty members from 30 schools of social work were surveyed about end-of-life care content in their own programs and about research on related topics. They reported that only a small proportion of students receive instruction in end-of-life issues and that it comes in small parts of courses on human behavior and the social environment, policy, and practice. It usually consists of one or two lectures. More comprehensive elective courses were taken by a minority of students. Only one-quarter of survey participants believed that their schools adequately prepared students for end-of-life work.

Research funding was a very scarce commodity: about one-quarter reported even modest monetary support for their ongoing research. They reported that they were aware of no money targeted specifically for end-of-life research in social work.

Opportunities for Improving Social Work End-of-Life Education

Some specific areas that could benefit from funding and development of programs are

- better undergraduate and master's level curricula in end-of-life care;
- innovative programs that integrate coursework with clinical work through alliances between schools and practice sites;
- accessible continuing education designed and provided by social work experts in end-of-life care; and
- collaborative educational programs with other professions working with dying patients and bereaved families.

Also key is funding earmarked for social work research to provide a better foundation for the development of innovative methods of care.

Ongoing Programs and Initiatives

The Project on Death in America has begun a program of Social Work Leadership Development Awards to promote innovative research and training projects for collaborations between schools of social work and practice sites that will advance the ongoing development of social work practice, education, and training in the care of the dying. The Hartford Foundation also provides support for gerontology social workers. The National Cancer Institute does not currently fund any social work education projects.

RECOMMENDATIONS FOR IMPROVING PROFESSIONAL EDUCATION FOR PHYSICIANS, NURSES, AND SOCIAL WORKERS IN END-OF-LIFE CARE

Leaders in medicine, nursing, and social work have recognized that training in end-of-life care has been inadequate. These leaders have systematically documented at least some of the shortcomings in the education process and continue to add to the information base. This has been effective both in broadening recognition among the professions of the need for improvements and in serving as a basis for determining what tasks must be accomplished to effect improvements. The work has been concentrated among a small group of experts nationwide, and funding has come almost exclusively from private foundations, which have catalyzed these movements. At this point, the groundwork has been laid for larger-scale activities, which could move quickly with significant funding from the federal government, in particular, the National Cancer Institute (NCI) and other National Institutes of Health.

Faculty Development

Few medical, nursing, or social work faculty, either at the undergraduate or graduate level, are knowledgeable and enthusiastic about end-of-life care and therefore are unlikely to be effective teachers. To compound this, little end-of-life care is included in the grand rounds, teaching conferences, or journals clubs of traditional continuing education programs. More intense faculty development programs should be offered to improve communication, mentoring, and other teaching skills.

Recommendation: NCI should fund a national oncology faculty development programs along the lines of the Project on Death in America Faculty Scholars Program.

Improved Educational Materials

New materials have to be created and existing materials improved for training new and practicing physicians, nurses, and social workers. This includes adding end-of-life content to textbooks, producing pocket guides and other references, and developing continuing education materials for practicing professionals.

Recommendation: NCI should make funding available for the development of appropriate materials, which could be pilot-tested by students and fellows in NCI-designated cancer centers. This could be accomplished through the "R25" mechanism, which was used to fund a small number of recent grants after a one-time call for proposals.

Coordination of Medical, Nursing, and Social Work Schools and Teaching Hospitals

Education takes place in a number of settings throughout the schooling process. Each medical, nursing, and social work school should develop a plan for teaching end-of-life care. This could be overseen by a committee with responsibility to review content across the entire curriculum, including preclinical and all phases of clinical education in outpatient, acute care hospital, long-term care, and home and hospice settings.

Coordination should also emphasize the need for interdisciplinary teamwork in caring for dying patients. Students should experience working together with physicians of different specialties, nurses, social workers, psychologists, other mental health workers, and clergy. They should also be instructed in caring for and have opportunities to interact with, dying patients and their families (Weissman et al., 1999).

Recommendation: In addition to coordination by the schools themselves, NCI should provide clinical training fellowship slots at all NCI-designated cancer centers that have clinical programs, including training in both clinical care and palliative or end-of-life care research for all of the relevant professions. Specific cancer centers could also be developed as "centers of excellence" for palliative and end-of-life care training and research.

Residency Program Guidelines

The residency review committees that establish guidelines for clinical training have generally not mandated the inclusion of end-of-life or palliative care instruction. Perhaps presaging change, however, the internal medicine residency review committee has revised its guidelines to require instruction in palliative care and recommend clinical experiences in hospice and home care.

Recommendation: All residency review committees should be canvassed to determine the status of end-of-life care in each set of guidelines. Each specialty should be encouraged to consider appropriate changes, and technical assistance should be offered, if necessary. This activity would not require large amounts of funding, but some money for coordination and consultation should be made available by either the government, academic institutions, or foundations.

Licensing and Certifying Examinations

Both undergraduate licensing and graduate certification examinations have begun to include more questions on end-of-life care, but the content is still minimal. More questions on these exams will likely promote appropriate additions to the curricula.

Recommendation: Licensing and certifying bodies should be encouraged and assisted in developing appropriate examination questions.

This should be coordinated with curriculum development and textbook revisions. A coordinating function might be helpful in ensuring communication among the key players, funded by public or private sector sources.

Improving the Research Base for Palliative Care Education

In addition to the many unanswered clinical questions surrounding end-of-life care, there is research to be done that could directly benefit the education process. The "epidemiology of dying" would describe where, how, and under whose care patients die in different settings, including the interactions of physicians, nurses, social workers, clergy, family, and other caregivers. Information about the effect on physicians and other caregivers of caring for dying patients could also help guide education.

The transition period of "prognostic uncertainty," when choices must be made in the face of an uncertain outcome, is relatively unstudied in terms of what the choices are for patients and physicians.

Recommendation: NCI should initiate a grant program for these activities by issuing a request for proposals in this area and by continuing such a program over the long term.

Activities of Professional Organizations

Medical societies of various kinds, as well as societies of medical educators, can take a leadership role in placing end-of-life care prominently on the educational agenda. They can assess the educational needs of their members, develop clinical practice guidelines, encourage research, highlight end-of-life care at annual and other meetings, and undertake other activities (Weissman et al., 1999).

Standard-setting organizations such as JCAHO can promote more comprehensive end-of-life care requirements for hospitals, nursing homes, and other institutions. They also can help to educate medical administrators about quality end-of-life care (Weissman et al., 1999).

Recommendation: Private sector organizations should be encouraged by government to undertake these activities and should be provided with technical assistance, if needed. Funding could come from either public or private sector sources.

REFERENCES

American Medical Association. The EPEC Project. 2000 Web page, http://222.ama-asn.org/ethic/epec/epec.htm.

Barnard D, Quill T, Hafferty FW, et al. Preparing the ground: contributions of the preclinical years to medical education for care near the end of life. *Academic Medicine* 1999;74:499-505.

Barzansky B, Veloski JJ, Miller R, Jonas HS. Palliative care and end-of-life education. *Academic Medicine* 1999;74(10):S102-104.

Begg L. National Cancer Institute, Cancer Training Branch. Personal communication, June 21, 2000.

Belani CP, Belcher AE, Sridhara R, Schimper SC. Instruction in the techniques and concept of supportive care in oncology. *Supportive Care Cancer.* 1994;2:50-55. Cited in Billings and Block (1997).

Berkow R, ed. 1992. *The Merck Manual of Diagnosis and Therapy. 16th ed.* Rahway, NJ: Merck Research Laboratories.

Billings, JS, Block S. Palliative care in undergraduate medical education. *JAMA* 1997;28:733-738.

Block SD, Bernier GM, Crawley LM. Incorporating palliative care into primary care education. *JGIM;* 1998;13:768-773.

Carron AT, Lynn J, Keaney P. End-of-life care in medical textbooks. *Arch Intern Med* 1999;130:82-6.

Christ GH, Sormanti M. Advancing social work practice in end-of-life care. *Social Work in Health Care* 1999;30(2):81-99.

Dickinson G, Sumner E, Frederick L. Death education in selected health professions. *Death Studies* 1992;16:281-289. Cited in Christ and Sormanti (1999).

Emanuel EJ. National Cancer Institute. Personal communication (unpublished data), 2000.

Ewald GA, McKenzie CR, eds. 1995. *Manual of Medical Therapeutics. 28th edition.* Boston: Little, Brown.

Ferrell BR, Grant M, Virani R. Strengthening nursing education to improve end-of-life care. *Nursing Outlook* 1999a;47:252-256.

Ferrell BR, McCaffery M. Nurses' knowledge about equianalgesia and opioid dosing. *Cancer Nursing* 1997;20(3):201-212.

Ferrell B, Virani R, Grant M. Analysis of end-of-life content in nursing textbooks. *Oncol Nurs Forum* 1999b;26(5):869-876.

Ferrell B, Virani R, Grant M, et al. Beyond the Supreme Court decision: nursing perspectives on end-of-life care. *Oncology Nursing Forum* 2000;27(3):445-455.

Foley KM. Competent care for the dying instead of physician-assisted suicide. *New England Journal of Medicine* 1997;336:54-58.

Gibson R. Robert Wood Johnson Foundation projects to promote professional education and training. Personal communication, June 2000.

Hilden JM, Emanuel EJ, Fairclough DL, Link MP, Foley KM, Clarridge BC, Schnipper LE, Mayer RJ. Attitudes and practices among pediatric oncologists regarding end-of-life care: results of the 1998 American Society of Clinical Oncology survey. *JCO* 2001;19:205-212.

Hill TP. Treating the dying patient: the challenge for medical education. *Arch Intern Med* 1995;155:1265-1269. Cited in Billings and Block (1997).

Holleman WL, Holleman MC, Gershenshorn S. Death education curricula in U.S. medical schools. *Teaching Learning Med* 1994;6:260-263. Cited in Billings and Block (1997).

Institute of Medicine (IOM). 1997. *Approaching Death: Improving Care at the End of Life,* Field MJ, Cassel CK, eds. Washington, D.C.: National Academy Press.

Isselbacher K, Martin W, Kasper F, eds. 1994. *Harrison's principles of internal medicine, 13th ed.* New York: McGraw-Hill.

Kovacs P, Bronstein L. Preparation for oncology settings: what hospice social workers say they need. *Social Work in Health Care* 1999;24(1):57-64. Cited in Christ and Sormanti (1999).

Kramer B. Preparing social workers for the inevitable: A preliminary investigation of a course on grief, death, and loss. *Journal of Social Work Education* 1998;34(2):1-17. Cited in Christ and Sormanti (1999).

Larson DE, ed. 1996. *Mayo Clinic Family Health Book. 2nd edition.* New York: W. Morrow.

McCaffery M, Ferrell BR. Nurses' knowledge about cancer pain: a survey of five countries. *Journal of Pain and Symptom Management* 1995;10(5):356-369.

Medical School Objectives Writing Group. Learning objectives for medical student education: guidelines for medical schools. Report I of the Medical School Objectives Project. *Academic Medicine* 1999;74:418-422.

Mermann AC, Gunn DB, Dickinson GE. Learning to care for the dying: a survey of medical schools and a model course. *Academic Medicine* 1991;66(1):25-28.

Osler W. 1899. *Principles and Practice of Medicine, 3rd edition.* New York: D. Appleton.

Rabow MW, Hadie GE, Fair JM, McPhee SJ. End-of-life care content in 50 textbooks from multiple specialties. *JAMA* 2000;283:771-778.

SAM-CD. 1994. *Scientific American Medicine on CD-ROM: A Comprehensive Knowledge-Base of Internal Medicine.* New York: Scientific American Medicine.

Sormanti M. Fieldwork instruction in oncology social work: supervisory issues. *Journal of Psychosocial Oncology* 1994;12(3):73-87. Cited in Christ and Sormanti (1999).

Weissman DE, Block SD, Blank L et al. Recommendations for incorporating palliative care education into the acute care hospital setting. *Academic Medicine* 1999;74:871-877.

Index

Animal models, 35, 246, 249, 254, 260

Anorexia and cachexia, 34, 35, 45, 108, 234, 237, 244, 248-251, 265
  see also Weight loss
  clinical trials, 250, 251, 267
  drug treatment, general, 249-250
  dyspnea, 254
  patient/family education, 133
  physicians' perceptions of, 46

Anxiety, 3, 5, 10, 30, 48, 108, 109-110, 184, 216-217, 233, 236, 237, 244, 255, 259, 259-261
  caregivers, 133, 135, 204, 215, 223, 240
  clinical practice guidelines, 21, 22, 200, 203, 204, 208, 209-214, 218, 221, 222-229 (passim)
  clinical trials, 234
  decisionmaking and, 109, 235
  drug treatment, 110, 216, 255, 259-261
  families, general, 133, 135, 204, 215, 223, 240
  gender factors, 109-110
  pain and, 106, 222, 223-225, 236-237, 238
  patient/family education, 133, 135, 204
  physicians, 46

Approaching Death: Improving Care at the End of Life, ix, 4, 12, 16, 40, 41, 203, 290

Association of American Medical Colleges, 279, 280-281

Association of Community Cancer Centers, 137

Attitudes
  see also Anxiety; Depression; Grief and bereavement
  African Americans, 154-156, 158
  family satisfaction, 123
  nurses, 300
  toward pain, 106, 222, 223-225, 236-237, 238
  patient beliefs about survival possibilities, 135, 237, 241
  patient satisfaction, 24, 25, 38, 67, 97, 115, 117-118, 119, 124, 150
  professionals, 46, 137, 221, 266, 288-289, 290, 291
  public opinion, 36, 41, 42, 106, 114, 140, 207
    African Americans, 155-156, 158

Autopsies, 92

B

Behavioral interventions, 83, 234, 236, 246-247, 258
  hypnosis, 246-247
  relaxation therapy, 246, 257

Bereavement, *see* Grief and bereavement

Black persons, *see* African Americans

Breast cancer, 78, 81, 84, 103, 185, 237, 248, 285-286
  depression, 109
  elderly women, 84
  patient/family education, 140, 143

Breathing difficulty, *see* Dyspnea

Bowel obstruction, 35, 224, 257, 258

C

Cachexia, *see* Anorexia and cachexia

Cancer Care Consortium, 202

Cancer Care, Inc., 142-143, 145, 147

Cancer Care Issues in the United States: Quality of Care, Quality of Life, 40, 42-43

Cancer Facts sheets, 139

Cancer Information Service, 139, 141

Cancer Pain Management, 242

Cancer Therapy Evaluation Program, 48

Cannabis, *see* Dronabinol

Capitation, 71, 91, 113

Cardiopulmonary resuscitation (CPR), 156, 240-241
  do-not-resuscitate orders, 38-39, 111, 112, 155, 189, 192, 241-242

Caring for the Patient with Cancer at Home, 28, 139

Case management, 20, 177-178, 183, 185-186, 301
  see also Clinical practice guidelines; Coordination of care; Referral to care; Social workers

Centers for Disease Control and Prevention, 63, 89

Chemotherapy, 19, 236, 237, 248
  cost of, 76-77, 78-79, 81, 82
  decisionmaking, 19, 111, 112, 113, 124
  dyspnea, 252
  nausea and vomiting, 257-258
  patient decisionmaking, 111, 112, 113, 124
  patient/family education, 141
  physicians' perceptions of, 47